PULMONARY AND RESPIRATORY DISEASES AND DISORDERS

PLEURAL EFFUSIONS

CAUSES, TYPES AND TREATMENT

PULMONARY AND RESPIRATORY DISEASES AND DISORDERS

Additional books and e-books in this series can be found on Nova's website under the Series tab.

PULMONARY AND RESPIRATORY DISEASES AND DISORDERS

PLEURAL EFFUSIONS

CAUSES, TYPES AND TREATMENT

RAHUL KHOSLA, MD, MBA
EDITOR

nova
Medicine & Health
New York

Library of Congress Cataloging-in-Publication Data

ISBN: 978-1-53614-683-7
Library of Congress Control Number: 2018961869

Published by Nova Science Publishers, Inc. † New York

CONTENTS

PREFACE

First Edition

There is extensive literature available on pleural effusions and in recent years there has been significant developments in their diagnostic evaluation. The use of point of care ultrasound, pleural manometry, and medical pleuroscopy has expanded over the last decade. The goal of writing this book was to become a source or reference for clinicians who manage patients with pleural effusions.

Pleural space contains minimal amount of fluid and physiological processes keep a constant equilibrium so that it remains as such. Pleural effusions develop as a result of processes that disrupt this fine balance, as in heart failure, infections, and malignancies, which account for majority of the pleural effusions. Besides these three common causes, pleural effusions cause symptoms in many other conditions, some of which are common regardless of the etiology of the pleural effusion, such as, dyspnea and cough. Diagnosing the etiology becomes important as management can vary depending upon the cause. In some situations, involvement of the pleural space portends a poor prognosis, such as in malignancies and treatment focuses on symptom relief.

The chapters in this book span go over a wide range of topics involving pleural effusions. Initial chapters focus on clinical presentation, radiology, diagnostic evaluation, and classification of pleural effusions. There is a chapter on malignant pleural effusions, pleural infections and empyema, rheumatological causes of pleural effusions and tubercular and fungal pleural effusions. Pleural manometry is an important tool in the work-up of a trapped lung and an entire chapter is dedicated to this topic. Another chapter focuses on interventional procedures including pleuroscopy. The last two chapters go over cases of pleural effusions which cover many of the topics covered in the book.

The book compiles recent literature on pleural effusions with an aim to help clinicians manage patients with pleural effusions effectively.

Rahul Khosla, MD, MBA
Washington, DC, USA

ACKNOWLEDGMENTS

I would like to thank all the authors who made excellent contributions to this book, the publisher for giving me an opportunity to compile and produce this work. Last, but not the least, my family, who gave me immense support and encouragement throughout the process.

In: Pleural Effusions: Causes, Types and Treatment
Editor: Rahul Khosla
ISBN: 978-1-53614-683-7

Chapter 1

Clinical Presentation and Imaging of Pleural Effusions

Rahul Khosla*[*], *MD Amandeep S. Bawa, MD and Kavita Vyas, MD
Pulmonary & CCM Section, Veterans Affairs Medical Center, Washington DC, US

Abstract

Pleural effusion is a manifestation of many disease processes and is commonly encountered by clinicians. The symptoms due to pleural effusion are non-specific including dyspnea, chest pain and cough. The physical examination has low sensitivity in determining the presence of effusion unless it is significant in size. There are various imaging modalities available and are used to diagnose a pleural effusion. Chest radiograph (Chest x-ray) is the initial radiological modality generally used as it is widely available, portable and practitioners are comfortable in interpreting basic radiographs. Computed Tomography (CT) scan of the chest is considered as the gold standard test to diagnose pleural effusions and other underlying thoracic abnormalities, but, it involves a larger dose of radiation, is not portable and requires a higher level of expertise to interpret the imaging. The ultrasound (US) is becoming a popular imaging technique as it is being used more often in clinical medicine by many practitioners of different specialties. It is portable, with no radiation exposure, dynamic and easy to learn technique that can be performed at the patient's bedside to detect pleural effusions. This chapter will discuss in detail the commonly used imaging techniques in clinical medicine to diagnose pleural effusions.

Keywords: pleural effusion, ultrasound, chest radiograph, computed tomography

Introduction

Pleural effusion occurs in approximately 1.5 million patients every year in United States [1]. The list of conditions causing pleural effusions is extensive. The patient presents

[*] Corresponding Author Email: Rahul.khosla@va.gov.

with symptoms which are similar to other diseases in the thorax. The bedside physical examination is also not very accurate in determining the presence of pleural effusion. Hence imaging plays a significant role in establishing the diagnosis and treatment of pleural effusions. There are multiple radiological modalities available but chest radiography remains the initial choice of examination. Depending upon the clinical scenario and abnormalities seen on chest x-ray, further imaging is most commonly done with the thoracic ultrasound and/or computed tomography of chest. The radiologically appearance of pleural effusion is variable depending upon the patient's position, size of effusion, underlying etiology and type of imaging used. In this chapter we will review characteristic appearance of pleural effusion on chest x-ray, ultrasound and CT scan of chest.

History and Physical Examination

For clinicians, history and physical examination are the initial steps in the diagnostic work-up of any ailment. Symptoms related to pleural effusion are non-specific, including cough, dyspnea and pleuritic chest pain. The size of the effusion determines the presence or absence of various symptoms and clinical signs related to the pleural effusion. Pleural effusions less than 300 mL in volume are difficult to detect on physical examination [18]. Common physical findings related to pleural effusions include tachypnea, decreased chest expansion, decreased breath sounds, tactile fremitus, mediastinal shift and egophony.

Signs and symptoms related to the underlying disease process can give a clue to the etiology of pleural effusion. Patients with pleural effusion secondary to lung cancer may have weight loss, chest pain, hemoptysis, enlarged lymph nodes and a history of tobacco use. Presence of fever, chills, rigors, cough productive of discolored sputum and an acute onset, suggest an infectious etiology in a patient with pleural effusion and on physical examination one may hear bronchial breath sounds secondary to parenchymal consolidation.

Compared to US, physical examination had a sensitivity ranging from 53% to 76% and a specificity ranging from 60% to71% [26]. Presence of normal vocal fremitus on physical examination was noted to have a high likelihood of ruling out a pleural effusion [29]. Dullness to percussion and asymmetric chest expansion on physical examination ruled in a pleural effusion with high accuracy in a systemic review [29].

Abnormal physical examination findings on a chest examination, such as those suggesting the presence of a pleural effusion, should always be confirmed with imaging. The choice of imaging examination is usually determined by local availability of the technique and expertise in interpreting the same. The three commonly used imaging techniques are US, chest x-ray and CT scan of the chest.

Chest Radiograph

The pleural space is not visualized on regular imaging [2, 15] and fluid accumulation in the pleural space indicates a disease process. Presence of pleural effusion can be confirmed by radiological imaging with chest x-ray as the initial imaging of choice. CT scan and ultrasound can be used to further characterize pleural effusion. Small volume of pleural fluid can be detected with lateral decubitus chest x-ray, CT scan or ultrasound.

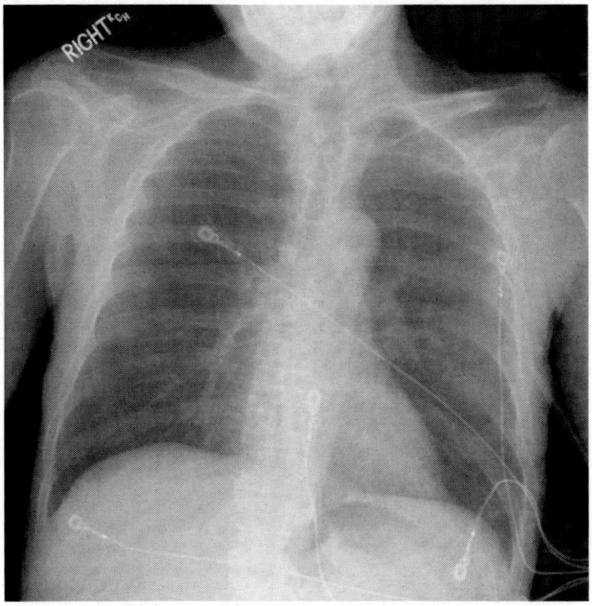

Figure 1. Normal Chest X-ray with sharp costophrenic angles.

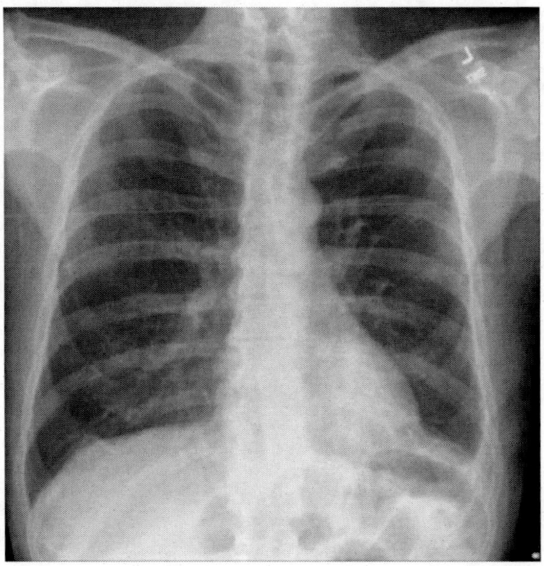

Figure 2a. Blunting of left costophrenic angle in PA view.

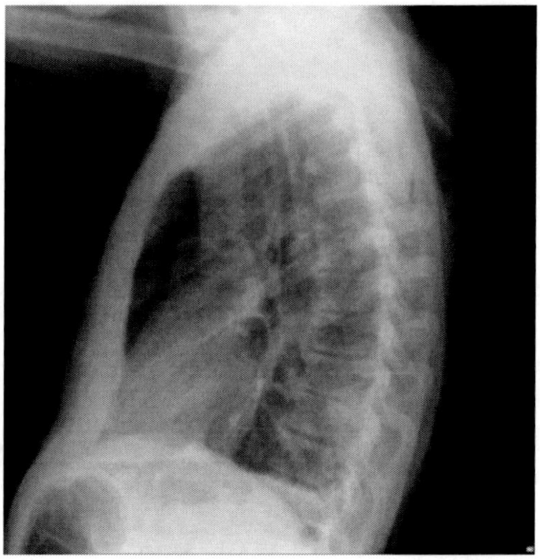

Figure 2b. Blunting of costophrenic angle in Lateral view.

Fluid accumulates in the thoracic cavity in gravity dependent locations. Fluid initially accumulates at the base of the hemithorax, between the diaphragm and inferior surface of lung [4, 6]. As fluid collection increases it fills the costophrenic sinuses followed by upward spread around the convex surface of lung. In a normal chest x-ray the costophrenic angles are sharp [Figure 1] and even 50 ml of pleural fluid can cause blunting [Figure 2b] of the posterior costophrenic angle on a lateral view [3, 11]. Collins et al. [5] injected saline into the pleural cavities of upright cadavers and showed that as little as 175 ml of fluid blunts the lateral costophrenic angle on a posterior-anterior (PA) view on a chest x-ray [Figure 2a]. But, in some cases even 525 ml of fluid did not show any evidence of such blunting, suggesting that the minimum volume of fluid required to cause blunting of the costophrenic angle can be variable.

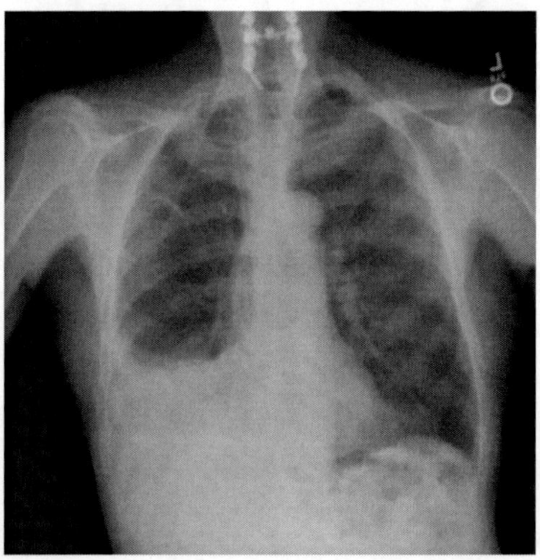

Figure 3a. PA view showing a "menisc" sign on right side.

In an erect chest x-ray presence of free fluid gives a classic appearance known as the "Menisc Sign" [Figure 3a and 3b]. It appears as a homogeneous opacity with a concave lateral upper border towards the chest well. The natural outward recoil of lung and positive hydrostatic intra-pleural pressure at the lung bases causes pleural fluid to rise against gravitational forces [8]. The true upper limit of free flowing pleural effusion is horizontal and not curved as suggested on a chest x-ray. The x-rays pass thorough a greater amount of fluid in the periphery giving it the raised radiographic line and hence the meniscus shape [7].

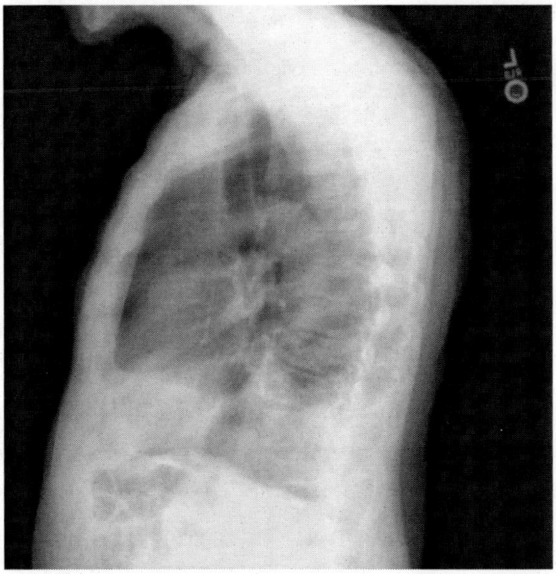

Figure 3b. Lateral view showing free flowing pleural fluid demonstrating a menisc sign.

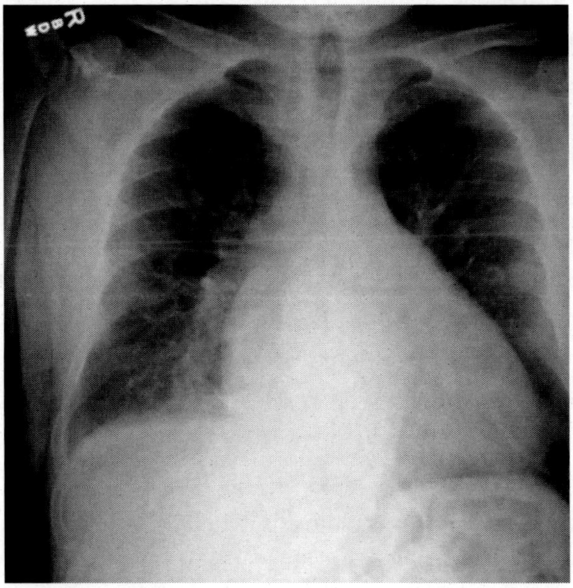

Figure 4a. Right sub-pulmonic effusion on a PA chest x-ray.

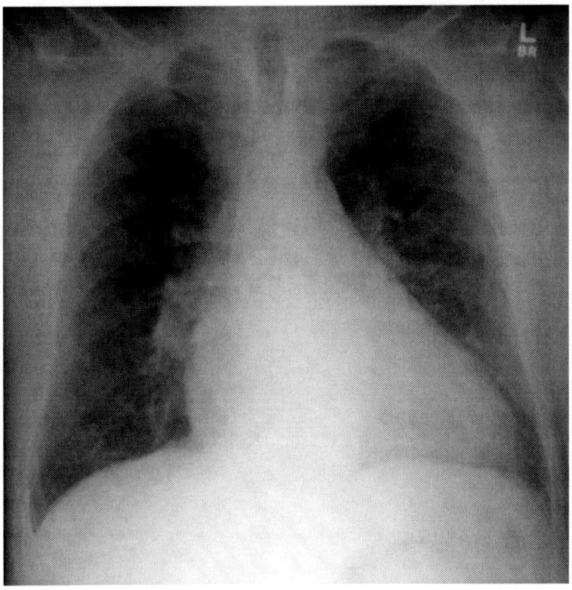

Figure 4b. Post thoracentesis in the same patient.

Sub-pulmonic effusions [Figure 4a] are difficult to detect on a PA film as pleural fluid is located between the diaphragmatic part of lung and diaphragm. The lung floats on this layer of fluid appearing as an elevated pseudo-diaphragm. On the PA view one sees a lateral peaking of the diaphragm, absence of lower intra-pulmonary vessels, an ill-defined costophrenic angle and more than 2 cm distance between left hemidiaphragm and gastric bubble [12].

A lateral decubitus view of chest is more sensitive than an erect view in detecting pleural effusions even those as small as 5 ml in volume [9, 10]. The free flowing pleural fluid is seen as a homogenous layer on the dependent chest wall [Figure 5].

On a supine chest x-ray pleural fluid layers posteriorly and produces a diffuse hazy opacity of hemithorax with preservation of bronchovascular markings [Figure 6)]. Supine films can underestimate the amount of pleural effusion present. One study determined that at least 175 ml of pleural fluid is required to be detected on a supine film [13]. When there is a significant accumulation of pleural fluid, a blunting of the lateral costophrenic angle can be seen. Other findings include, an elevation of the hemidiaphragm, absence of normal diaphragm silhouette, decreased visibility of lower intrapulmonary vessels below the level of hemidiaphragm and prominence of minor fissure.

On imaging a pleural effusion can be described as massive, large, moderate, small or very small in size. If no abnormality is seen on a PA view and fluid is seen only on a lateral or a decubitus image, the volume is classified as "very small". An effusion causing a minimal blunting of the lateral costophrenic angle on a PA view is considered "small". An effusion is considered "moderate" in size if it occupies the lower hemithorax up to the fourth anterior rib on the PA view. An effusion is considered "large" if it extends beyond the fourth anterior rib on a PA view [13]. Massive effusions occupy more than half of hemithorax obscuring the cardiac border and causing a contralateral shift of the mediastinum [Figure 7]. If a mediastinal shift is absent in a massive effusion [Figures 8 and 9] then an endobronchial obstruction or mediastinal fixation should be suspected [14].

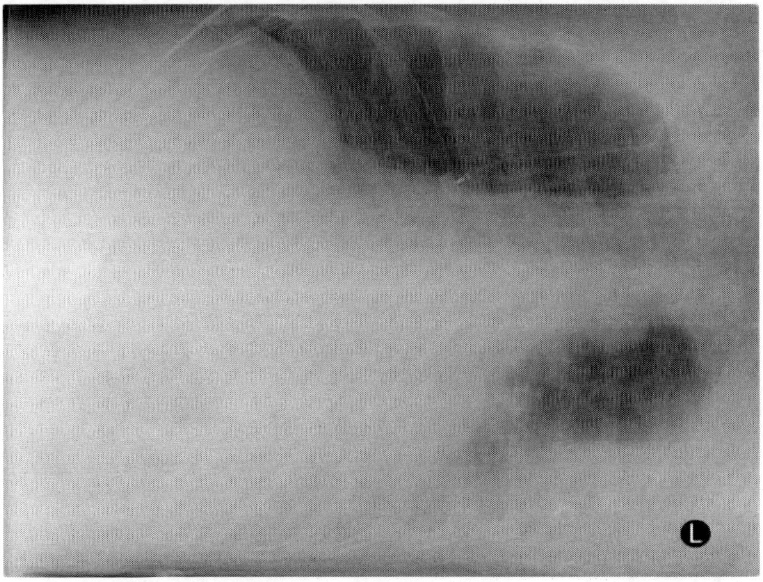

Figure 5. Layering of pleural fluid on left lateral decubitus.

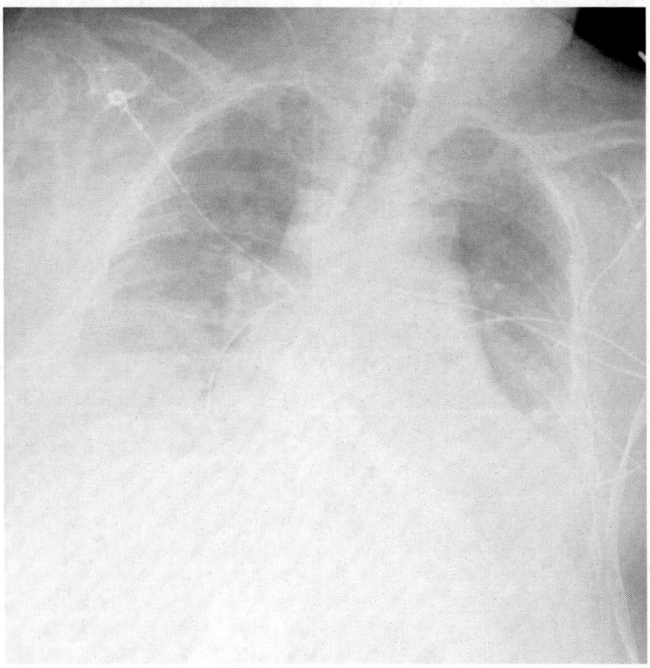

Figure 6. Supine film showing a hazy opacity of hemithorax with preservation of bronchovascular markings.

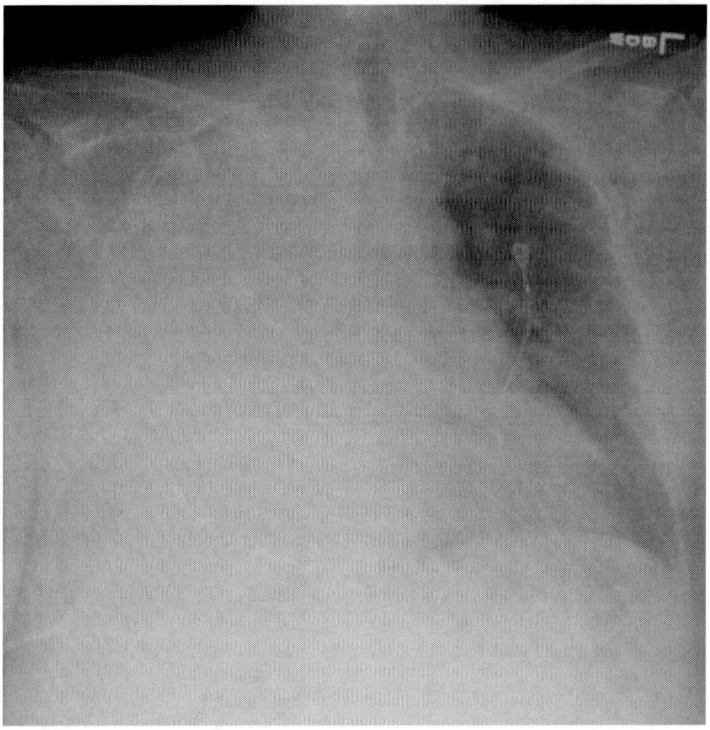

Figure 7. Massive right pleural effusion with a mediastinal shift to the left.

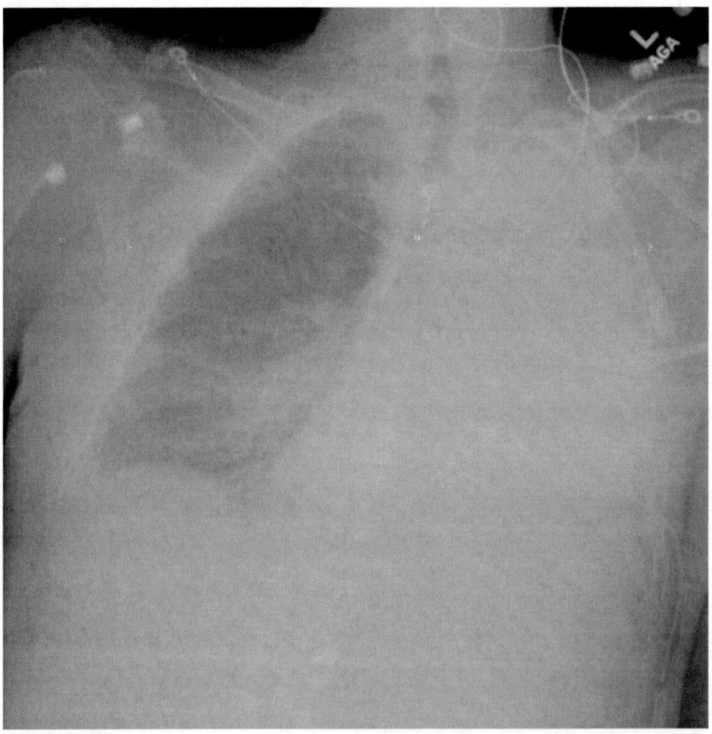

Figure 8. Massive left pleural effusion without a mediastinal shift.

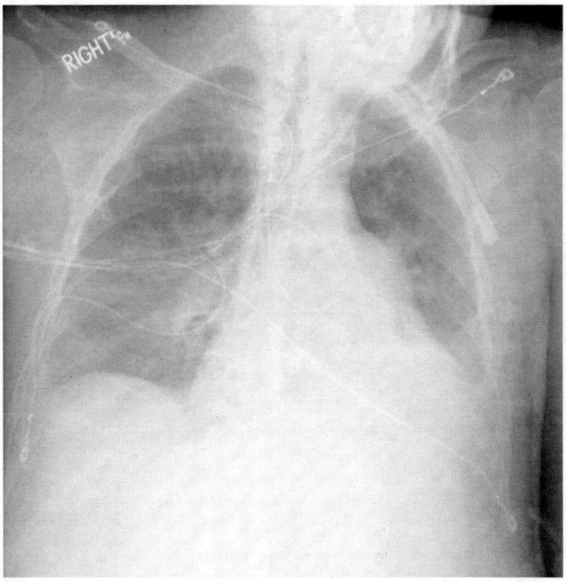

Figure 9. Post left side thoracentesis in the same patient.

Pleural fluid can accumulate within fissures producing a characteristic appearance on the chest x-ray. This depends upon the direction of the x-ray beam and the fissure involved. It commonly presents as a rounded, or an oval opacity, giving a mass like appearance on the PA view [Figure 10]. The fluid in the fissure can be absorbed spontaneously, hence described as a vanishing tumor or a "pseudotumor". On a lateral view it presents as a lenticular opacity within the fissure.

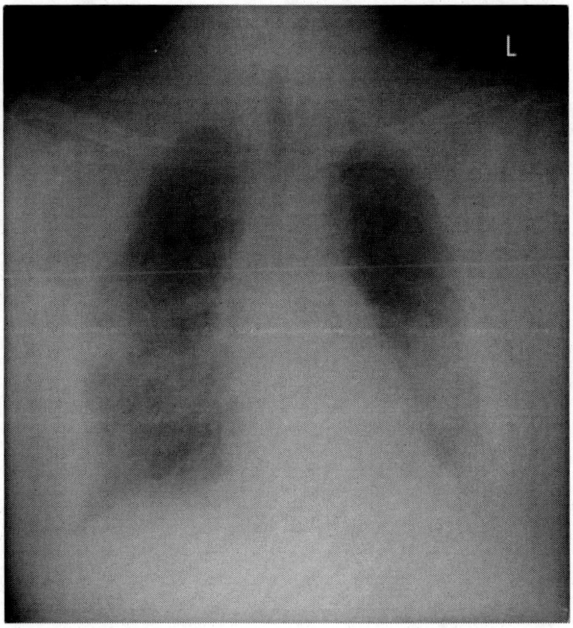

Figure 10. Rounded opacity seen in the right mid zone.

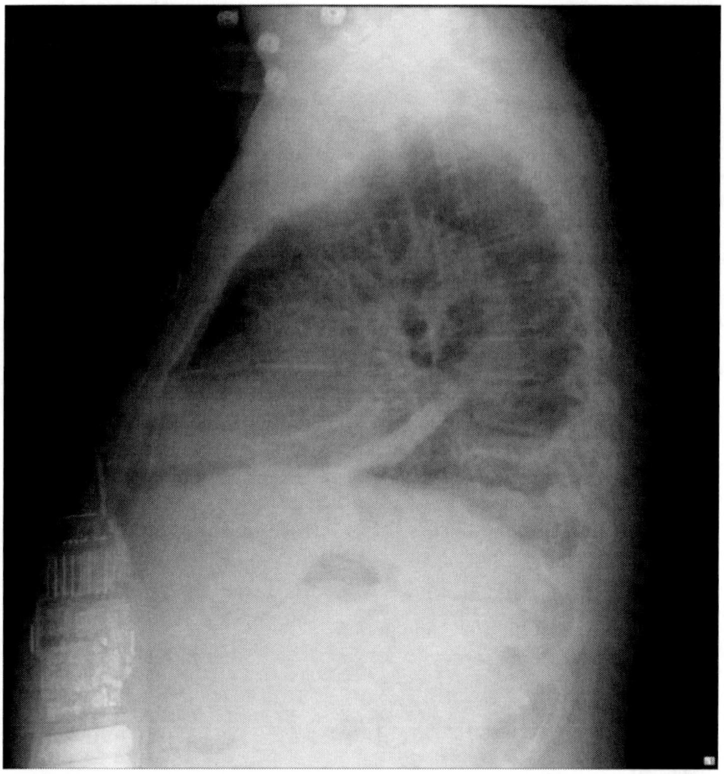

Figure 11. Fluid in the right major fissure.

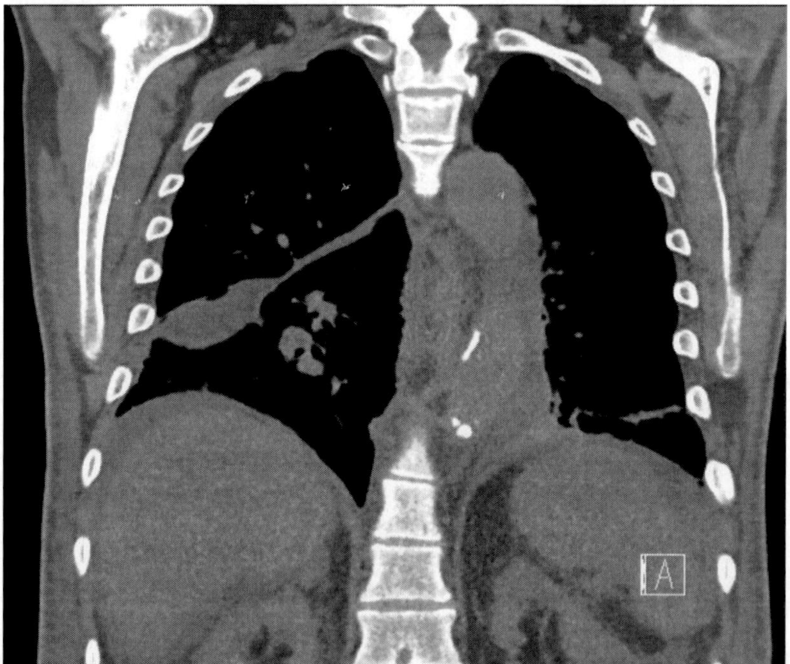

Figure 12. Fluid in the right major fissure. This is more clearly seen on the coronal cuts on CT scan in the same patient.

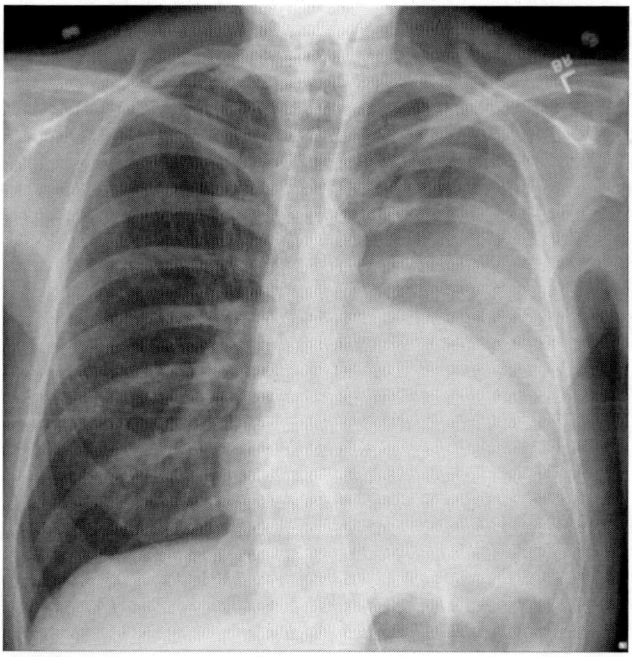

Figure 13. Loculated effusion on left (PA view).

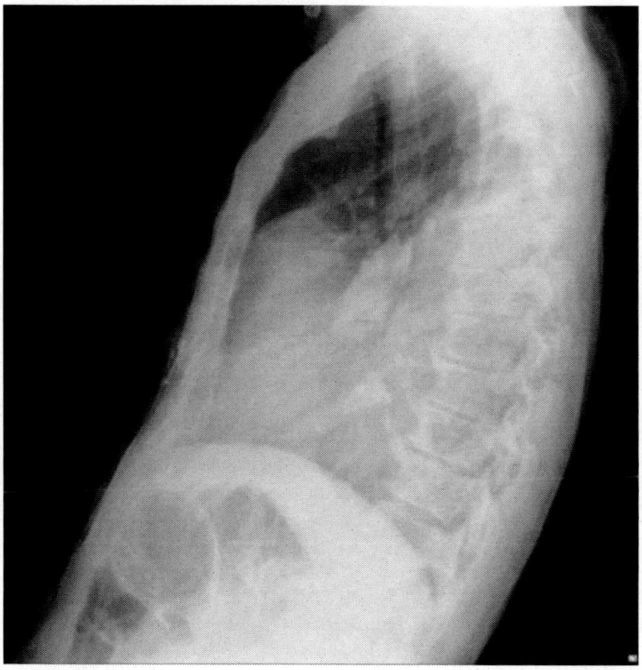

Figure 14. Loculated effusion on left side (Lateral view).

Loculated effusion develops when there are adhesions between the visceral and parietal pleural surfaces. The fluid does not move freely with the characteristic menisc sign is not seen and the [Figures 13, 14 and 15] fluid fails to layer on a lateral decubitus film.

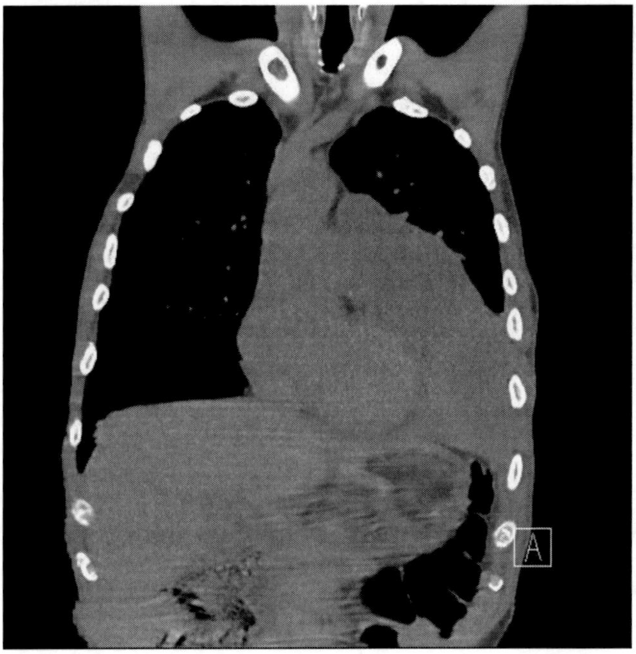

Figure 15. CT scan chest (coronal cuts), loculated effusion in the same patient.

Computed Tomography

CT scan is the best imaging modality to visualize intrathoracic structures and abnormalities, including pleural effusions. They can determine the location, extent and nature of pleural fluid. Normally the visceral and parietal pleurae are not visualized on CT scan and at the fissures the pleura is sharply defined with a thickness of less than 1 mm. The patient lies supine during a CT scan and the free fluid initially accumulates in the deep lateral and posterior recesses [15]. The dependent collection of free flowing fluid is seen as a sickle shaped opacity [Figure 16].

The ascitic fluid can be differentiated from pleural fluid by certain radiological signs. The "diaphragm sign" arises due to different distribution of pleural versus intraabdominal fluid in relation to diaphragm [Figure 17]. The lung and pleura are adjacent and peripheral to the convexity of hemidiaphragm whereas intraabdominal fluid lies adjacent and central to the hemidiaphragm [9]. In the "displaced crus sign" there is an anterior displacement of the diaphragmatic crus by pleural fluid interposed between the crus and the vertebral column. This is absent in an ascitic fluid collection. The "interface sign" represents the interface between fluid and the liver or spleen. It is ill-defined in a pleural fluid collection and sharp in ascites. The "bare area" is the portion of the right lobe of liver which doesn't have peritoneal covering and is attached directly to posterior abdominal wall. The ascitic fluid does not extend here unlike pleural fluid, which does produce the "bare area sign" [Figure 18].

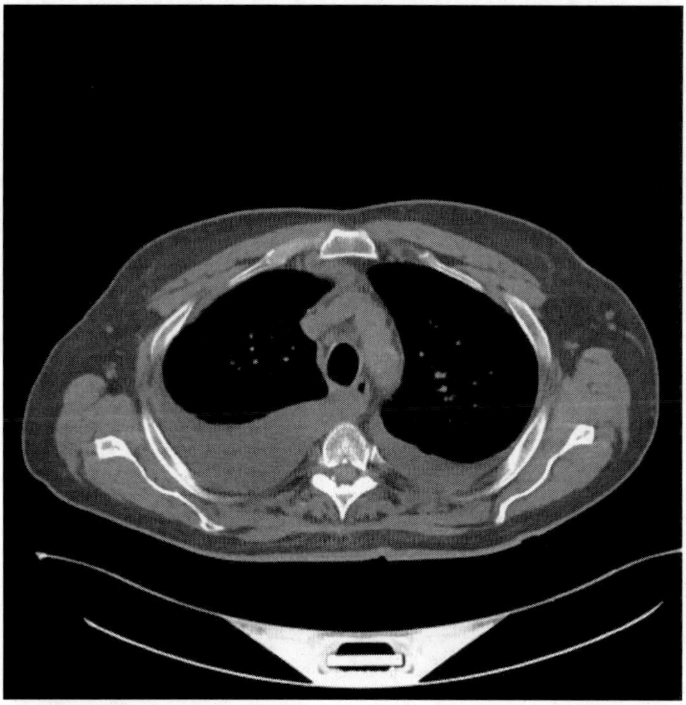

Figure 16. Free flowing pleural fluid forms a sickle shape opacity.

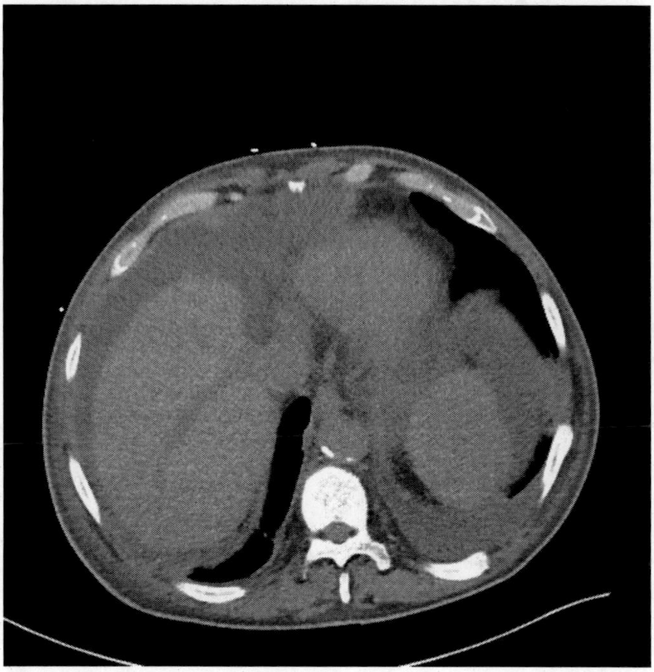

Figure 17. Pleural fluid lies peripheral to the hemidiaphragm and extends posterior to the bare area of the liver. There is an ill-defined interface between the pleural fluid and spleen.

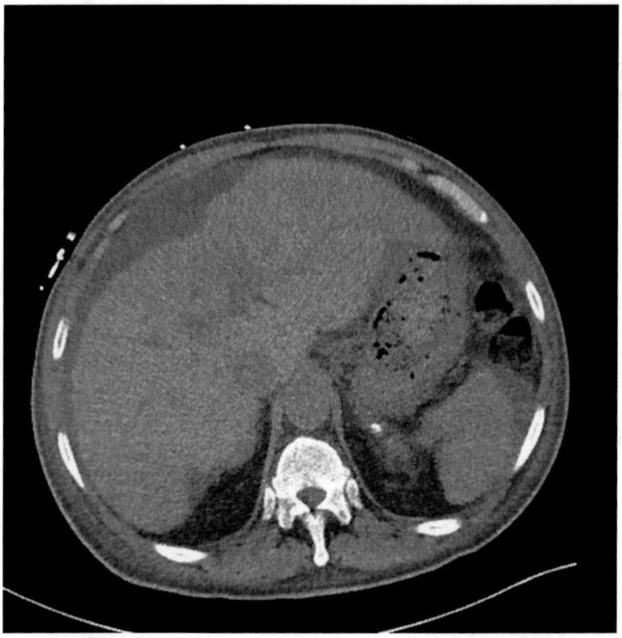

Figure 18. In the same patient as in Figure 17, the ascitic fluid does not extend posteriorly to the bare area of liver. There is a sharp interface between the ascitic fluid with spleen.

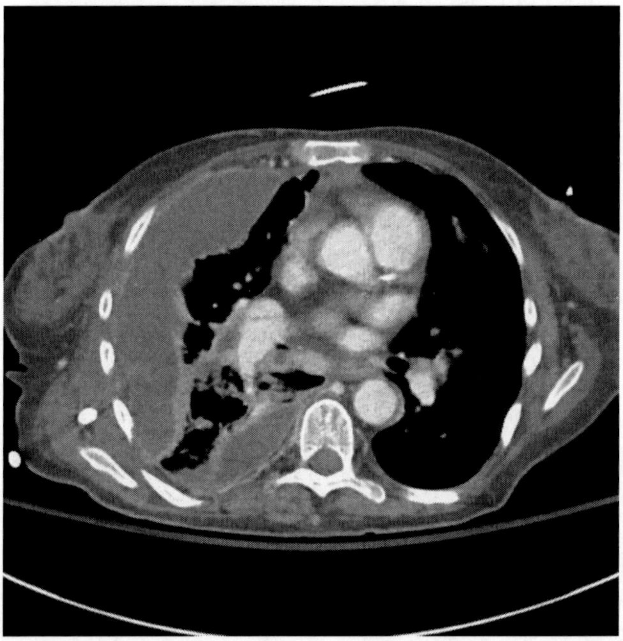

Figure 19. CT scan shows a right sided loculated effusion with split pleura sign and contrast enhancement of visceral and parietal pleura.

CT scan is an excellent tool to identify loculated pleural effusions. They appear as lenticular opacity with smooth margins and homogenous attenuation. In empyema the contrast enhanced CT scan demonstrates parietal and visceral pleural enhancement resulting in the “split-pleura” sign [Figure 19]. The septations are not that well visualized on a CT-scan, unlike on ultrasound imaging.

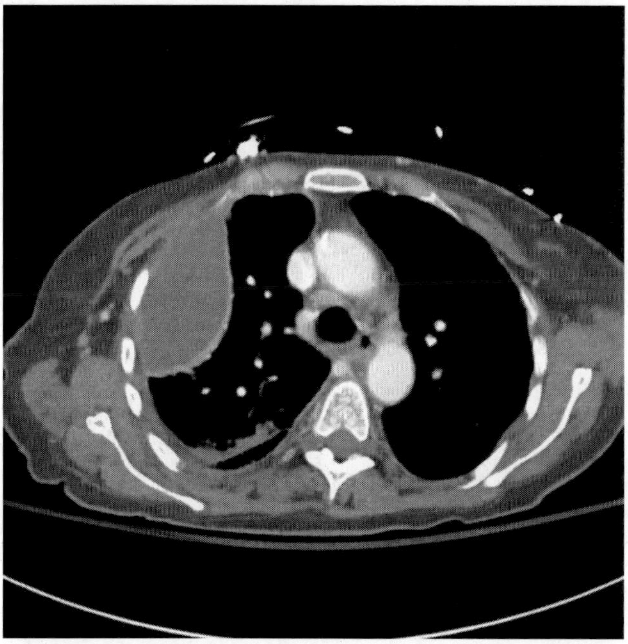

Figure 20. CT scan shows a right side loculated effusion forming an obtuse angle with the chest wall.

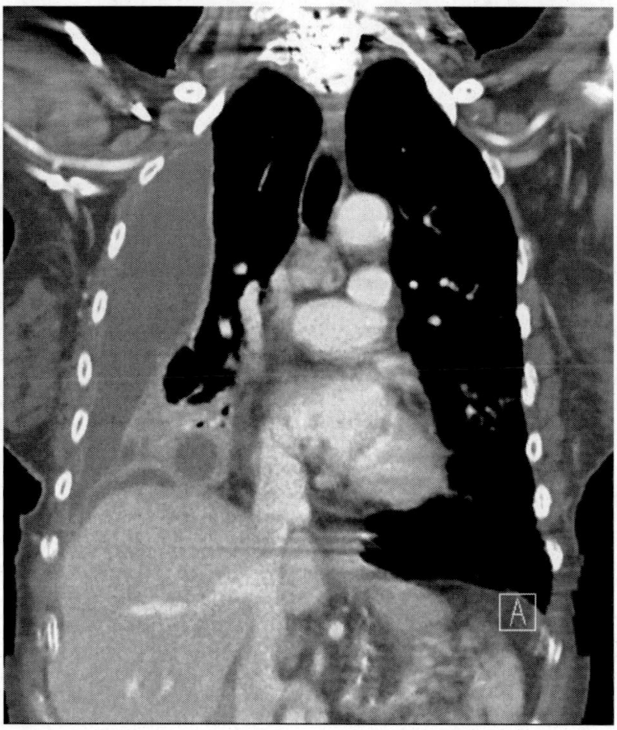

Figure 21. Coronal cuts in the same patient showing a loculated effusion.

CT scan also helps in differentiating between empyema and pulmonary abscesses which abut the pleura. On CT scan an abscess will appear as a spherical, thick walled lesion with abrupt vessel cut off and displacement of the surrounding parenchyma. It also makes an acute angle with chest wall, unlike an empyema which creates an obtuse angle [Figures 20 and 21].

Ultrasound

Free flowing fluid in the pleural space accumulates in the dependent portion of the thoracic cavity. Depending on the clinical condition and comfort, the patient can be in a sitting, supine, semi-recumbent or in a lateral decubitus position [Figure 23 a-d]. The goal should be to examine as much of the hemithorax as possible to be able to detect small or loculated pleural effusions. There are three important findings that are helpful in diagnosing a pleural effusion with the help of US [Figure 22]:

1. Anatomic boundaries of pleural effusions: chest wall, diaphragm, lung, sub-diaphragmatic organs and the ribs.

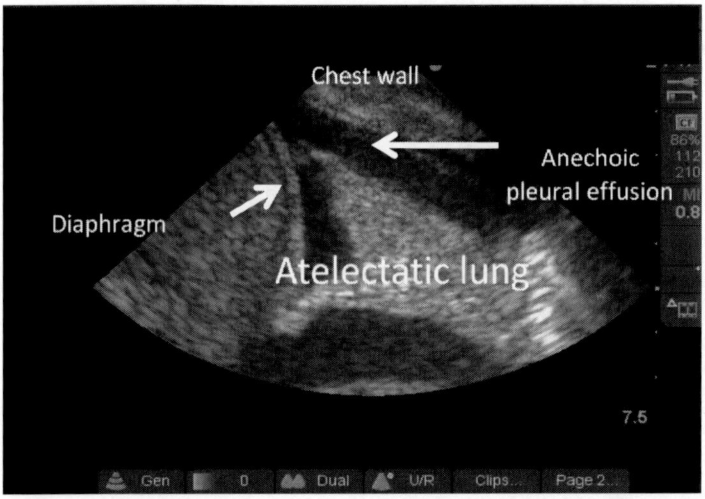

Figure 22. Pleural effusion is present as an anechoic space with anatomic boundaries made up of chest wall, diaphragm and atelectatic lung.

2. Presence of anechoic space (black) between the visceral and parietal pleura.
3. Dynamic changes.

The examiner should place the probe in a cranio-caudal direction and confirm orientation by looking at the probe marker on the US screen. First step is to identify the diaphragm as a curvilinear hyperechoic structure that moves with respiration. Pleural fluid in general is visualized as hypoechoic or anechoic collection above the diaphragm [Figure 22].

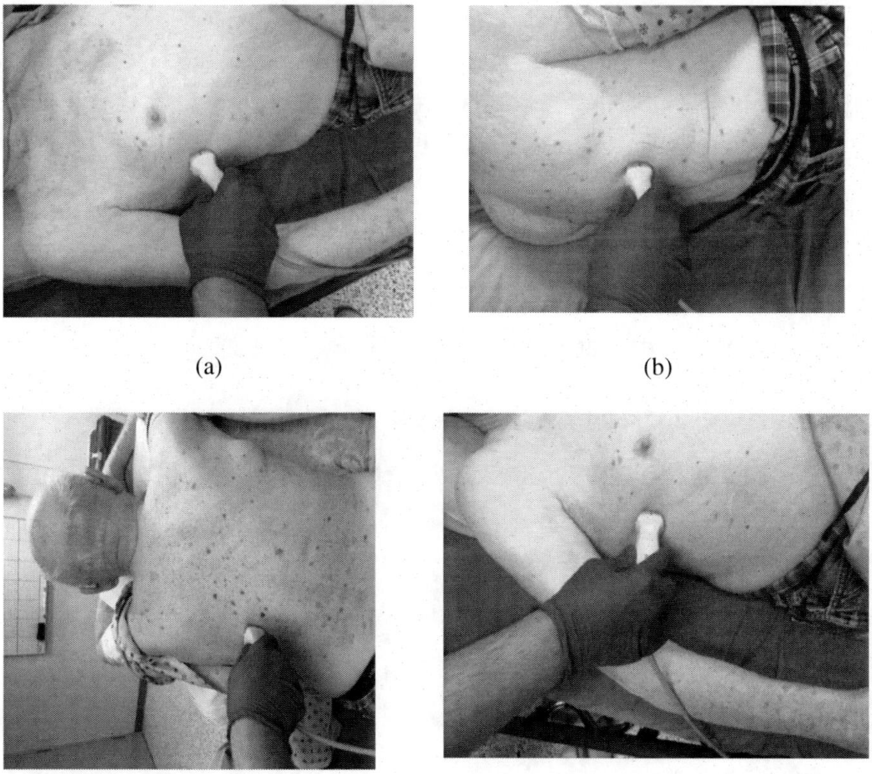

(a) (b)

(c) (d)

Figure 23. (a) Supine, (b) laterally rotated, (c) sitting and (d) semi-recumbent.

The utility of US for diagnosing pleural effusion is well established. US can detect pleural effusions as small as 3-5 mL in volume [20]. Physical examination is not very accurate in detecting pleural effusions and is likely not helpful for effusions less than 300 mL [18, 28]. US has a diagnostic accuracy of 93% when compared with CT scan in detecting a pleural effusion [21]. At times it can be challenging to distinguish a pleural effusion from other findings on chest x-ray. US has been shown to be a better imaging modality than chest radiograph in distinguishing pleural thickening, atelectasis, pleural effusion, parenchymal infiltrates or a combination of these findings [20].

There are many methods for estimating the volume of pleural effusions and require several measurements. Knowing the exact amount of fluid has limited usefulness in clinical practice and a qualitative approach might be better suited by classifying the effusion as small: seen in one probe range, moderate: seen in two probe range and large: greater than two probe range [16, 19].

In moderate to large pleural effusions, the adjacent lung may become atelectatic and appears as tissue like structure flapping in the pleural effusion, a dynamic sign on US called the "flapping lung" or the "jellyfish sign" [32]. The compressed lung has an echogenicity similar to that of the liver, and this is termed as sonographic hepatization of the lung [Figure 22]. When the effusion is small, aerated lung can be seen moving with inspiration into the costophrenic angle, but, the lateral diaphragm is still seen, causing an abnormal "curtain sign" [34]. The movement of the visceral pleural towards or away from the chest wall with inspiration and expiration creates a sinusoidal waveform pattern on the M-mode US [Figure 25]. This is called the "sinusoid sign", which again is a dynamic sign and very specific for the diagnosis of pleural effusion. It is helpful in distinguishing small pleural effusions from pleural thickening [33]. The "quad sign" too helps to detect small pleural effusions and the pleural effusion is seen as an anechoic space between the dark rib shadows and the lung and the parietal pleura [Figure 24] [33].

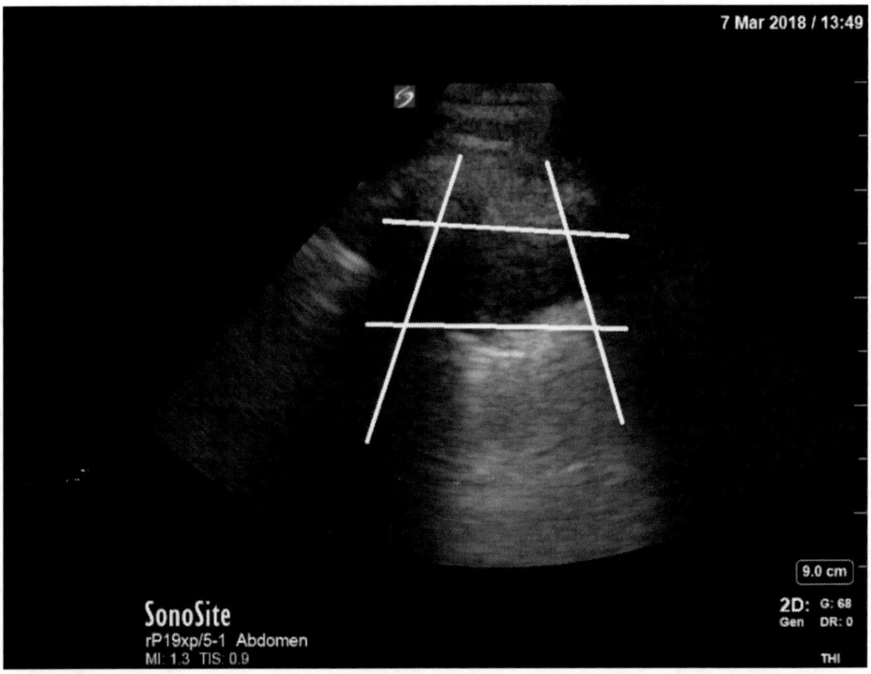

Figure 24. Quad sign: pleural effusion is seen as an anechoic space between two rib shadows (vertical white lines), parietal pleura (upper horizontal line) and the lung line (lower horizontal line).

Cellular or proteinaceous debris in the pleural fluid can be agitated by respiratory or cardiac motion creating a swirling pattern, which is called the "plankton sign" or the "swirl sign" [17]. Fibrin strands may be present and seen floating in the effusion or connected to each other in a lattice like pattern. Cellular debris in the effusion may settle down due to gravity, this creates an echogenic layering effect (hypocellular hypoechoic top layer with a cellular hyperechoic bottom layer) called the "hematocrit sign" [32].

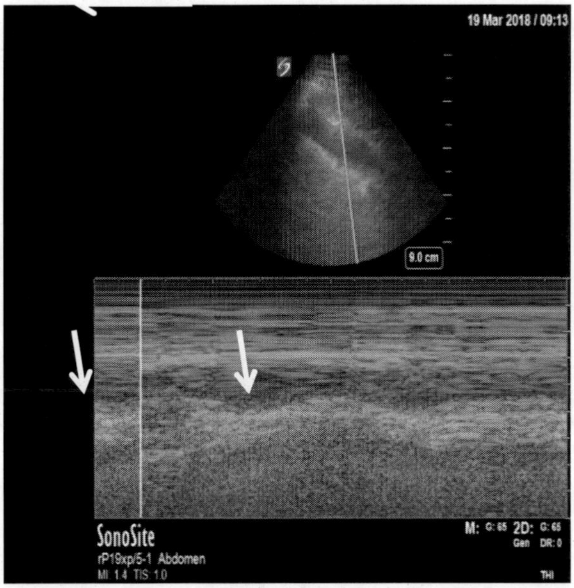

Figure 25. Sinusoid sign on M-mode (arrows).

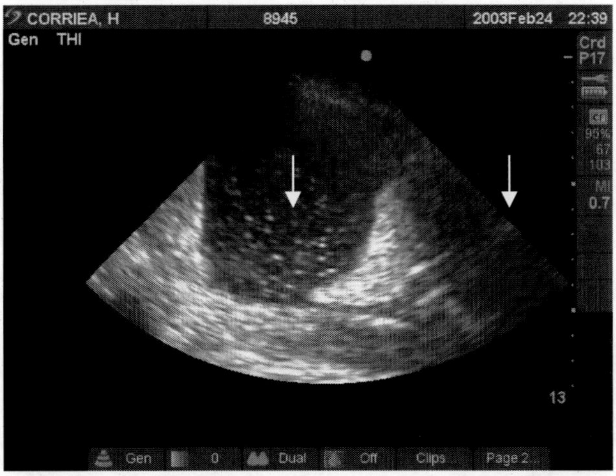

Figure 26. Complex non-septated pleural effusion.

Sonographic characteristics of the pleural fluid have been used to distinguish transudates from exudates. Effusions can have one of the following sonographic patterns, (1) anechoic: echo-free (black) space between the visceral and parietal pleura (2) complex non-septated: echogenic material is present in a non-homogenous pattern without septations [Figure 26]. (3) complex septated: floating fibrin strands or septae in a lattice like pattern are present [Figure 27]. This can be seen in parapneumonic effusions, empyema's, and malignant effusions. US has been shown to be superior to CT scan in detecting septations in pleural effusions [24], and (4) homogenously echogenic: very cellular echogenic material is strewn homogenously in the effusion, as in an empyema or hemorrhagic effusions [Figure 28]. Transudates are almost always anechoic [30]. Exudates on the other hand can have any of the four patterns. Although a definitive diagnosis of a transudate or an exudate requires a thoracentesis to identify the true nature of a pleural effusion by using Lights criteria or other laboratory tests [6].

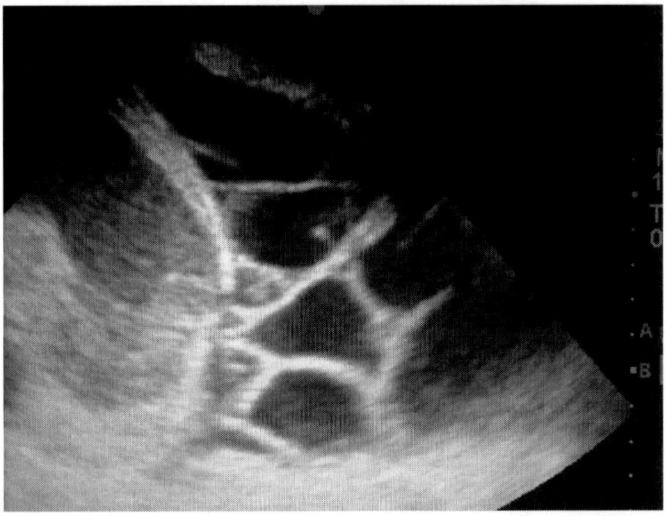

Figure 27. Complex septated pleural effusion.

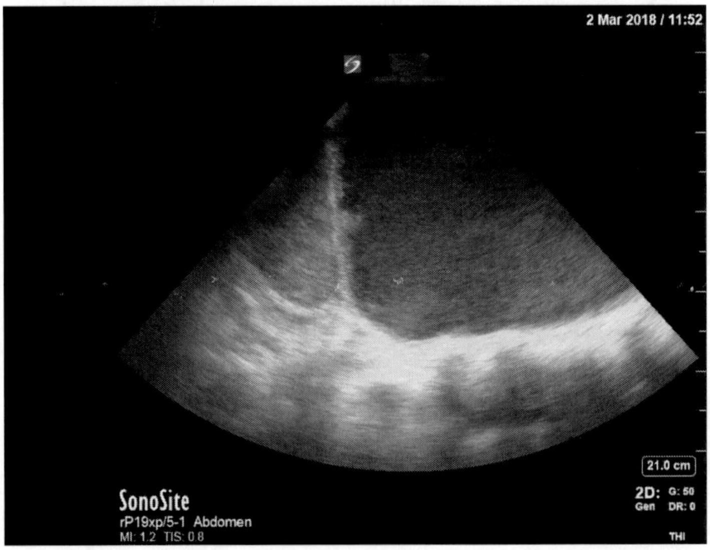

Figure 28. Homogenously echogenic pleural effusion.

Additional findings on US may be helpful to assess the etiology of pleural effusions [22, 27]. Echogenic swirling patterns or the presence of pleural nodules are suggestive of malignant effusions [17]. The presence of adjacent consolidated lung with an irregular interface, the “shred sign”, between the consolidated and normal lung [Figure 29] and/or mobile hyperechoic air bronchograms, the “dynamic air-bronchogram” sign, indicates an effusion of infectious origin [23]. The presence of bilateral pleural sliding with diffuse B lines suggests transudative effusion during heart failure [21, 25, 27].

Loculated pleural effusions may be missed if the entire hemithorax is not examined, as they can be in nondependent areas. They do not change with body position, can be circular or elongated, with thick pleural linings.

US is very helpful in determining the cause of a complete white out of a hemithorax [Figure 30]. US allows the distinction between effusion, atelectasis and lung consolidations [31].

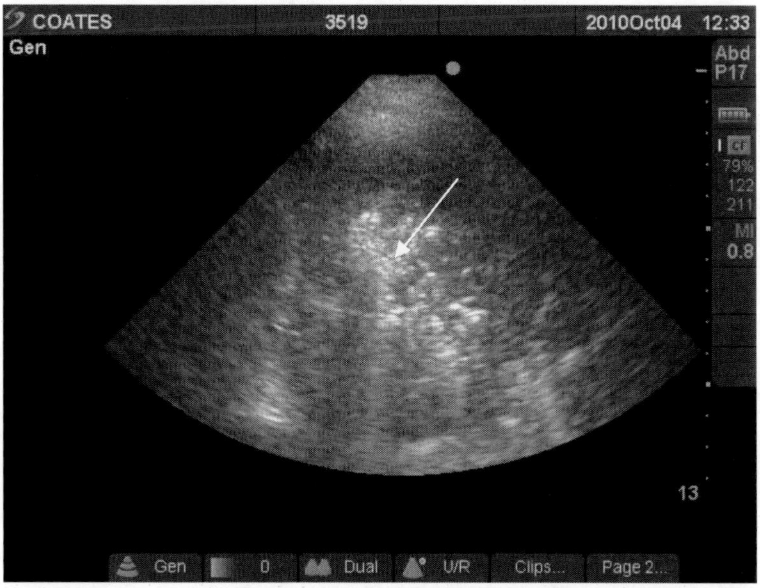

Figure 29. Consolidated adjacent lung with the “shred sign” (arrow), suggesting a parapneumonic effusion.

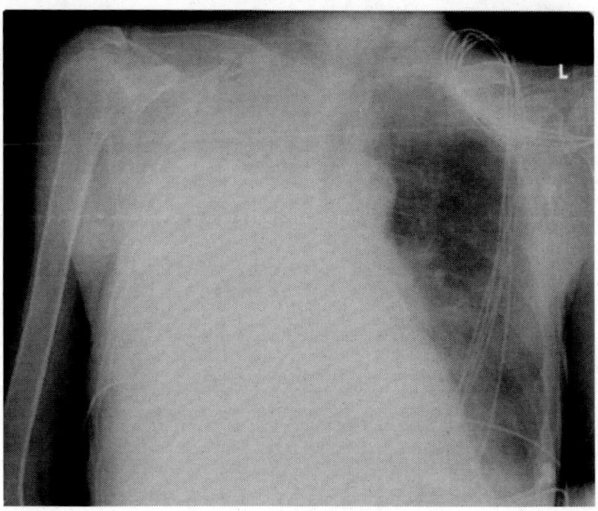

Figure 30. White out of right hemithorax on chest radiograph.

Conclusion

Pleural effusions are commonly encountered by clinicians as manifestations of many disease processes. History and physical examination have low diagnostic performance in detecting pleural effusions making it is important for clinicians to be familiar with commonly used imaging modalities to diagnose pleural effusions. Chest x-ray, US and CT scan of the chest are the most commonly used imaging modalities for detecting pleural effusions. Depending upon the etiology of the effusion they can present in various sizes, shapes and patterns. Clinicians should be familiar with the different presentations of pleural effusions on various imaging techniques to help them confidently diagnose pleural effusions and also the possible underlying cause of the same.

References

[1] Feller-Kopman, David; Richard, Light. "Pleural Disease." *New England Journal of Medicine*, 378, no. 8, (02, 2018), 740-51. doi:10.1056/nejmra1403503.

[2] Qureshi, Nagmi R; Fergus, V. Gleeson. "Imaging of Pleural Disease." *Clinics in Chest Medicine*, 27, no. 2, (2006), 193-213. doi:10.1016/j.ccm.2006.02.001.

[3] Saguil, A; Wyrick, K; Hallgren, J. 2014. "Diagnostic Approach to Pleural Effusion." *American Family Physician*, 90 (2), 99-104. doi:d10960 [pii].

[4] Yalcin, NG; Choong, CK; Eizenberg, N. 2013. "Anatomy and Pathophysiology of the Pleura and Pleural Space." *Thoracic Surgery Clinics*, 23 (1), 10, v. doi:10.1016/j.thorsurg.2012.10.008 [doi].

[5] Colins, JD; Burwell, D; Furmanski, S; Lorber, P; Steckel, RJ. 1972. "Minimal Detectable Pleural Effusions. A Roentgen Pathology Model." *Radiology*, 105 (1), 51-53. doi:10.1148/105.1.51 [doi].

[6] Light, Richard W. *Pleural Diseases*. Philadelphia: Wolters Kluwer/Lippincott Williams & Wilkins Health, 2013.

[7] Davis, S; Gardner, F; Qvist, G. 1963. "The Shape of a Pleural Effusion." *British Medical Journal*, 1 (5328), 436-437.

[8] Ilsen, Bart; Frederik, Vandenbroucke; Cathérine, Beigelman-Aubry; Carola, Brussaard; Johan, De Mey. "Comparative Interpretation of CT and Standard Radiography of the Pleura." *Journal of the Belgian Society of Radiology*, 100, no. 1, (11, 2016). doi:10.5334/jbr-btr.1229.

[9] Muller, NL. 1993. "Imaging of the Pleura." *Radiology*, 186 (2), 297-309. doi:10.1148/radiology.186.2.8421723 [doi].

[10] Moskowitz, H; Platt, RT; Schachar, R; Mellins, H. 1973. "Roentgen Visualization of Minute Pleural Effusion. an Experimental Study to Determine the Minimum Amount

of Pleural Fluid Visible on a Radiograph." *Radiology*, 109 (1), 33-35. doi:10.1148/109.1.33 [doi].

[11] Hooper, C; Lee, YC; Maskell, N. BTS Pleural Guideline Group. 2010. "Investigation of a Unilateral Pleural Effusion in Adults: British Thoracic Society Pleural Disease Guideline 2010." *Thorax*, 65, Suppl 2, 17. doi:10.1136/thx.2010.136978 [doi].

[12] Muniz, S; Hernandez, P; Olmedilla Arregui, A; Garcia de Vicente, V; Quintana, S; Moron Hodge, S; Alonso, Roca; Albillos Merino, JC. "Imaging review of pleural effusion: diagnosis and intervention." *ESTI*, 2014. doi: 10.1594/esti2014/P-0058 [doi].

[13] Woodring, JH. 1984. "Recognition of Pleural Effusion on Supine Radiographs: How Much Fluid is Required?" *AJR. American Journal of Roentgenology*, 142 (1), 59-64. doi:10.2214/ajr.142.1.59 [doi].

[14] Na, MJ. 2014. "Diagnostic Tools of Pleural Effusion." *Tuberculosis and Respiratory Diseases*, 76 (5), 199-210. doi:10.4046/trd.2014.76. 5.199 [doi].

[15] Hallifax, Rj; Talwar, A; Wrightson, Jm; Edey, A; Gleeson, Fv. "State-of-the-art: Radiological Investigation of Pleural Disease." *Respiratory Medicine*, 124, (03 2017), 88-99. doi:10.1016/ j.rmed.2017.02.013.

[16] Blackmore, C. Craig; William, C. Black; Robert, V. Dallas; Harte, C. Crow. "Pleural fluid volume estimation: A chest radiograph prediction rule." *Academic Radiology*, 3, no. 2 (1996), 103-09. doi:10.1016/s1076-6332(05)80373-3.

[17] Chian, Chih-Feng; Wen-Lin, Su; Li-Hui, Soh; Horng-Chin, Yan; Wann-Cherng, Perng; Chin-Pyng, Wu. "Echogenic Swirling Pattern as a Predictor of Malignant Pleural Effusions in Patients With Malignancies." *Chest*, 126, no. 1, (2004), 129-34. doi:10.1378/chest. 126.1.129.

[18] Diacon, Andreas H; Martin, H. Brutsche; Markus, Solèr. "Accuracy of Pleural Puncture Sites*." *Chest*, 123, no. 2, (2003), 436-41. doi:10.1378/chest.123.2.436.

[19] Eibenberger, KL; Dock, WI; Ammann, ME; Dorffner, R; Hörmann, MF; Grabenwöger, F. "Quantification of pleural effusions: sonography versus radiography." *Radiology*, 191, no. 3, (1994), 681-84. doi:10.1148/radiology.191.3.8184046.

[20] Gryminski, Janusz; Pawel, Krakówka; Grazyna, Lypacewicz. "The Diagnosis of Pleural Effusion by Ultrasonic and Radiologic Techniques." *Chest*, 70, no. 1, (1976), 33-37. doi:10.1378/chest. 70.1.33.

[21] Lichtenstein, Daniel; Ivan, Goldstein; Eric, Mourgeon; Philippe, Cluzel; Philippe, Grenier; Jean-Jacques, Rouby. "Comparative Diagnostic Performances of Auscultation, Chest Radiography, and Lung Ultrasonography in Acute Respiratory Distress Syndrome." *Anesthesiology*, 100, no. 1, (2004), 9-15. doi:10.1097/00000542-200401000-00006.

[22] Lichtenstein, Daniel A; Gilbert, A. Mezière. "Relevance of Lung Ultrasound in the Diagnosis of Acute Respiratory Failure*: The BLUE Protocol." *Chest*, 134, no. 1, (2008), 117-25. doi:10.1378/ chest.07-2800.

[23] Lichtenstein, Daniel; Gilbert, Mezière; Julien, Seitz. "The Dynamic Air Bronchogram." *Chest*, 135, no. 6, (2009), 1421-425. doi:10.1378/ chest.08-2281.

[24] Mcloud, TC; Flower, CD. "Imaging the pleura: sonography, CT, and MR imaging." *American Journal of Roentgenology*, 156, no. 6, (1991), 1145-153. doi:10.2214/ ajr.156.6.2028857.

[25] Noble, Vicki E; Alice, F. Murray; Roberta, Capp; Mary, H. Sylvia-Reardon; David, Jr. Steele; Andrew, Liteplo. "Ultrasound Assessment for Extravascular Lung Water in Patients Undergoing Hemodialysis." *Chest*, 135, no. 6, (2009), 1433-439. doi:10. 1378/chest.08-1811.

[26] Patterson, La; Costantino, Tg; Satz, Wa. "Diagnosing pleural effusion: A prospective comparison of physical examination with bedside thoracic ultrasonography." *Annals of Emergency Medicine*, 44, no. 4, (2004). doi:10.1016/j.annemergmed.2004.07.364.

[27] Prosen, Gregor; Petra, Klemen; Matej, Strnad; Štefek, Grmec. Combination of lung ultrasound (a comet-tail sign) and N-terminal pro-brain natriuretic peptide in differentiating acute heart failure from chronic obstructive pulmonary disease and asthma as cause of acute dyspnea in prehospital emergency setting." *Critical Care*, 15, no. 6, (2011), 450. doi:10.1186/cc10511.

[28] Rolston, D; Diaz-Guzman, E; Budev, MM. "Accuracy of the physical examination in evaluating pleural effusion." *Cleveland Clinic Journal of Medicine*, *75*, no. 4, (January 2008), 297–303. doi:10.3949/ccjm.75.4.297.

[29] Wong, Camilla L. "Does This Patient Have a Pleural Effusion?" *Jama*, 301, no. 3, (2009), 309. doi:10.1001/jama.2008.937.

[30] Yang, PC; Luh, KT; Chang, DB; Wu, HD; Yu, CJ; Kuo, SH. "Value of sonography in determining the nature of pleural effusion: analysis of 320 cases." *American Journal of Roentgenology*, 159, no. 1, (1992), 29-33. doi:10.2214/ajr.159.1.1609716.

[31] Yu, Chong-Jen; Pan-Chyr, Yang; Huey-Dong, Wu; Dun-Bing, Chang; Sow-Hsong, Kuo; Kwen-Tay, Luh. "Ultrasound Study in Unilateral Hemithorax Opacification: Image Comparison with Computed Tomography." *American Review of Respiratory Disease*, 147, no. 2, (1993), 430-34. doi:10.1164/ajrccm/147.2.430.

[32] Cardenas-Garcia, Jose; Paul, H. Mayo; Erik, Folch. "Ultrasonographic Evaluation of the Pleura." *Pleura*, 2, (2015), 237399751561027. doi:10.1177/2373997515610270.

[33] Lichtenstein, Daniel A. "Lung Ultrasound in the Critically Ill Neonate." *Lung Ultrasound in the Critically Ill*, 2016, 277-85. doi:10.1007/978-3-319-15371-1_32.

[34] Lee, Francis Chun Yue. "The Curtain Sign in Lung Ultrasound." *Journal of Medical Ultrasound*, 25, no. 2, (2017), 101-04. doi:10. 1016/j.jmu.2017.04.005.

In: Pleural Effusions: Causes, Types and Treatment ISBN: 978-1-53614-683-7
Editor: Rahul Khosla

Chapter 2

ETIOLOGY AND DIAGNOSTIC WORK-UP OF PLEURAL EFFUSIONS

Amandeep S. Bawa[1,*], MD
and Montserrat Diaz-Abad[2], MD
[1]Pulmonary and Critical Care Medicine, Veterans Affairs Medical Center, The George Washington University, Washington DC, US
[2]Pulmonary and Critical Care Medicine, University of Maryland Medical Center, University of Maryland School of Medicine,
Baltimore, MD, US

ABSTRACT

Pleural effusions are a common medical problem with an extensive list of known causes. Pleural effusion develops in about 1.5 million patients each year in the United States [1]. The three most common causes of pleural effusions include heart failure, pneumonia and malignancy. In patients with clinical history and examination suggestive of congestive heart failure, aspiration of fluid is not warranted. However, in most other cases analysis of pleural fluid is required to delineate the etiology. Pleural effusions are characterized into two groups as transudate or an exudate based on the fluid's laboratory characteristics using the Light's criteria. Point of care ultrasound has increased the safety of thoracentesis and decreased the need for multiple attempts.

Keywords: pleural effusion, thoracentesis, Light's criteria, transudate, exudate

INTRODUCTION

The pleura is a thin membrane lining the lung and the chest cavity creating a potential pleural space. The pleural space normally contains very small amount of fluid, about 8.4 ±

* Corresponding Author Email: Amandeep.Bawa@va.gov.

4.3 ml each side [22], which assist in the movement of the lungs over chest wall during respiration by providing lubrication [20]. The increased fluid accumulation in the pleural space manifests as pleural effusion and this is a common medical problem seen in clinical medicine. The list of causes for pleural effusion is extensive and clinical history is helpful in determining the etiology in certain conditions like congestive heart failure. The biochemical analysis of pleural fluid assists in forming the differential diagnosis. The Light's criteria have been well established since 1972 to dichotomize the effusions into transudates and exudates.

Anatomy and Pathogenesis

The thoracic cavity is divided into two compartments of pleural cavities on either side of mediastinum. Each pleural cavity encloses a lung with associated anatomical structures and do not communicate with each other. The pleura is a serous membrane lining the interior of thoracic cavity and consists of two layers, the parietal and the visceral pleura, and is a thin membrane lined with a single layer of mesothelial cells overlying a thin layer of connective tissue [2]. The parietal pleura lines the inner surface of the thoracic cavity while the visceral pleura is adherent to the lung and follows the interlobar fissures. The pleural space formed between the two layers of pleura is a closed space and surrounds the lung except at the hilum where the visceral pleura is contiguous with the parietal pleura [2, 3]. This maintains apposition during respiration. This potential space contains small physiologic amount of pleural fluid (0.1 ml/kg) normally [5]. The pleural membranes assist in movement of the lungs over the chest wall and diaphragm with the pleural fluid acting as a lubricant.

The arterial supply of the parietal pleura is from the systemic circulation via the intercostal arteries with venous drainage through intercostal veins. The parietal pleura lymphatics are in the sub-mesothelial connective tissue and they drain into the intercostal, parasternal, diaphragmatic and posterior mediastinal nodes. The arterial supply of the visceral pleura is from bronchial circulation, like the lung parenchyma. The visceral pleura venous drainage is by pulmonary veins except from the hilum which drains into bronchial veins [3, 20]. The visceral pleura lymphatics drain towards the nodes of the lungs.

The parietal pleura is innervated by intercostal and phrenic nerve. This somatic innervation of parietal pleura makes them highly sensitive to pain. On the other hand, the visceral pleura is innervated by autonomic nerves which are insensitive to pain.

The pleural fluid is primarily formed from the capillaries located in the sub-mesothelial connective tissue on parietal pleura and normally produced at a rate of approximately 0.01ml/kg/h. The fluid is removed via stomata on the parietal pleura which drains into the lymphatics at the same rate to maintain a constant volume in the pleural space. In the presence of excessive pleural fluid formation, the lymphatic vessels in the parietal pleura can increase the resorption of pleural fluid by 30-fold to a rate of approximately 0.28 ml/kg/h [2, 13, 20]. On the other hand, no stomas are present in the visceral pleura.

The formation of pleural fluid is determined by the difference in the hydrostatic and oncotic pressures between the pleural space and the parietal and visceral capillaries. The hydrostatic pressure in the microcirculation is much higher in the parietal pleural than the visceral pleura while the oncotic pressures are similar, thus the pleural fluid is primarily formed from the parietal surface. The parietal pleura mesothelium has similar permeability like capillary endothelium for small solutes, thus the pleural fluid formed from the parietal pleura capillaries has the composition of plasma filtrate with low protein content. The Starling law explains the movement of solute and fluid across the microcirculation. This is determined by the transmembrane hydrostatic pressure gradient, osmotic pressure gradient and the permeability of the membrane [10]. The Starling equation for the movement of solute and fluid across the pleural microcirculation and pleural mesothelium is stated as below [8, 20, 21]:

$$Q_F = L_P \times A\,[(P_{CAP}-P_{PL})-\sigma_D\,(\pi_{CAP}-\pi_{PL})]$$

where,

Q_F is the pleural fluid movement,

L_P is the hydraulic conductivity (measures water permeability), A is the surface area of the pleura, the product of Lp and A is the filtration coefficient,

σ_D is reflection coefficient for protein movement across the pleural ($_{PL}$) mesothelium,

P_{CAP} is the hydrostatic pressure (P) in the subpleural capillaries ($_{CAP}$),

π_{PL} is the oncotic pressure (π) of pleural ($_{PL}$) space.

In general, the pleural fluid would accumulate when fluid formation for any reason overwhelms the lymphatics capabilities to clear fluid. Pleural fluid accumulates from one or more of the following mechanism [19]:

a) Increased hydrostatic pressures in microcirculation from increased systemic venous pressure and increased pulmonary capillary pressure. Most common example is congestive heart failure.
b) Decreased oncotic pressure in microcirculation, as in hypoproteinemia.
c) Decreased pleural space pressure. A good example is atelectasis causing increased negative intrapleural pressure.
d) Increased permeability in microcirculation. Examples are inflammation in parapneumonic effusion and malignant effusion.
e) Lymphatic flow impairment from obstruction. Examples include fibrosis or malignancy.
f) Translocation of ascitic fluid from the peritoneum via diaphragmatic holes, as in hepatic hydrothorax.

Etiology of Pleural Effusion

Most cases of pleural effusion occur due to heart failure, infection and malignancy. The differential diagnosis of etiology of pleural effusion is exhaustive (Tables 1 and 2). Pleural effusions that develops in the presence of intact capillary barrier occurs from increased hydrostatic pressure (e.g., congestive heart failure) or decreased oncotic pressure (e.g., hypoalbuminemia). The fluid is characterized as transudate, which generally indicates that the pleural membranes are normal. Transudate can also occur in cases with decrease in the pleural pressures (e.g., atelectasis, trapped lung) and trans-diaphragmatic movement of fluid from the peritoneal cavity (e.g., hepatic hydrothorax). The exudative pleural fluid accumulates due to increased permeability from altered capillary barrier from underlying inflammatory and malignant causes [4, 11, 17].

The causes of transudative effusion are limited whereas those for exudative effusion are extensive. A list of potential causes is listed below (Table 1 and Table 2) [1, 4, 13, 15]. Congestive heart failure is the most common cause of transudative effusion and along with hepatic hydrothorax accounts for majority of transudative effusion. Parapneumonic effusions are the most common cause of exudative effusion followed by malignant effusions and pulmonary embolism.

Table 1. Transudative causes

- Congestive heart failure.
- Hepatic (cirrhosis) hydrothorax
- Nephrotic syndrome
- Hypoalbuminemia
- Superior vena cava obstruction
- Urinothorax
- Hypothyroidism
- Peritoneal dialysis
- Cerebrospinal fluid leak to pleura
- Atelectasis
- Pulmonary embolism

History and physical examination is helpful in diagnosing the causes of effusion. This is especially important in patient's presenting with dyspnea, orthopnea, paroxysmal nocturnal dyspnea, bilateral lower extremities swelling and associated with jugular venous distention, S_3 gallop, bilateral crackles and bilateral pleural effusion. This is all suggestive for congestive heart failure and in the absence of chest pain and fever, a trial of diuretic should be considered. In three fourth of such cases pleural effusion should resolve within 48 hours of starting diuretics.

Table 2. Exudative causes

• Infections (bacterial, viral, fungal, mycobacterial and parasitic) • Malignancy (metastatic, mesothelioma, primary body cavity lymphoma) • Pulmonary embolism • Cardiac diseases (post-cardiac injury syndrome, post-coronary artery bypass graft surgery, catheter ablation procedures, pulmonary vein stenosis) • Gastrointestinal disease (Esophageal perforation, pancreatitis, intra-abdominal abscess, post-abdominal surgery) • Rheumatological disorders (rheumatoid arthritis, systemic lupus erythematosus, sjogren's syndrome, eosinophilic granulomatosis, granulomatosis with polyangiitis) • Genitourinary (endometriosis, Meigs' syndrome, ovarian hyperstimulation syndrome) • Medications (amiodarone, methotrexate, nitrofurantoin, phenytoin, beta blockers, bromocriptine) • Chylothorax • Pseudochylothorax (cholesterol effusions) • Hemothorax • Miscellaneous causes: sarcoidosis, asbestos exposure, electric burn, radiation therapy, amyloidosis, uremia, yellow nail syndrome, trapped lung, iatrogenic effusion.

Chest x-rays are usually the initial radiological modality used to determine the presence and size of pleural effusion. The blunting of the lateral costo-phrenic angle is suggestive of 175 ml of pleural fluid. [2]. If the diaphragm is obscured then at least 500 ml of pleural fluid is present and if it extends to the anterior fourth rib then the estimated volume of pleural fluid is at least 1000 ml. Smaller amount of pleural fluid as little as 5 ml can be detected on the lateral decubitus film. Point of care ultrasound and computed tomography (CT) scan of the chest further help in delineating the size and characteristics of pleural effusion, especially if it is loculated.

Diagnostic thoracentesis, which involves aspiration off a small volume of pleural fluid (50 to 100 ml), is indicated when the underlying ideology is unclear. Therapeutic or larger volume aspiration, up to 1500 ml is done for treatment of symptomatic effusion. Though the initial thoracentesis should aim for both the diagnostic evaluation and therapeutic management of pleural effusion. Diagnostic thoracentesis should be considered if the thickness of pleural fluid on the decubitus chest x-ray, CT scan or ultrasound is greater than 10 mm. The British Thoracic Society guidelines highly recommend thoracentesis under ultrasound guidance [6]. The use of ultrasound increases the probability of successful aspiration, decreases the incidence of pneumothorax and is associated with lower hospital costs [16, 18]. One of the worrisome complication after the thoracentesis is lung puncture causing pneumothorax. It has been reported in 4% to 30% of cases in procedure done blindly without the use of ultrasound, though in one study less than half of those who developed post thoracentesis pneumothorax ended up with chest tube placement [14]. The incidence of pneumothorax is significantly reduced with the use of ultrasound guidance with rates varying between 1.3% and 6.7%. Thoracentesis under ultrasound guidance remains a safe procedure even in mechanically ventilated patients when compared to patients not on mechanical ventilation. Post procedure point of care ultrasound can rapidly detect pneumothorax and has higher sensitivity than chest x-ray. On ultrasound if B lines and lung sliding sign are seen then the pneumothorax can be reliably excluded with 100% negative predictive value [18, 47].

Other complications include cough, chest pain, vasovagal response, bleeding, re-expansion pulmonary edema, organ laceration, and infection [7, 14]. Post procedure chest x-ray is not indicated unless symptoms develops [5, 14]. Aspiration of air during thoracentesis is highly associated with development of subsequent pneumothorax. Also, the use of vacuum bottle for drainage likely prevented the identification of free air during the procedure and was associated with increased risk of post procedure pneumothorax [14]. Hence manual aspiration of pleural fluid is highly recommended.

Pleural Fluid Analysis

One of the initial step in management of pleural effusion is to determine if it is a transudate (non-inflammatory) or an exudate (inflammatory) using the Light's criteria (Table 3). They were first described in 1972 and remains the most commonly used criteria [25]. The protein and lactate dehydrogenase (LDH) levels help in differentiating transudates from exudates. The pleural fluid LDH correlates with degree of pleural inflammation and increases with the inflammation of pleural surface or the capillaries. The increase in pleural fluid protein correlates with increased permeability of the capillaries [17].

An exudate is defined if any one of the following criteria is present while none are present in transudate: (1) a ratio of pleural fluid protein to serum protein greater than 0.5; (2) a ratio of pleural fluid LDH to serum LDH greater than 0.6; and (3) a pleural fluid LDH level greater than 200 IU/L or greater than two third of the upper limit of the normal range for serum LDH level. It has a sensitivity of 98% for exudative effusions though the specificity is slightly lower at 83% [9].

Table 3. Light's criteria

(Exudate: if one or more are present; Transudate: if all three are absent)
1) Ratio of pleural fluid to serum protein > 0.5
2) Ratio of pleural fluid to serum LDH > 0.6
3) Pleural fluid LDH > 2/3rd the upper limit of normal for serum LDH level.

In patients with congestive heart failure (CHF) on diuretics, using Light's criteria can incorrectly classify the effusion as an exudate in 25% of cases. In these patients, the serum to pleural protein gap greater than 3.1 g/dL or a serum to pleural albumin gap greater than 1.2 g/dL helps in identifying transudates which have been incorrectly labelled as exudates. Between the two, the albumin gap has more accuracy than protein gap in identifying pseudo-exudates [17]. Pleural fluid N-terminal pro-brain natriuretic peptide (NT-pro-BNP) levels higher than 1300 pg/mL has been also used to accurately identify pleural effusions from CHF. The serum BNP shows close correlation with pleural fluid NT-pro-BNP, advocating the use of serum levels along with clinical assessment as a more readily available test.

The albumin gap should not be used alone as initial criteria to differentiate exudates and transudates as it can misidentify 13% of exudates as transudate [9] and is best used in conjunction with Light's criteria. Pleural fluid cholesterol greater than 45 mg/dL or pleural fluid protein greater than 3 g/L indicates exudative effusion as accurately as Light's criteria [13]. They have not been found superior when compared to original Light's criteria [17].

Gross Appearance of Pleural Fluid

The gross appearance of pleural fluid provides clinical clues. If the fluid has a bloody appearance then in order to diagnose a hemothorax the pleural fluid hematocrit should be compared with peripheral hematocrit. If it is greater than 50% of peripheral blood, it is suggestive of hemothorax. If it is between 1 and 20%, it could be seen in cancer, pulmonary embolism and trauma. If it is less than 1%, than it is clinically not significant.

Turbidity of fluid is seen in the presence of cells, debris, or high lipid levels. The fluid should undergo centrifugation, if it clears then its due to the presence of cells or debris in pleural fluid. If the turbidity persists then it's from high lipid levels, triglyceride or cholesterol.

The odor of pleural fluid can be helpful in certain diseases. Putrid odor in seen with anaerobic infection while smell of urine seen in urinothorax [7, 9].

Pleural Fluid Total Cell Count and Differential

The cellular content of pleural fluid was measured in a study [22] done on healthy humans who underwent thorocoscopic sympatholysis surgery for severe essential hyperhidrosis. A pleural lavage was done to evaluate for the volume and cellular content of pleural fluid. In this study about 1,700 cells/μL of total white blood cell (WBC) count were seen with predominant macrophages (75%), lymphocytes (23%) and mesothelial cell (1%).

In most cases the total nucleated cell count is not helpful in identifying a specific diagnosis. The transudates generally have less than 1000 total nucleated cell/μL, whereas exudates have more than 1000 nucleated cell/μL. In the presence of greater than 10,000 nucleated cell/μL, the likely causes include uncomplicated parapneumonic effusion, acute pancreatitis, pulmonary infarction, lupus pleuritis, acute rheumatoid pleurisy and post cardiac injury syndrome. In complicated parapneumonic effusions including empyema the cell count exceeds 50,000 nucleated cell/μL [2, 12, 50].

On the other hand, the differential cell count is highly useful in limiting the differential diagnosis in exudative pleural effusions [6]. The presence and predominance of neutrophils suggests an acute process while that of mononuclear cells suggests a chronic process. [9]. Pleural effusions with neutrophils predominance (defined as >50% nucleated cells being neutrophils) is seen in acute conditions, such as, parapneumonic effusion, pulmonary embolism, acute tuberculosis, benign asbestos pleural effusion, viral infection or pancreatitis.

The pleural effusions with lymphocytic predominance (defined as >50% nucleated cells being lymphocytes) generally suggests a chronic process. Common causes include malignancy, tuberculosis, lymphoma, congestive heart failure, rheumatoid effusion, uremia, sarcoidosis, chylothorax, yellow nail syndrome, and post-coronary artery bypass graft. Though the two most common causes of lymphocytic effusions include malignancy and tuberculosis. The presence of mesothelial cells in lymphocytic effusion makes the possibility of tuberculosis highly unlikely. Light et al. evaluated pleural fluids from 182 patients prospectively and found that all with tuberculous pleural effusion had less than 1% of mesothelial cell, whereas nontuberculous effusions had at least 5% mesothelial cells [50]. However, the absence of mesothelial cells in pleural fluid is not diagnostic for tuberculosis as it can be seen in conditions with extensive pleural surface involvement, like in empyema in which the pleura is coated with fibrin.

Pleural fluid eosinophilia (defined at 10% or more nucleated cells being eosinophils) in majority of the cases is seen in the presence of air (pneumothorax) or blood (hemothorax) in the pleural space [23]. Other uncommon causes include drug reactions (e.g., nitrofurantoin and propylthiouracil), asbestos exposure, pulmonary infarction, parasitic infections (e.g., paragonimasis), fungal diseases (e.g., histoplasmosis, cryptococcosis and coccidioidomycosis) and malignancy (carcinoma and lymphoma).

Pleural Fluid Lactate Dehydrogenase (LDH) Level

As mentioned earlier, the pleural fluid LDH correlates with the degree of pleural inflammation and increases with the inflammation of pleural surface or the capillaries. LDH is an intracellular enzyme and its normal serum level is less than 200 IU/L. Very high LDH levels (> 1000 IU/L) in pleural effusion analysis are seen in empyema, rheumatoid pleurisy, paragonimiasis, and malignancy [2, 17].

Pleural Fluid Total Protein Level

As previously explained, the pleural fluid has the composition of plasma filtrate with low protein content. Majority of the transudates have protein level less than 3.0 g/dL. This may be falsely high in patient on diuretics. On the contrary, exudates have higher protein levels and is due to increased permeability of the capillaries. In pleural tuberculosis, the protein level is generally more than 4.0 gm/dL in the pleural effusion [2, 4].

Pleural Fluid pH

Measurement of the pleural fluid pH is indicated if malignant or parapneumonic pleural effusions are suspected. Use of a blood gas analyzer is more accurate and the preferred method of measurement. The pH should be measured within one hour of sampling without exposure to air or anesthetic [7]. In a patient suspected of having a parapneumonic effusion a pH < 7.20 indicates the presence of a complicated paraneumonic pleural effusion, and a possible need for chest tube placement [26]. Patients with malignant pleural effusion and pH $\leq$ 7.28 have lower survival [27] and lower pH may also be associated with less successful pleuredesis in these patients [28]. Common additional causes of low pH pleural effusions include tuberculosis, collagen vascular disease, esophageal rupture, and hemothorax [29].

Pleural Fluid Glucose

Pleural fluid glucose concentration is normally the same as blood. A low pleural fluid (< 60 mg/dL or a pleural fluid to glucose ratio < 0.50) is associated with complicated parapneumonic effusion, rheumatoid arthritis and esophageal rupture, and less frequently with malignancy, tuberculosis and lupus pleuritis [12, 30].

Pleural Fluid Amylase

Measurement of pleural fluid amylase is not routinely performed. Isoenzyme (salivary or pancreatic) measurement while helpful, is not readily available in many centers. Elevated amylase (higher than the upper limit of normal in serum or pleural fluid to serum ratio > 1.0) occurs in acute and chronic pancreatitis, esophageal rupture, pleural malignancy (most frequently lung cancer), and pneumonia [6, 31].

Pleural Fluid Lipids

When pleural effusions appear milky, diagnosis include chylothorax and cholesterol effusions. Accumulation of chyle in the pleural space due to damage to the thoracic duct causes a chylothorax, while a cholesterol effusion is a long-standing effusion associated with increased cholesterol and thickening of the pleura. A chylothorax is diagnosed with the pleural fluid triglyceride level is > 110 mg/dL and pleural fluid triglycerides of < 50 g/dL excludes it. For intermediate values (50-110 mg/dL) lipoprotein analysis is necessary for chylomicron analysis to make a diagnosis of chylothorax. In cholesterol effusions, the cholesterol level is > 200 mg/dL. Malignancy and trauma are the major causes of chylothorax, while tuberculosis and rheumatoid arthritis are the major causes for cholesterol effusions. Chylothoraces have lymphocyte predominance, while cholesterol effusions have neutrophilic predominance [32, 33].

Pleural Fluid Adenosine Deaminase (ADA) and Interferon Gamma

Adenosine deaminase (ADA) catalyzes the conversion of adenosine to inosine and its major value in pleural fluid analysis is in the diagnosis of tuberculosis. Pleural fluid ADA > 35 IU/L is a very accurate test for the diagnosis of tuberculous pleural effusions: in patients with lymphocytic exudates, an ADA level above 35 IU/L had a sensitivity of 93% and a specificity of 90% for diagnosis [34]. A pleural fluid LDH/ADA ratio ≥ 16.2 is highly predictive of tuberculous pleural effusion as opposed to parapneumonic effusion [35]. Conversely, extremely high levels of pleural fluid ADA (> 250 IU/L) is more suggestive of empyema or lymphoma than tuberculosis [34].

Interferon gamma is also a useful marker for tuberculous pleural effusion, although not more accurate than ADA. A metaanalysis of 22 studies showed elevated interferon gamma had a sensitivity of 89% and a specificity of 97% for tuberculous pleural effusion [36].

Pleural Fluid Creatinine

Urinothorax is a very rare cause of transudative pleural effusion due to obstructive uropathy. Very few cases have been reported [37]. The urine tracts through the retroperitoneum to the pleural space. It is usually resolved with relief of the urinary obstruction. Diagnosis is based on pleural fluid creatinine > serum creatinine [6].

Pleural Fluid Bilirubin

Bilious pleural effusions are an extremely rare condition. A review from 2016 identified 12 cases reported in the medical literature [38]. It is associated with liver diseases, sub-hepatic and sub-phrenic abscesses, biliary peritonitis, percutaneous biliary drainage or liver biopsy. While diagnosis of bilious pleural effusion is based on pleural total bilirubin to serum total bilirubin ratio > 1, in this review, the sensitivity of this ratio was 77% and increased to 100% when it was combined with pleural glycoholic acid measurement.

Pleural Fluid Procalcitonin (PCT) and C-Reactive Protein(CRP)

Pleural fluid procalcitonin is a biological marker and has a reasonable diagnostic accuracy for bacterial parapneumonic pleural effusions. But, it is far from perfect and despite many studies a definite cut-off value has not been identified. PCT can be an adjunct to other tests along with the clinical scenario that fits an infectious etiology to help in diagnosing a bacterial parapneumonic pleural effusion. PCT is not useful in making a diagnosis of pleural effusions from viral, fungal and mycobacterial causes. Zou et al. conducted a systemic review and meta-analysis of the diagnostic performances of pleural fluid PCT and CRP in differentiating parapneumonic effusions [39]. In their meta-analysis, they found 6 studies that met their quality standards for inclusion with a total of 780 patients with suspected parapneumonic effusions and 306 confirmed cases of the same. All six studies examined the diagnostic performance of pleural fluid PCT, also tested for serum PCT, and another 3 tested for serum CRP. Based on their meta-analysis of studies done prior to 2012 the authors suggested that in the existing literature both serum and pleural fluid PCT have low sensitivity and specificity for differentiating parapneumonic effusion from other causes of pleural effusion. In 2017, He et al. published a meta-analysis of 11 studies involving 1320 patients, comprising 463 with parapneumonic effusions and 857 controls [46]. They concluded that both serum and pleural fluid PCT have a modest performance in diagnosing parapneumonic effusions. Of note, all the six studies include in the meta-analysis published by Zou et al. were a part of this meta-analysis.

Pleural Fluid ANA and RF

Rheumatoid factor (RF) levels in pleural effusion are usually equal or higher than serum levels and strongly suggestive of rheumatoid arthritis as the cause of the effusion [40]. Antinuclear antibody (ANA) testing in pleural fluid is very sensitive but nonspecific for systemic lupus erythematosus (SLE) associated pleural effusions. It has been associated also with malignancy in patients without SLE [41].

Pleural Fluid Cultures

Gram stain and culture in both aerobic and anaerobic media should be obtained to diagnose empyema. The use of blood culture bottles increases the yield in patients with empyema. In one study, adding blood cultures to standard pleural fluid cultures increased positive cultures from 38% to 59% [42]. Forty percent of cultures may be falsely negative in empyema, likely related in part to prior use of antibiotic therapy [11]. Pleural fluid smear and culture yield are very low in pleural tuberculosis: 6 and 36%, respectively. The yield can increase in patients with human immunodeficiency virus infection [43].

Pleural Fluid Cytology

When malignancy is in the differential diagnosis, cytology of the pleural fluid may provide the diagnosis. Mean sensitivity is on average 60% with increased yield if a second sample is sent. If lymphoma is suspected, flow cytometry should be performed [6]. Tumor type affects the yield, with a recent study showing higher rates of positive cytology for adenocarcinoma (88%) and lower for mesothelioma (46%) [45]. Combination of cytology with cell block examination increased the yield in a study from 61% for cytology alone to 71% when both methods were combined [44].

Large amounts of fluid appear to not increase significantly the yield for diagnosis of malignant pleural effusion. One study suggested a minimum sample of 25 ml and that between 25 and 50 ml of fluid was enough for adequate assessment of pleural effusions for malignancy [48]. A recent study of 74 samples from 60 patients did not show any significant difference in the detection of malignant cells comparing 25 ml, 50 ml, and 150 ml samples; sensitivities were 88.5%, 96.2%, and 100.0%, respectively ($P = 0.16$). Although no statistically significant difference was found, there might be added value in isolated cases for larger samples than the minimum requirement of 25 ml: two cases in this series that were negative with 25 ml were positive with 50 ml and 150 ml and one case negative in the 25 ml and 50 ml was positive in the 150 ml sample [49].

CONCLUSION

Pleural effusions are very common diagnoses. Even after four decades since its initial description, the Light's criteria have stood the test of time as a starting point in the diagnostic evaluation of pleural effusions. There is an increasing interest in developing more sophisticated methods to diagnose pleural disease. Many changes have occurred recently in the evaluation of pleural disease. Ultrasound has become standard of care to guide thoracentesis. Newer tests have significantly impacted the diagnosis of pleural disease, such as ADA for pleural tuberculosis with the potential for newer tumor markers to facilitate diagnosis of malignancy. Clinical prediction models are being developed to facilitate diagnosis. Increased interest in pleuroscopy in training programs may facilitate diagnosis further. Timely and accurate diagnosis of pleural effusions is of the upmost importance.

REFERENCES

[1] Light, R. W. 2011. "Pleural Effusions." *Medical Clinics of North America* 95, no. 6 (2011): 1055-1070. doi:10.1016/j.mcna.2011.08.005.

[2] Yalcin, Nilay Gamze, Cliff K. c. Choong, and Norman Eizenberg. "Anatomy and Pathophysiology of the Pleura and Pleural Space." *Thoracic Surgery Clinics* 23, no. 1 (2013): 1-10. doi:10.1016/j.thorsurg.2012.10.008. doi:10.1016/j.thorsurg.2012.10.008.

[3] Standring, Susan, and Henry Gray. *Gray's Anatomy: The Anatomical Basis of Clinical Practice*. Philadelphia: Elsevier, 2016.

[4] Broaddus, V. Courtney., Robert J. Mason, Joel D. Ernst, Talmadge E. King, Stephen C. Lazarus, John F. Murray, Jay A. Nadel, Arthur Samuel Slutsky, and Michael B. Gotway. *Murray & Nadel's Textbook of Respiratory Medicine*. Philadelphia: Elsevier Saunders, 2016.

[5] Saguil, A., K. Wyrick, and J. Hallgren. 2014. "Diagnostic Approach to Pleural Effusion." *American Family Physician* 90 (2): 99-104. doi:d10960 [pii].

[6] Hooper, C., Y. C. G. Lee, and N. Maskell. "Investigation of a Unilateral Pleural Effusion in Adults: British Thoracic Society Pleural Disease Guideline 2010." *Thorax* 65, no. Suppl 2 (2010): Ii4-i17. doi:10.1136/thx.2010.136978.

[7] Na, Moon Jun. "Diagnostic Tools of Pleural Effusion." *Tuberculosis and Respiratory Diseases* 76, no. 5 (2014): 199. doi:10.4046/trd.2014.76.5.199.

[8] Mitrouska, Ioanna, and Demosthenes Bouros. "The Trans-Exudative Pleural Effusion." *Chest* 122, no. 5 (2002): 1503-505. doi:10.1378/chest.122.5.1503.

[9] Light, Richard W. "Pleural Effusion." *New England Journal of Medicine* 346, no. 25 (2002): 1971-977. doi:10.1056/nejmcp010731.

[10] Mcgrath, E. E., and P. B. Anderson. "Diagnosis of Pleural Effusion: A Systematic Approach." *American Journal of Critical Care* 20, no. 2 (2011): 119-28. doi:10.4037/ajcc2011685.

[11] Porcel, José M. "Diagnosis of Pleural Effusions." *Hospital Medicine Clinics* 2, no. 3 (2013). doi:10.1016/j.ehmc.2013.02.001.

[12] Sahn, Steven A. "Getting the Most from Pleural Fluid Analysis." *Respirology* 17, no. 2 (2012): 270-77. doi:10.1111/j.1440-1843.2011.02100.x.

[13] Feller-Kopman, David, and Richard Light. "Pleural Disease." *New England Journal of Medicine* 378, no. 8 (2018): 740-51. doi:10.1056/nejmra1403503.

[14] Petersen, William G., and Robert Zimmerman. "Limited Utility of Chest Radiograph After Thoracentesis." *Chest* 117, no. 4 (2000): 1038-042. doi:10.1378/chest.117.4.1038.

[15] Light, Richard W. *Pleural Diseases*. Philadelphia: Wolters Kluwer/Lippincott Williams & Wilkins Health, 2013.

[16] Mercaldi, Catherine J., and Stephan F. Lanes. "Ultrasound Guidance Decreases Complications and Improves the Cost of Care Among Patients Undergoing Thoracentesis and Paracentesis." *Chest* 143, no. 2 (2013): 532-38. doi:10.1378/chest.12-0447.

[17] Light, Richard W. "The Light Criteria." *Clinics in Chest Medicine* 34, no. 1 (2013): 21-26. doi:10.1016/j.ccm.2012.11.006.

[18] Sachdeva, Ashutosh, Ray Wesley Shepherd, and Hans J. Lee. 2013. "Thoracentesis and Thoracic Ultrasound." *Clinics in Chest Medicine* 34 (1): 1–9. doi:10.1016/j.ccm.2012.11.005.

[19] Muller, N. L. 1993. "Imaging of the Pleura." *Radiology* 186 (2): 297-309. doi:10.1148/radiology.186.2.8421723 [doi].

[20] Zocchi, L. "Physiology and Pathophysiology of Pleural Fluid Turnover." *European Respiratory Journal* 20, no. 6 (2002): 1545-558. doi:10.1183/09031936.02.00062102.

[21] Miserocchi, G. "Mechanisms Controlling the Volume of Pleural Fluid and Extravascular Lung Water." *European Respiratory Review* 18, no. 114 (2009): 244-52. doi:10.1183/09059180.00002709.

[22] Noppen, Marc, Marc De Waele, Rong Li, Kristien Vander Gucht, Jan Dhaese, Erik Gerlo, and Walter Vincken. "Volume and Cellular Content of Normal Pleural Fluid in Humans Examined by Pleural Lavage." *American Journal of Respiratory and Critical Care Medicine* 162, no. 3 (2000): 1023-026. doi:10.1164/ajrccm.162.3.9910050.

[23] Kalomenidis, Ioannis, and Richard W. Light. "Eosinophilic Pleural Effusions." *Current Opinion in Pulmonary Medicine* 9, no. 4 (2003): 254-60. doi:10.1097/00063198-200307000-00002.

[24] Sahn, Steven A. "Pleural Fluid PH in Malignant Effusions." *Annals of Internal Medicine* 108, no. 3 (1988): 345. doi:10.7326/0003-4819-108-3-345.

[25] Light, Richard W. "Pleural Effusions: The Diagnostic Separation of Transudates and Exudates." *Annals of Internal Medicine* 77, no. 4 (1972): 507. doi:10.7326/0003-4819-77-4-507.

[26] Heffner, J. E., L. K. Brown, C. Barbieri, and J. M. Deleo. "Pleural Fluid Chemical Analysis in Parapneumonic Effusions. A Meta-analysis." *American Journal of Respiratory and Critical Care Medicine* 151, no. 6 (1995): 1700-708. doi:10.1164/ajrccm.151.6.7767510.

[27] Heffner, John E., Paul J. Nietert, and Celia Barbieri. "Pleural Fluid PH as a Predictor of Survival for Patients with Malignant Pleural Effusions." *Chest* 117, no. 1 (2000): 79-86. doi:10.1378/chest.117.1.79.

[28] Heffner, John E., John N. Heffner, and Lee K. Brown. "Multilevel and Continuous Pleural Fluid PH Likelihood Ratios for Evaluating Malignant Pleural Effusionsa." *Chest* 123, no. 6 (2003): 1887-894. doi:10.1378/chest.123.6.1887.

[29] Good, James T., David A. Taryle, Robert M. Maulitz, Robin L. Kaplan, and Steven A. Sahn. "The Diagnostic Value of Pleural Fluid PH." *Chest* 78, no. 1 (1980): 55-59. doi:10.1378/chest.78.1.55.

[30] Sahn, Steven. "The Diagnostic Value of Pleural Fluid Analysis." *Seminars in Respiratory and Critical Care Medicine* 16, no. 04 (1995): 269-78. doi:10.1055/s-2007-1009837.

[31] Joseph, Jose, Steve Viney, Beter Beck, Charlie Strange, Steven A. Sahn, and Gurnam S. Basran. "A Prospective Study of Amylase-rich Pleural Effusions with Special Reference to Amylase Isoenzyme Analysis." *Chest* 102, no. 5 (1992): 1455-459. doi:10.1378/chest.102.5.1455.

[32] Agrawal, Vishal, and Steven A. Sahn. "Lipid Pleural Effusions." *The American Journal of the Medical Sciences* 335, no. 1 (2008): 16-20. doi:10.1097/maj.0b013e31815d2634.

[33] Maskell, N. A., and R. J. A. Butland. "BTS Guidelines for the Investigation of a Unilateral Pleural Effusion in Adults." *Thorax* 58, no. Supplement 2 (2003): Ii8-i17. doi:10.1136/thx.58.suppl_2.ii8.

[34] Porcel, José M., Aureli Esquerda, and Silvia Bielsa. "Diagnostic Performance of Adenosine Deaminase Activity in Pleural Fluid: A Single-center Experience with over 2100 Consecutive Patients." *European Journal of Internal Medicine* 21, no. 5 (2010): 419-23. doi:10.1016/j.ejim.2010.03.011.

[35] Wang, Jinlin, Jun Liu, Xiaohong Xie, Panxiao Shen, Jianxing He, and Yunxiang Zeng. "The Pleural Fluid Lactate Dehydrogenase/adenosine Deaminase Ratio Differentiates between Tuberculous and Parapneumonic Pleural Effusions." *BMC Pulmonary Medicine* 17, no. 1 (2017). doi:10.1186/s12890-017-0526-z.

[36] Jiang, Jing, Huan-Zhong Shi, Qiu-Li Liang, Shou-Ming Qin, and Xue-Jun Qin. "Diagnostic Value of Interferon-γ in Tuberculous Pleurisy." *Chest* 131, no. 4 (2007): 1133-141. doi:10.1378/chest.06-2273.

[37] Garcia-Pachon, Eduardo, and Isabel Padilla-Navas. "Urinothorax: Case Report and Review of the Literature with Emphasis on Biochemical Diagnosis." *Respiration* 71, no. 5 (2004): 533-36. doi:10.1159/000080642.

[38] Saraya, Takeshi, Richard W. Light, Sho Sakuma, Yasuo Nakamoto, Shoko Wada, Manabu Ishida, Toshiya Inui, Takashi Koide, Haruyuki Ishii, and Hajime Takizawa. "A New Diagnostic Approach for Bilious Pleural Effusion." *Respiratory Investigation* 54, no. 5 (2016): 364-68. doi:10.1016/j.resinv.2016.03.009.

[39] Zou, Ming-Xiang, Rong-Rong Zhou, Wen-Jun Wu, Ning-Jie Zhang, Wen-En Liu, and Xue-Gong Fan. "The Use of Pleural Fluid Procalcitonin and C-reactive Protein in the Diagnosis of Parapneumonic Pleural Effusions: A Systemic Review and Meta-analysis." *The American Journal of Emergency Medicine* 30, no. 9 (2012): 1907-914. doi:10.1016/j.ajem.2012.04.004.

[40] Amital, Anat, David Shitrit, and Yochai Adir. "The Lung in Rheumatoid Arthritis." *La Presse Médicale* 40, no. 1 (2011). doi:10.1016/j.lpm.2010.11.003.

[41] Wang, Der-Yuan. "Diagnosis and Management of Lupus Pleuritis." *Current Opinion in Pulmonary Medicine* 8, no. 4 (2002): 312-16. doi:10.1097/00063198-200207000-00012.

[42] Menzies, S. M., N. M. Rahman, J. M. Wrightson, H. E. Davies, R. Shorten, S. H. Gillespie, C. W. H. Davies, N. A. Maskell, A. A. Jeffrey, Y. C. G. Lee, and R. J. O. Davies. "Blood Culture Bottle Culture of Pleural Fluid in Pleural Infection." *Thorax* 66, no. 8 (2011): 658-62. doi:10.1136/thx.2010.157842.

[43] Porcel, José M. "Advances in the Diagnosis of Tuberculous Pleuritis." *Annals of Translational Medicine* 4, no. 15 (2016): 282. doi:10.21037/atm.2016.07.23.

[44] Assawasaksakul, Theerada, Viboon Boonsarngsuk, and Pimpin Incharoen. "A Comparative Study of Conventional Cytology and Cell Block Method in the Diagnosis of Pleural Effusion." *Journal of Thoracic Disease* 9, no. 9 (2017): 3161-167. doi:10.21037/jtd.2017.08.52.

[45] Loveland, Paula, Micheal Christie, Gary Hammerschlag, Louis Irving, and Daniel Steinfort. "Diagnostic Yield of Pleural Fluid Cytology in Malignant Effusions: An Australian Tertiary Centre Experience." *Internal Medicine Journal*, 2018. doi:10.1111/imj.13991.

[46] He, C., Wang, B., Li, D., Xu, H., & Shen, Y. (2017). Performance of procalcitonin in diagnosing parapneumonic pleural effusions. *Medicine, 96*(33).

[47] Lichtenstein, D., Mezière, G., Lascols, N., Biderman, P., Courret, J., Gepner, A., Goldstein, I. and Tenoudji-Cohen, M. (2005). Ultrasound diagnosis of occult pneumothorax*. *Critical Care Medicine*, 33(6), pp.1231-1238.

[48] Thomas, S. C., L. R. R. Davidson, and M. E. Mckean. "An Investigation of Adequate Volume for the Diagnosis of Malignancy in Pleural Fluids." *Cytopathology* 22, no. 3 (2011): 179-83. doi:10.1111/j.1365-2303.2010.00786.x.

[49] Wu, Huimin, Rahul Khosla, Prashant K. Rohatgi, Sumans Chauhan, Edina Paal, and Wen Chen. "The Minimum Volume of Pleural Fluid Required to Diagnose Malignant Pleural Effusion: A Retrospective Study." *Lung India* 34, no. 1 (2017): 34. doi:10.4103/0970-2113.197120.

[50] Light, Richard W., Yener S. Erozan, and Wilmot C. Ball, Jr. "Cells in Pleural Fluid." *Archives of Internal Medicine* 132, no. 6 (1973): 854. doi:10.1001/archinte.1973.03650120060011.

In: Pleural Effusions: Causes, Types and Treatment
Editor: Rahul Khosla
ISBN: 978-1-53614-683-7

Chapter 3

TRANSUDATIVE PLEURAL EFFUSIONS

Kavita Vyas**, MD, Amandeep S. Bawa, MD and Rahul Khosla, MD

Pulmonary and CCM Section, Veterans Affairs Medical Center, Washington DC, US

ABSTRACT

Pleural effusions are classified as either transudative or exudative depending on the fluid analysis. Transudates are non-inflammatory and contain low protein, lactate dehydrogenase and cholesterol when compared to serum. The most common etiology of a transudative effusion is heart failure and a thoracentesis may not be necessary. Any unilateral effusion without an obvious source requires investigation including a hepatic hydrothorax, hypoalbuminemia, peritoneal dialysis and urinothorax.

Keywords: transudate, Starling, Light's criteria, congestive heart failure, hepatic hydrothorax, nephrotic syndrome, hypoalbuminemia, peritoneal dialysis, urinothorax

INTRODUCTION

Pleural effusions are common findings on chest radiographs (CXR) and a thoracentesis is not needed if the etiology is apparent. However, if any doubt remains, an ultrasound guided thoracentesis is the standard of care. Once pleural fluid has been obtained, the next step is to distinguish between a transudate and an exudate. A transudative effusion occurs due to either overproduction of fluid and movement into the pleural space (via increased

* Corresponding Author Email: Kavita.vyas@va.gov.

hydrostatic or decreased oncotic pressure) or decreased absorption. These factors can be described by the Starling forces and the following equation [15]:

$$QF = Lp \times A\,[(Pcap - Ppl) - \sigma D\,(\pi cap - \pi pl)]$$

QF is the flow of fluid

Lp is the filtration coefficient

A is the surface area of the pleura

Pcap is the hydrostatic pressure of the pulmonary capillary bed

Ppl is the hydrostatic pressure of the pleural space

σD is the reflection coefficient for protein movement across the pleura. This ranges from 0, meaning completely permeable to 1, which is completely impermeable.

πcap is the oncotic pressure of the capillary bed

πpl is the oncotic pressure of the pleural space

The pulmonary capillary membrane and the surrounding structures remain intact in a transudate compared to the inflammatory nature of an exudative effusion. Therefore, there is less filtration of proteins and larger molecules.

Classically, Light's criteria published in 1972 have been used to distinguish between a transudate and exudate [1]. The criteria include:

1. Pleural fluid to serum protein ratio less than 0.5
2. Pleural fluid to serum lactate dehydrogenase (LDH) ratio less than 0.6.
3. Pleural fluid LDH less than 2/3 the upper limit of normal for serum.

If all three parameters are met, the effusion is classified as a transudate. Light's criteria is very sensitive for exudates but less specific i.e.: transudates can be incorrectly labeled as an exudate. This is an accepted consequence of the above cutoff values as the diagnosis of an exudate requires further intervention and/or treatment.

Light's criteria have been criticized for its use of LDH in 2 out of the 3 parameters thus decreasing its specificity. Additionally, a blood draw is required to obtain concurrent serum values of protein and LDH. Two additional criteria have been proposed to circumvent these deficiencies as follows [2]:

Two-test Rule

1. Pleural fluid LDH less than 0.45 times the upper limit of normal for serum.
2. Pleural fluid cholesterol less than 45 mg/dL.

If both criteria are met, the fluid is a transudate.

Three-test rule

1. Pleural fluid LDH less than 0.45 times the upper limit of normal for serum.
2. Pleural fluid cholesterol less than 45 mg/dL.
3. Pleural fluid protein less than 2.9 g/dL.

If all three criteria are met, the fluid is classified as a transudate.

Newer studies have shown that pleural fluid viscosity can be used to differentiate between a transudate and exudate however cutoff values are unknown [3]. This remains an interesting avenue of inquiry as viscosity measurement is simple, quick and cost-effective.

Congestive Heart Failure

Congestive heart failure due to left ventricular dysfunction is the leading cause of transudative pleural effusions. The lymphatics of the parietal pleura and not the visceral pleura is responsible for pleural fluid reabsorption based on sheep studies [4]. They can increase the rate of absorption of the pleural fluid to 0.28 mL/kg/hr which is 28 times the baseline. Only after overwhelming this drainage system does the effusion begin to form [4]. Multiple hypotheses pertaining to the etiology of the effusion exist. First, left heart failure leads to an increase in pulmonary capillary bed pressure (Pcap), specifically in the systemic and pulmonary venous circulation. Therefore, there is increased filtration from both the parietal pleura and visceral pleura into the pleural space. This would result in very low pleural fluid protein concentrations with a pleural fluid to serum protein ratio less than 0.15. Most transudative effusions due to heart failure have ratios between 0.4 and 0.5 making this theory less convincing [5]. The arterial circulation is thought to play a very small role in pleural fluid formation due to high resistance and arteriolar tone preventing fluid leakage.

The second possibility is that the increased interstitial edema (from alveolar capillaries) leads to elevated hydrostatic pressures and movement of the fluid across the visceral pleura into the pleural space [5]. Due to direct leakage of the fluid from the pleura, it is more protein rich. However, this would result in pleural fluid to serum protein ratios much greater than 0.5. It is therefore the combination of elevated systemic and pulmonary venous pressures leading to increased filtration and interstitial edema with direct flow of fluid into the pleural space which forms the effusion.

$$QF = Lp \times A \, [(\mathbf{Pcap} - Ppl) - \sigma D \, (\pi cap - \pi pl)]$$

Thoracentesis for a patient with obvious congestive heart failure (elevated jugular venous distention, peripheral edema) and bilateral pleural effusions is not necessary unless treatment with diuresis does not result in resolution over a couple days. Of note, effusions due to heart failure can be one sided in about 10% of patients [9]. A diagnostic thoracentesis can then be performed to determine if the effusion is actually an exudate.

An effusion due to heart failure may become an exudate by Light's criteria after aggressive diuresis due to concentration of pleural fluid proteins [6]. In this clinical setting, a serum-effusion albumin gradient can be calculated. A value greater than 1.2 g/dL is consistent with a transudate. A series of 59 consecutive patients with pleural effusions showed that although Light's criteria is very sensitive for exudates, the albumin gradient is more specific for congestive heart failure [7]. Pleural fluid amino-terminal fragment of pro-brain natriuretic peptide (NT-pro BNP) can also be obtained and compared to the serum value although the correlation coefficient for serum and pleural NT-pro BNP is 0.93 [7]. It may be sufficient to obtain a serum value and assume it to be similar in the pleural fluid.

If the effusion is an exudate according to Lights' criteria and has an albumin gradient <1.2 g/dL, further investigation with imaging and cytology should be completed.

If the effusion is large and causing symptoms the treatment includes thoracentesis followed by diuresis to prevent re-accumulation and standard medical management of heart failure.

HEPATIC HYDROTHORAX

A pleural effusion due to decompensated cirrhosis is a known complication and typically occurs in conjunction with massive ascites. The effusions tend to be large, > 500 mL, and therefore symptomatic with complaints ranging from dyspnea at rest, cough, nausea and pleuritic chest pain [23]. The effusion tends to be right sided in most cases (approx. 75%) but bilateral or left sided effusions can also occur [10].

The pathophysiology of the pleural effusion is from the direct communication of the ascites up through perforations in the diaphragm, especially via the medial tendinous portion, into the pleural cavity. Negative intrathoracic pressure coupled with the increased intra-abdominal pressure due to ascites leads to the flow of fluid from the peritoneal cavity into the pleural space. It is the negative intra-thoracic pressure which promotes pleural fluid accumulation in patients with minimal ascites. In fact, a radioisotope study involving the injection of 99mTC-sulphur colloid into the peritoneal cavity followed by visualization in the thorax can be used to confirm a hepatic hydrothorax [11]. The left hemidiaphragm is more muscular and with less perforations which prevents left sided effusions. A thoracentesis must be performed in all patients with a suspected hepatic hydrothorax as up to 20% of patients will have an alternate etiology [12]. Coagulopathy is not a contraindication for a thoracentesis.

A hepatic hydrothorax is a diagnosis of exclusion and therefore infection, heart failure and malignancy must be ruled out. Pleural fluid should be analyzed for protein, LDH, cell count and differential, gram stain and culture, bilirubin, pH and cytology. In an uncomplicated hepatic hydrothorax, nucleated cells are common but polymorphonuclear cell

(PMN) count is less than 250 cells/mm^3 and there is a lymphocyte and mononuclear cell predominance. If a serum to pleural fluid albumin gradient (SPAG) is obtained, it should be greater than 1.1 g/dL and should mirror the serum to ascites fluid albumin gradient (SAAG). In a case series of 77 patients with hepatic hydrothorax, all the subjects had a SPAG > 1.1 g/dL and the average was 2.1 [22]. SPAG is therefore very useful in the diagnosis.

Up to 15% of patients with suspected hepatic hydrothorax may have spontaneous bacterial empyema (SBE) due to concurrent migration of abdominal pathogens [15]. Diagnostic criteria include:

1. No underlying pneumonia on imaging.
2. Positive pleural fluid culture and PMN count greater than 250 cells/mm^3.
3. Negative pleural fluid culture and PMN count greater than 500 cells/mm^3.

Culture positive SBE tends to grow Escherichia coli, Enterococcus, Klebsiella, Streptococcus species and Pseudomonas and 50% occur in conjunction with spontaneous bacterial peritonitis (SBP) [13]. Treatment is with ceftriaxone or levofloxacin in penicillin allergic patients and should be started immediately. SBE portends a poor prognosis with a mortality up to 20%.

Treatment of the hepatic hydrothorax is similar to that of ascites and includes therapeutic thoracentesis for symptom management, sodium restricted diet and diuresis. Repeated thoracentesis will result in quick re-accumulation of the fluid due to the presence of ascites and depletion of protein. Those with refractory ascites may require evaluation for transjugular intrahepatic portosystemic shunt (TIPS) placement, surgical repair of the diaphragmatic defect and/or liver transplantation. Pleurodesis is difficult to achieve due to rapid movement of fluid from the abdomen into the thorax which prevents the two pleural surfaces from fusing [13]. Chest tubes are typically not recommended due to risk of protein and electrolyte depletion and infection risk [14]. In a small study involving 17 patients who received a chest tube for a hepatic hydrothorax, 16 developed an infection and required prolonged hospitalization [13]. Liver transplantation is definitive treatment and should be considered due to increased mortality. Most importantly, all patients should be advised to stop alcohol consumption.

Nephrotic Syndrome/ Hypoproteinemia/Hypoalbuminemia

Small pleural effusions are common in patients with hypoprotenienmia due to decreased plasma oncotic pressures but tend to be larger with concurrent hypoalbuminemia [16].

$$QF = Lp \times A\,[(Pcap - Ppl) - \sigma D\,(\boldsymbol{\pi cap} - \pi pl)]$$

The size of the effusion is inversely correlated with the albumin concentration. In a series of patients with acquired immune deficiency syndrome (AIDS), those with pleural effusions had significantly lower albumin levels [16].

Patients with nephrotic syndrome typically also experience peripheral edema and ascites due to primary renal sodium retention. Treatment should be aimed at decreasing protein loss by treating the underlying cause. If this is not possible, lowering intra-glomerular pressure will in turn decrease protein loss. This can be achieved with the administration of either angiotensin-converting enzyme (ACE) inhibitor or angiotensin receptor blockers (ARBs). Additional treatment includes sodium restriction and diuretics. Excessive diuresis can lead to a hypovolemic state and therefore these patients needs to be managed closely. Recurrent, large, symptomatic effusions can be treated with pleurodesis.

Atelectasis

Atelectasis leads to a decrease in pleural pressure (Ppl) leading to increased filtration of low protein fluid and the formation of a transudate.

$$QF = Lp \times A\,[(Pcap - \mathbf{Ppl}) - \sigma D\,(\pi cap - \pi pl)]$$

These effusions tend to be small and do not require extensive work up. Fluid will continue to accumulate until the atelectasis is resolved.

Peritoneal Dialysis

Continuous ambulatory peritoneal dialysis (CAPD) can lead to multiple complications and therefore infection, heart failure and systemic volume overload due to incomplete dialysis must be excluded. Unilateral, right sided pleural effusion similar to a hepatic hydrothorax should prompt a diagnosis of a pleuroperitoneal communication and leak. Negative intrathoracic pressure coupled with increased pressure in the abdomen due to the dialysate leads to the transfer of fluid from the peritoneal space to the pleural space. Either congenital malformation or acquired defects in the diaphragm allow movement of the fluid [17]. Patients may present with shortness of breath and inability to achieve appropriate ultrafiltration however many are asymptomatic [18]. Most effusions are unilateral, right sided (up to 90 percent of cases) and found within 30 days of starting peritoneal dialysis [17].

Diagnosis can be made by multiple modalities including peritoneal scintigraphy which injects technetium 99m isotope into the abdominal cavity and followed by visualization of the radioactive material in the pleural space [19]. A thoracentesis can also be performed if an adequate amount of fluid is seen with an ultrasound. The pleural fluid should be sent for cell count and culture to rule out infection, glucose, LDH protein and L and D isomers of lactate if possible. In the setting of a hydrothorax, cultures will be negative, glucose concentration will be higher than plasma and LDH and protein concentrations will be in the transudate range. Additionally, as D lactate is not endogenous but is found in dialysate, its presence confirms a hydrothorax [20].

Treatment is based on the size of pleural effusion, the degree of symptoms and the patient's desire to continue peritoneal dialysis. Majority of the time, stopping peritoneal dialysis for the night to allow the pleural space to drain and then resuming while the patient is upright (non-supine) is sufficient. Chemical pleurodesis was effective in 67% patients according to a review article and therefore can be offered as an option to patients who insist on CAPD [21]. Finally, if a diaphragmatic defect is seen on imaging, surgical repair may be attempted. However, this does require a thoracotomy and recovery can be prolonged. Verification of the defect with thoracoscopy should be performed first. Despite these treatment modalities, most patients need to switch from CAPD to hemodialysis [17].

URINOTHORAX

A urinothorax is very uncommon and consequently underdiagnosed. It occurs when there is obstruction (i.e.: malignancy, stone or stricture) or trauma (iatrogenic due to a procedure or injury) to the genitourinary (GU) tract. The pleural effusion typically forms on the ipsilateral side of the obstruction and occurs within 2 days of the precipitating event [22]. Fluid travels from the ureter to the pleural space via either direct communication from the abdomen or via the retroperitoneal and pleural lymphatic system. First, the urine accumulates locally in the perirenal space creating a urinoma. The urinoma can then rupture into the pleural space due to increased pressure in the abdomen and move through diaphragmatic pores.

On thoracentesis, an urinothorax is classically described as a pauci-cellular transudate with low pH, < 7.4 and pleural fluid to serum (PF/S) creatinine ratio > 1.0 [22]. The PF/S is highly specific for a urinothorax. CT scan should be obtained to identify a cause for urine in the pleural cavity. Although the above characteristics easily distinguish an urinothorax from other etiologies, these patients tend to be complicated. They may have multiple co-morbidities which can also contribute to a pleural effusion including heart failure and therefore PF/S creatinine ratio maybe low. A technetium-99m renal scan can help by following the labeled albumin from the GU tract to the pleural space however a high level of suspicion must be present.

Treatment is aimed at correcting the underlying cause as this leads to rapid resolution of the urinothorax. A therapeutic and diagnostic thoracentesis should be completed to drain the pleural space and prevent infection. Surgical closure of diaphragmatic defects or pleurodesis is not recommended as treatment of the GU tract obstruction is sufficient [22].

CONCLUSION

Pleural effusions are commonly seen on chest radiographs and computed tomography and do not require further investigation if it is small, asymptomatic and the underlying etiology is known. If a thoracentesis is done, ultrasound should be used for guidance followed by laboratory studies to distinguish it from an exudate. Light's criteria, although not perfect, have stood the test of time and classify transudates with excellent specificity. Transudates are a result of either increased formation or decreased absorption of pleural fluid due to systemic factors without involvement of the pleural surfaces. Heart failure is the most common cause of a transudate followed by nephrotic syndrome and hepatic hydrothorax. Other rarer causes include peritoneal dialysis and urinothorax and high clinical suspicion must be present. Treatment is symptom management with therapeutic thoracentesis and management of the underlying disease.

REFERENCES

[1] Light, Richard W. "Pleural Effusions: The Diagnostic Separation of Transudates and Exudates." *Annals of Internal Medicine* 77, no. 4 (1972): 507. doi:10.7326/0003-4819-77-4-507.

[2] Heffner, John E., Lee K. Brown, and Celia A. Barbieri. "Diagnostic Value of Tests That Discriminate Between Exudative and Transudative Pleural Effusions." *Chest* 111, no. 4 (1997): 970-80. doi:10.1378/chest.111.4.970.

[3] Yetkin, Ozkan, Ibrahim Tek, Akin Kaya, Aydin Ciledag, and Numan Numanoglu. "A Simple Laboratory Measurement for Discrimination of Transudative and Exudative Pleural Effusion: Pleural Viscosity." *Respiratory Medicine* 100, no. 7 (2006): 1286-290. doi:10.1016/j.rmed.2005.10.010.

[4] Broaddus, V. C., J. P. Wiener-Kronish, Y. Berthiaume, and N. C. Staub. "Removal of Pleural Liquid and Protein by Lymphatics in Awake Sheep." *Journal of Applied Physiology* 64, no. 1 (1988): 384-90. doi:10.1152/jappl.1988.64.1.384.

[5] Broaddus, V. C., J. P. Wiener-Kronish, and N. C. Staub. "Clearance of Lung Edema into the Pleural Space of Volume-loaded Anesthetized Sheep." *Journal of Applied Physiology* 68, no. 6 (1990): 2623-630. doi:10.1152/jappl.1990.68.6.2623.

[6] Shinto, Richard A., and Richard W. Light. "Effects of Diuresis on the Characteristics of Pleural Fluid in Patients with Congestive Heart Failure." *The American Journal of Medicine* 88, no. 3 (1990): 230-34. doi:10.1016/0002-9343(90)90147-6.

[7] Roth, Bernard J., Thomas F. Omeara, and W. Hal Cragun. "The Serum-Effusion Albumin Gradient in the Evaluation of Pleural Effusions." *Chest* 98, no. 3 (1990): 546-49. doi:10.1378/chest.98.3.546.

[8] Porcel, José Manuel, Manuel Vives, Gonzalo Cao, Aureli Esquerda, Manuel Rubio, and M.carmen Rivas. "Measurement of Pro-brain Natriuretic Peptide in Pleural Fluid for the Diagnosis of Pleural Effusions Due to Heart Failure." *The American Journal of Medicine* 116, no. 6 (2004): 417-20. doi:10.1016/j.amjmed.2003.11.008.

[9] Race, George A., Charles H. Scheifley, and Jesse E. Edwards. "Hydrothorax in Congestive Heart Failure." *The American Journal of Medicine* 22, no. 1 (1957): 83-89. doi:10.1016/0002-9343(57)90339-x.

[10] Lieberman, Fred L. "Pathogenesis and Treatment of Hydrothorax Complicating Cirrhosis with Ascites." *Annals of Internal Medicine* 64, no. 2 (1966): 341. doi:10.7326/0003-4819-64-2-341.

[11] Benet, A., F. Vidal, R. Toda, R. Siurana, C. M. De Virgala, and C. Richart. "Diagnosis of Hepatic Hydrothorax in the Absence of Ascites by Intraperitoneal Injection of 99m-Tc-Fluor Colloid." *Postgraduate Medical Journal* 68, no. 796 (1992): 153. doi:10.1136/pgmj.68.796.153.

[12] Xiol, Xavier, Jose Castellote, Ricart Cortes-Beut, Mercedes Delgado, Jordi Guardiola, and Eva Sesé. "Usefulness and Complications of Thoracentesis in Cirrhotic Patients." *The American Journal of Medicine* 111, no. 1 (2001): 67-69. doi:10.1016/s00
02-9343(01)00744-6.

[13] Falchuk, K. R., I. Jacoby, W. S. Colucci, and M. E. Rybak. "Tetracycline-induced Pleural Symphysis for Recurrent Hydrothorax Complicating Cirrhosis. A New Approach to Treatment. A New Approach to Treatment." *Gastroenterology* 72, no. 2 (February 1977): 319-21.

[14] Chen, Chia-Hung, Chuen-Ming Shih, Jen-Wei Chou, Yi-Heng Liu, Liang-Wen Hang, Te-Chun Hsia, Wu-Huei Hsu, and Chih-Yen Tu. "Outcome Predictors of Cirrhotic Patients with Spontaneous Bacterial Empyema." *Liver International* 31, no. 3 (2011): 417-24. doi:10.1111/j.1478-3231.2010.02447.x.

[15] Mitrouska, Ioanna, and Demosthenes Bouros. "The Trans-Exudative Pleural Effusion." *Chest* 122, no. 5 (2002): 1503-505. doi:10.1378/chest.122.5.1503.

[16] Joseph, Jose. "Pleural Effusions in Hospitalized Patients with AIDS." *Annals of Internal Medicine* 118, no. 11 (1993): 856. doi:10.7326/0003-4819-118-11-199306010-00005.

[17] Lew, S. Q. "Hydrothorax: Pleural Effusion Associated With Peritoneal Dialysis." *Peritoneal Dialysis International* 30, no. 1 (2010): 13-18. doi:10.3747/pdi.2008.00168.

[18] Nomoto, Yasuo, Takao Suga, Keiko Nakajima, Hideto Sakai, Gengo Osawa, Kazuo Ota, Yoshindo Kawaguchi, Tadasu Sakai, Shinji Sakai, Masao Shibat, and Susumu Takahashi. "Acute Hydrothorax in Continuous Ambulatory Peritoneal Dialysis – A Collaborative Study of 161 Centers." *American Journal of Nephrology* 9, no. 5 (1989): 363-67. doi:10.1159/000167997.

[19] Berman, Claudia, Michael G. Velchik, Neil Shusterman, and Abass Alavi. "The Clinical Utility of the Tc-99m SC Intraperitoneal Scan in CAPD Patients." *Clinical Nuclear Medicine* 14, no. 6 (1989): 405-09. doi:10.1097/00003072-198906000-00002.

[20] Benz, Robert L., and Charles R. Schleifer. "Hydrothorax in Continuous Ambulatory Peritoneal Dialysis: Successful Treatment With Intrapleural Tetracycline and a Review of the Literature." *American Journal of Kidney Diseases* 5, no. 2 (1985): 136-40. doi:10.1016/s0272-6386(85)80011-1.

[21] Sudduth, C. David, and Steven A. Sahn. "Pleurodesis for Nonmalignant Pleural Effusions." *Chest* 102, no. 6 (1992): 1855-860. doi:10.1378/chest.102.6.1855.

[22] Toubes, María E., Adriana Lama, Lucía Ferreiro, Antonio Golpe, José M. Álvarez-Dobaño, Francisco J. González-Barcala, Esther San José, Nuria Rodríguez-Núñez, Carlos Rábade, Tamara Lourido, and Luis Valdés. "Urinothorax: A Systematic Review." *Journal of Thoracic Disease* 9, no. 5 (2017): 1209-218. doi:10.21037/jtd.2017.04.22.

[23] Badillo, Ricardo, and Don C. Rockey. "Hepatic Hydrothorax." *Medicine* 93, no. 3 (2014): 135-42. doi:10.1097/md.0000000000000025.

In: Pleural Effusions: Causes, Types and Treatment
Editor: Rahul Khosla
ISBN: 978-1-53614-683-7

Chapter 4

PARAPNEUMONIC EFFUSIONS AND EMPYEMA

Warren Naselsky[1], MD, Van K. Holden[2], MD, Lindsey B. Black[1], Ashutosh Sachdeva[2*], MBBS and Edward M. Pickering[2], MD

[1]Division of Thoracic Surgery, Department of Surgery,
University of Maryland School of Medicine, Baltimore, MD, US
[2]Section of Interventional Pulmonology, Division of Pulmonary, Critical Care,
and Sleep Medicine, Department of Medicine,
University of Maryland School of Medicine, Baltimore, MD, US

ABSTRACT

Parapneumonic effusions and empyema are the most common cause of exudative pleural effusions, with an increasing incidence in an aging population and result in significant morbidity and mortality despite advances in antimicrobial therapy. All patients suspected of having a parapneumonic effusion or empyema require prompt attention and clinical, radiographic, and pleural fluid analysis for risk stratification. Selecting the appropriate workup and management of these conditions remains challenging for many clinicians. While chest radiographs and computed tomography scans continue to be important in the radiologic evaluation of these conditions, the role of point-of-care ultrasonography in characterizing effusions and aiding with intervention has become standard of care. Early and complete drainage of the infected space remains the mainstay of treatment. Ultrasound-guided small-bore chest tube placement is recommended as an initial step given low risk of complications. Many patients will require adjunct therapies, such as intra-pleural fibrinolytic/mucolytic combination to facilitate resolution of parapneumonic effusions and reduce the need for surgical procedures. Despite these advances, some patients still require surgical intervention for complicated pleural spaces or empyemas. It is important for clinicians to stratify patients who are likely to fail medical treatment, and early surgical consultation is suggested. Finally, a multidisciplinary

[*]Corresponding Author Email: asachdeva@som.umaryland.edu.

approach involving physicians, advance care practitioners, nurses, and ancillary staff is essential to provide optimal care for these patients.

Keywords: parapneumonic effusions, empyema, fibrinolytic therapy, decortication

INTRODUCTION

Parapneumonic effusions (PPEs), commonly defined as pleural effusions in the presence of pneumonia or lung abscess, remains the most common cause of exudative pleural effusions and are associated with significant morbidity and mortality [1]. Empyema refers to frank infection or pus in the pleural space, and the importance of its early drainage has been long recognized [2]. The clinical relevance of these conditions stems from an increasing incidence and expanded pool of patients affected; young and old, healthy and chronically ill, as well as hospitalized and outpatients [3]. It is estimated that over 500 million US dollars each year is spent in the work-up and management of these conditions [4].

Incidence and Epidemiology

As many as 40% of patients with community acquired pneumonia (CAP) develop an effusion consistent with PPE and 10% of these patients will progress to empyema [5]. Recent reviews indicate that an upwards of 80,000 patients are diagnosed with empyema each year [3]. This also accounts for patients who develop PPE or empyema in the hospital. As many as 1 million people are hospitalized with pneumonia in the United States each year [6], and an estimated 25-40% of these patients will also develop PPE [7, 8]. Several risk factors have been identified that are associated with the development of PPE and empyema including chronic lung disease and diabetes [9]. In addition, certain patient populations are more likely to present with PPE or empyema. Up to 8% of pneumonias in pregnancy are complicated by empyema [10]. Patients with chronic alcohol use or intravenous drug abuse (IVDA) are 3 to 4 times more likely to have PPE or empyema on initial presentation [11]. Importantly however, as many as 30% of patients diagnosed with empyema have no identifiable risk factors [12].

Although the advent and wide spread use of antibiotic therapy initially decreased both the overall occurrence of PPEs and the rate of subsequent progression to empyema, these conditions remain prevalent [13, 14]. Even more concerning, several recent studies have shown that rates for both PPEs and empyema have risen over the past few decades [3]. One study showed that for the past two decades, rates of pleural space infections in the United States have increased by 3% per year on an average [4]. Hospitalizations for empyema, have also doubled over the past two decades [15].

It is unclear why rates of these conditions are on the rise. Some postulate that this may be due to an increasing proportion of elderly population with multiple comorbidities, predisposing them to pneumonia and its complications [16]. While this theory may account for some of the increase in the overall number of observed cases, it is important to note that this higher rate of diagnosis is also found across all age groups [15]. Several studies have noted the changing bacteriology of pleural infections, a phenomenon that may predispose patients to an increasing proportion of antibiotic-resistant bacteria or virulent strains more likely to induce empyema formation [17].

Prognosis

PPEs and empyema are associated with worse outcomes as compared to patients presenting with pneumonia without these complications [18, 19]. It is estimated that unilateral PPE increases mortality by at least 3-fold and that the presence of bilateral effusions estimates a 6.5-times increase in mortality compared to patients with pneumonia without effusion [18]. One study found that for those patients who had early failure of medical therapy due to the presence of empyema, mortality may be increased by upwards of 11-fold [19]. Mortality is significantly increased in patients who develop empyema while hospitalized compared to those who present with community acquired pneumonia [20]. Overall, mortality in patients hospitalized with empyema is estimated anywhere from 6% to as high as around 20% in some groups of patients, specifically those with delayed treatment [6, 21]. As the incidence of PPEs and empyema are on the rise, so appears to be the morbidity and mortality of these conditions. In one recent review of state medical records, there was a 6-fold increase in mortality of empyema in the years after 2000 as compared to those before 1975 in the absence of influenza pandemic [22]. This increased mortality despite advances in therapy is likely related to an overall older population of patients and the increasing prevalence of more pathogenic infection.

Bacteriology of Empyema

A variety of organisms have been isolated and implicated in empyema. Pleural fluid is a potent bacterial medium and facilitates the growth of bacteria, in-particular *Streptococcus pneumonia* [23]. Historically, aerobic organisms were the most common, followed by anaerobic organisms, then mixtures of both. The most common aerobic organisms were gram positive organisms, in particular *Streptococcus pneumoniae* and *Staphylococcus aureus*; gram negative organisms were less common, though the most common of these isolates were *Escherichia coli*, *Klebsiella pneumoniae*, and *Haemophilus influenzae* [24]. Frequently isolated anaerobic organisms included *Prevotella spp*, *Porphyromonas spp*,

Bacteroides spp, and *Fusobacterium spp*. Anaerobic infection was more often associated with aspiration and abscess formation [24]. However, in more recent analyses, the incidence of aerobic gram-negative organisms, in particular *Klebsiella pneumoniae* is becoming more common especially in patients who have diabetes mellitus as a comorbidity [25]. Anaerobic infections have also risen in incidence and fungal pleural space infections are being reported in immunosuppressed populations, in particular patients with neoplasms undergoing treatment [26]. Tuberculosis remains a frequent cause of pleural effusions worldwide [27], but is still seen in non-endemic regions as well, most commonly associated with immunosuppression from HIV [28], or anti-neoplastic treatment [26].

Clinical Presentation

Patients with PPE and empyema present with symptoms of fever, cough, dyspnea, and pleuritic chest pain. Based solely upon clinical features, it is difficult to differentiate PPEs and empyema from pneumonia [8]. It is also challenging to determine which patients will progress from a simple pneumonia to a PPE and/or empyema. Elderly patients often do not present with classic features, but instead anemia, fatigue, dyspnea, and weight loss; often resulting in a delayed presentation [29].

The development of a PPEs or empyema is often the result of an unrecognized or undertreated infection. In a large series, empyema developed in less than 2% of patients hospitalized with CAP who received appropriate antibiotics [30]. Conversely, in a series of patients ultimately diagnosed with empyema, patients presented to a general practitioner 5 days after symptom onset and were not hospitalized until an average of 13 days later. Despite this interval, over one-quarter of the patients were diagnosed after one week or more into the hospital stay [12].

Imaging Evaluation

Radiological evaluation of patients presenting with clinical symptoms of pneumonia is critical to appropriately diagnose PPE of empyema.

Chest Radiography

Although plain radiographs just show forms, extent, and opacity, their nature, development and anatomic correlates provide meaningful information to the clinicians in their approach to pulmonary infection [31]. As such, chest radiograph is usually the first imaging study in the work up of patients with suspected pneumonia. While effusions seen on chest radiographs are often non-specific, there are some imaging characteristics that may indicate the presence of a PPEs or empyema. For example, an atypical meniscus or spherical like fluid collection may indicate the presence of loculated fluid. The presence of air fluid levels may hint at the presence of collections with infected material. Figure 1 demonstrates an air-fluid level in a complex appearing left chest process.

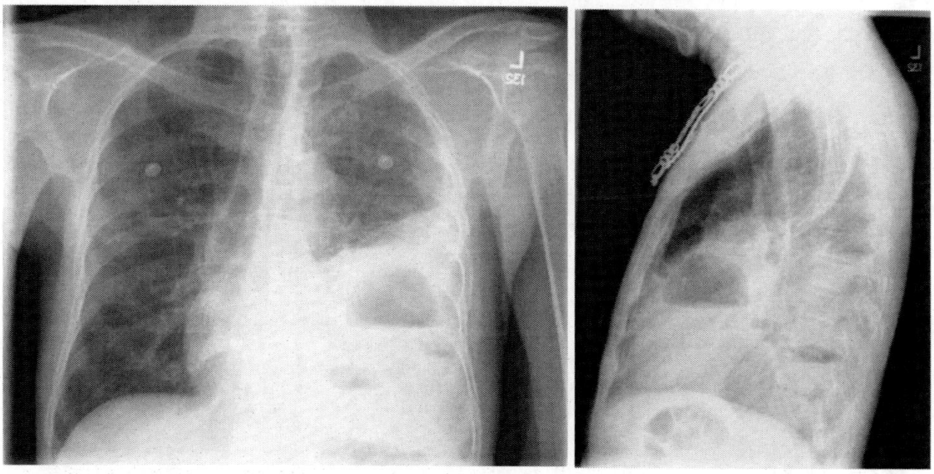

(a) (b)

Figure 1. (a) Postero-anterior view of chest radiograph in a patient diagnosed with empyema. (b) Lateral view in the same patient demostrating air-fluid level, above the diaphragm.

There are several significant limitations of chest radiography in the imaging of PPEs and empyema. Chest radiographs are unable to specifically identify septations in the pleural space or pleural thickening and thus have no significant predictive value in identifying complex PPEs [32-34]. Also, chest radiographs are limited in the minimum volume of effusion they can detect, typically estimated as 175-200 mL [35, 36]. Although original recommendations from the American Thoracic Society indicated that lateral decubitus imaging is necessary to improve the sensitivity of these studies [37], recent data has shown that different forms of chest radiography are likely equally efficacious as an initial imaging modality [38, 39]. As such, chest radiography as a sole imaging modality is generally insufficient to fully evaluate a parapneumonic effusion or empyema.

Computerized Tomography of the Chest

Computerized tomogroaphy (CT) scan of the chest with contrast is helpful in differentiating empyema from parenchymal lung abscess, which is a critical determination as it impacts management strategy. The wall of an empyema is uniform, smooth and relatively thin; whereas, lung abscesses have thick and irregular walls. Empyemas, especially if large can cause compression of the surrounding lung parenchyma and vessels [40]. They tend to be lenticular in shape with obtuse angles to the chest wall [Figure 2].

Lung abscesses are often round with acute chest wall angles [Figure 3] and have an indistinct boundary between the lung parenchyma and fluid collection [41]. On the other hand, the "split pleura" sign, caused by separation and enhancement of both the thickened parietal and visceral pleural surfaces [Figure 4], is characteristic of empyema. When it is present with a ≥3 cm pleural effusion, the sign had a 79% sensitivity and 81% specificity for differentiating complicated PPE/empyema from a simple parapneumonic effusion [42]. Other CT findings that can be found in patients with empyema are thickening of the parietal pleura or extra-pleural subcostal tissues and increased attenuation of extra-pleural fat [43].

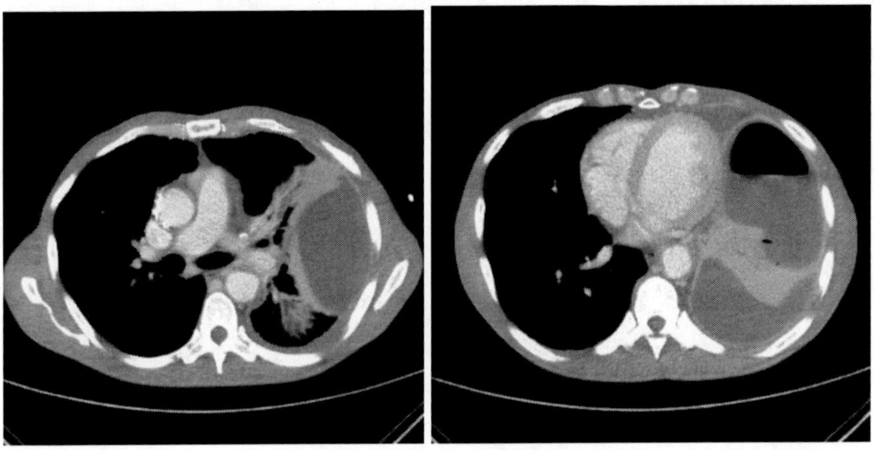

(a) (b)

Figure 2. CT imaging in a patient with left empyema. Note the "lenticular" shape and obtuse angle with the chest wall.

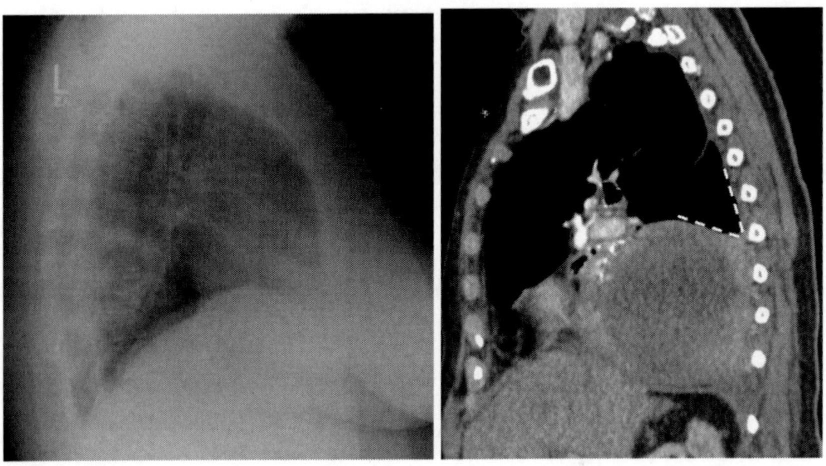

(a) (b)

Figure 3. (a) Lateral view of chest radiograph demonstrating cavitary lung process. (b) Sagittal view of CT imaging demonstrating a lung abscess forming an acute angle with the chest wall (dashed lines).

Further, CT scan is useful in demonstrating full extent of an effusion, degree of loculations, and guiding pleural catheter insertion. Loculations are defined by any one of the following: failure of the effusion to layer on decubitus films, fixed fluid in abnormal locations, septations, air-fluid levels, or irregular scalloped appearance of the effusion contour. This finding suggests progression from the exudative to the fibrinopurulent stage of a PPE. It also offers prognostic information as patients with loculated effusions had longer hospitalizations and may require multiple pleural tubes or decortication [44].

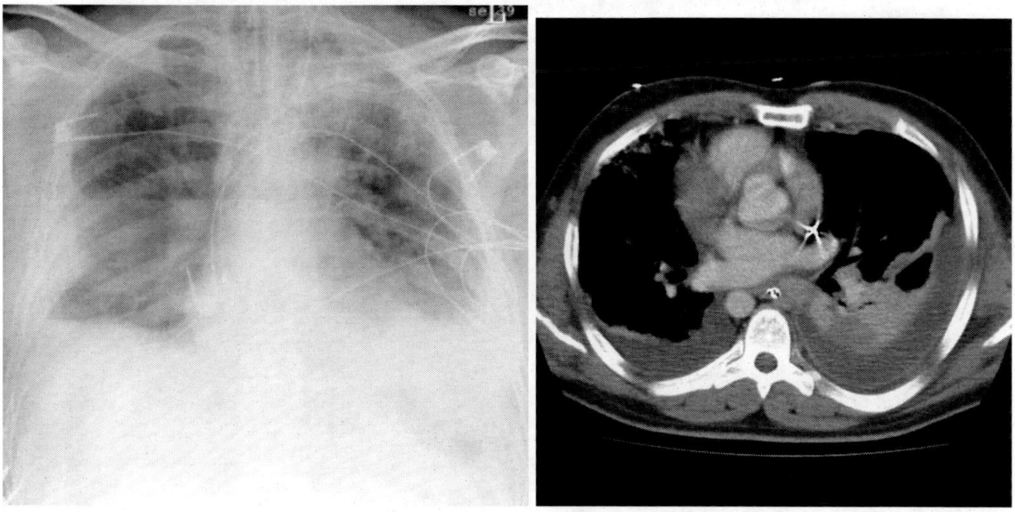

(a) (b)

Figure 4. (a) Chest radiograph demonstrating loculated plerual effusion; (b) CT imaging on the same patient demonstrating a "split-pleura" sign.

Ultrasonography of the Chest

Ultrasonography of the pleural space has unique position in diagnosis and management of PPEs and empyemas. It is superior to chest radiographs in both differentiating pleural fluid from other lung opacities and as a means of localizing fluid [45]. To help characterize PPEs, four different patterns of ultrasound features have been described: a) anechoic; b) complex non-septate; c) complex septate; and d) echogenic, in order of increasing complexity [46] [Figure 5]. Exudative effusions of varying etiology typically exhibit complex echogenicity and infected collections are frequently septated [47, 48]. It is important to recognize that while ultrasonography is helpful in identifying exudative effusions and predicting complexity of PPEs, the appearances of fluid do not correlate with biochemical parameters or outcome measures [32, 49].

Ultrasound technology has its limitations. There is a learning curve for interpretation of images and misinterpretation may result in inadvertent complications. Additionally, ultrasound evaluation may be limited by inability to properly position the patient, crowded intercostal spaces, and presence of subcutaneous emphysema.

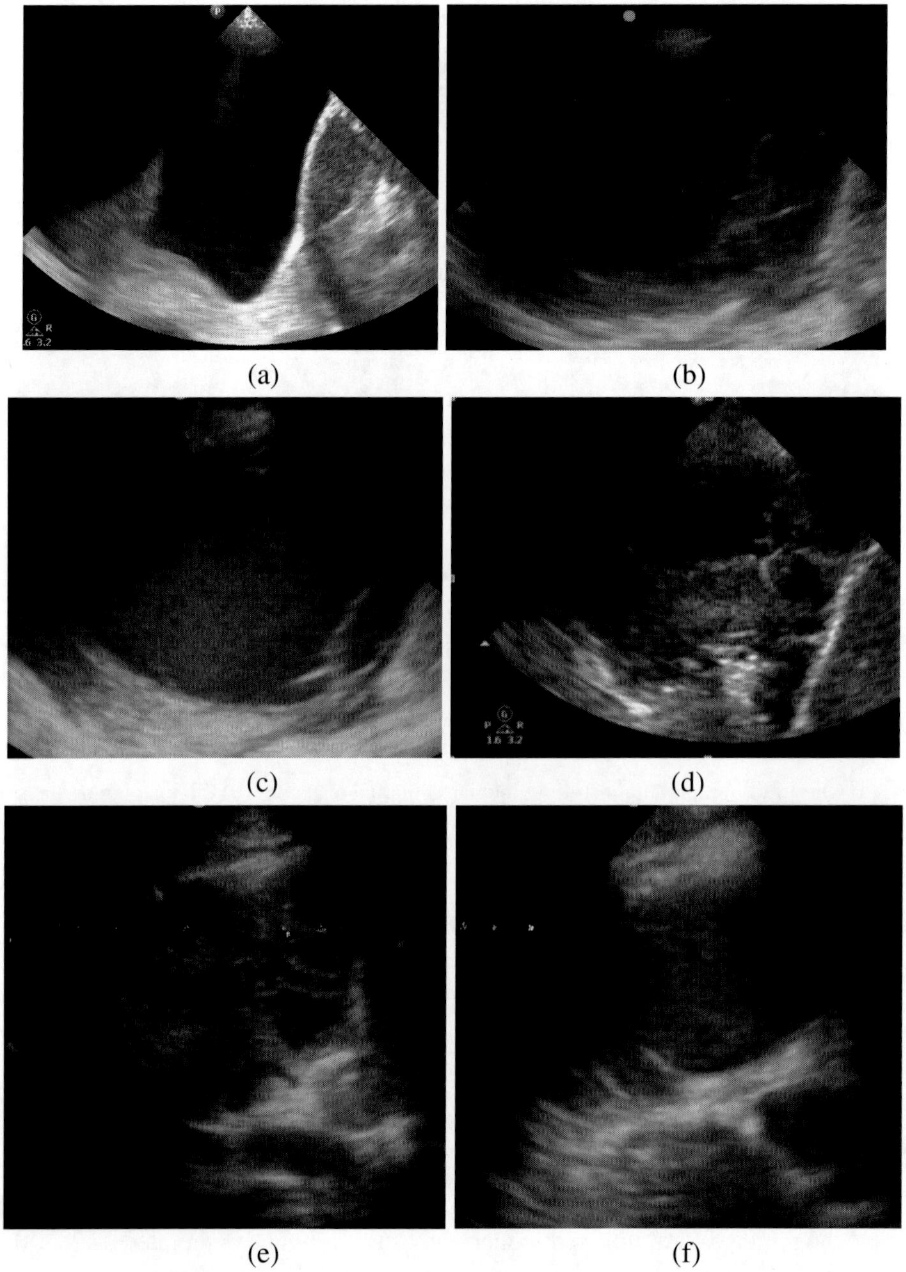

Figure 5. (a) Anechoic simple parapneumonic effusion. (b) Complex non-septate with "sails" suggesting fibrin strands. (c) Complex non-septate in a patient with empyema. Note the increased echogenicity. (d) Evolution into complex septate. (e) Complex septate pleural effusion. (f) Complex loculated and "echogenic" effusion.

Pleural Fluid Analysis

Pleural fluid analysis provides critical information and helps risk stratify patients with PPE. It begins with gross appearance of the fluid as it is aspirated or evacuated from the pleural space. Clear, serous fluid indicates either a transudate or a pauci-cellular exudative effusion. Cloudy fluid or pus suggests empyema and should prompt consideration of placement of tube thoracostomy. Serosanguinous or bloody fluid may be encountered in PPEs especially in patients who are on anticoagulant or antiplatelet therapy.

Determining whether the pleural fluid is a transudate (non-inflammatory) or exudate (inflammatory) is the next step in diagnosis and treatment. In the sentinel article by Light et al. [50], protein and lactate dehydrogenase (LDH) concentrations are measured in both the serum and pleural fluid. Using Light's criteria the fluid is classified as an exudate if any of the following criteria are met:

1. Pleural fluid to serum total protein ratio >0.5
2. Pleural fluid LDH >2/3rd upper limit of normal serum LDH
3. Pleural fluid to serum LDH >0.6

Use of these criteria approaches sensitivity of 100% for identifying exudative effusions. However, the specificity is much lower, thereby classifying some transudative effusions as exudative. One such example is in patients with congestive heart failure receiving diuretic therapy. In scenarios such as this, an albumin gradient value (serum albumin-pleural albumin) <1.2 has a sensitivity and specificity of 95% and 100%, respectively, for the diagnosis of exudates [51]. In addition, the further the values are from the above criteria, the more likely the fluid will be correctly identified as a transudate or exudate [52].

In parapneumonic effusions, which are nearly always exudative, additional criteria are used to further stratify patients based upon predicted outcomes and need for definitive drainage. Using pleural values of pH, LDH, glucose and gram stain/culture, a PPE can be classified as 1) uncomplicated (UPPE) and 2) complicated (CPPE) [53]. Similar categories are proposed by the American College of Chest Physicians (ACCP) [4] and the British Thoracic Society (BTS) [9]. Importantly, pH must be determined using a blood gas analyzer as litmus paper has been shown to be unreliable [9,54]. Empyema, in which frank pus is aspirated, always requires drainage, either via tube thoracostomy or surgical evacuation.

UPPE or effusions in the low risk category are likely to resolve with antibiotics and initial drainage via thoracentesis. Pleural fluid studies in these patients have a pH > 7.2, LDH < 1000 IU/L, and glucose >60 mg/dL, as well as negative gram stain and culture.

CPPE or patients in the high-risk category for poor outcomes have pleural studies with pH < 7.2, LDH >1000 IU/L, glucose less than 60 mg/dL, and/or positive gram stain/culture.

These findings are based largely upon the meta-analysis from Heffner et al. [54], which showed that an acidic pleural space is the greatest predictor of the need for further drainage. The AACP and BTS guidelines both recommend definitive drainage in these cases. These recommendations are supported by more recent studies indicating a 98% sensitivity for identifying CPPE, though the specificity was ~60%, suggesting some effusions classified as CPPE were more akin to UPPE [55].

Pathogenesis and Disease Evolution

There is usually a small volume of pleural fluid in humans to provide lubricating membrane between visceral and parietal pleural surfaces. The amount of the fluid that accumulates depends upon hydrostatic-oncotic pressures and pleuro-lymphatic drainage. An effusion occurs when the resorptive capacity of the pleural space is exceeded.

The transmigration of the bacteria through mesothelial cells into the pleural space is one mechanism for development of empyema. In addition, elevated levels of intrapleural IL-8, VEGF, MCP-1, TNF-alpha levels have been demonstrated in a mouse model of empyema [56]. Bacterial invasion of the pleural space can activate the coagulation cascade, leading to increased levels of plasminogen activator inhibitors and decreased tissue-type plasminogen activator. This inhibits fibrin clearance, thus promoting fibrin deposition and the formation of septations [57].

The progression to empyema has been described to occur in three phases: the exudative, fibrinopurulent, and organizing phases [58]. The *exudative* phase is characterized by increased permeability of local tissue and regional capillaries due to inflammation from pneumonia. This leads to the accumulation of fluid in the pleural space, which is usually free-flowing and easily drained at first. Pleural fluid analysis demonstrates negative bacterial cultures, neutrophil predominance, glucose level > 60 mg/dL, pH > 7.20, and LDH level less than three times the upper limit of normal.

With ongoing inflammation, fibrin clots and fibrin membranes ("sails") are deposited in the pleural space, leading to the formation of loculations. The pleural fluid becomes more viscous and purulent in this *fibrinopurulent* phase, which can cause complete drainage to be difficult. Bacterial invasion of the pleural space occurs. Pleural fluid analysis is characterized by positive bacterial cultures, glucose level < 60 mg/dL, pH < 7.20, and LDH level more than three times the upper limit of normal.

If the effusion remains undrained, fibroblasts proliferate and deposit around the lung in the organizing phase. This creates a thickened fibrous pleural peel that encases the lung and prevents lung expansion ("trapped lung"). Functionally, gas exchange is often severely impaired thus surgical intervention is often needed.

Table 1. Categories of parapneumonic effusions based on both ACCP and BTS guidelines, adapted and modified

Effusion Category	Pleural Space Anatomy	Macroscopic Appearance	Pleural Fluid Chemistry*	Pleural Fluid Bacteriology	Drainage
Uncomplicated or simple parapneumonic	Minimal, free-flowing effusion (<10 mm on lateral decubitus chest radiograph)				Not necessary
	Small to moderate, free-flowing effusion (>10 mm but less than half hemothorax on chest radiograph)	Clear or cloudy/turbid	$pH \geq 7.20$ Glucose ≥60 mg/dL LDH < 1000 IU/L	Gram stain and Culture – both negative	Drain, if symptomatic relief is required
Complicated parapneumonic	Large, free-flowing effusion (≥one half hemithorax of chest radiograph), loculated effusion, or effusion with parietal pleura thickening	Clear or cloudy/turbid	$pH < 7.20$ Glucose <60 mg/dL LDH > 1000 IU/L	Gram stain and/or culture may be positive	Tube thoracostomy
Empyema	Large or loculated effusion; split-pleura sign	Purulent/pus	Not indicated If performed, resemble complicated parapneumonic effusion	Gram stain and/ or culture likely positive	Tube thoracostomy

*BTS guidelines use a glucose cut-off value of 40 mg/dL.

These phases are often regarded as a continuum of events. The ACCP further risk stratified parapneumonic effusions into four categories based on pleural space anatomy and pleural fluid bacteriology and chemistry (Table 1) [4, 59]. The BTS also differentiated stages of parapneumonic effusions based on pleural fluid characteristics (Table 1) [9, 59].

Identification of patients with PPEs or empyema who are at high-risk for poor outcomes can help clinicians triage patients into more aggressive therapies. Using clinical, ultrasonographic, and biochemical parameters, these patients can be identified, though the ideal or optimal treatment algorithm has yet to be determined.

Clinical

Severity score have previously been used to identify high-risk patients presenting with pneumonia. However, earlier attempts to risk stratify patients with pleural infection based on clinical criteria have been less successful [60]. More recent studies have shown that factors such as diet or hospital acquired infections impact outcomes [11, 20]. In a study by Rahman et al. a scoring system called RAPID (renal function, age, purulence, infection source, dietary factors) was used to identify patients at risk for poor outcomes at the time of presentation (Table 2) [61]. Patients with scores of 0-2 were considered low risk, while those with 3-4 were medium and 5-7 high. Those in the high-risk group had mortality rates of at least 31% at 3 months. Using this scoring system, similar results were found in 2 subsequent studies [62, 63].

Table 2. RAPID [Renal function, Age, Purulence of pleural fluid, Infection, Dietary factors] scoring system

Category	Value	Score
BUN, mg/dL	<14	0
	14-22.4	1
	>22.4	2
Age, yr	<50	0
	50-70	1
	>70	2
Purulence of Pleural Fluid	Purulent	0
	Nonpurulent	1
Infection Source	Community	0
	Hospital	1
Albumin, g/dL	≥2.7	0
	<2.7	1

A validated scoring model used to predict 3-month mortality in patients with pleural infection. Patients classified into one of the 3 risk groups based on this cumulative scoring: low risk [0-2, 1-3% mortality], medium risk [3-4, 9-12% mortality], high risk [31-51%] mortality. Adapted from Rahman et al. [61].

Ultrasonography

Point-of-care ultrasonography may provide important information regarding clinical outcomes and treatment efficacy. The presence of loculations are suggestive of lower pH and glucose and indicative of worse outcomes including length of stay, need for surgery, and mortality [44]. Patients with septations on pleural ultrasound have an increased length of stay and longer duration of chest tube drainage. They are also more likely to have incomplete drainage and undergo surgical intervention [64, 65]. However, ultrasonographic features have not been shown to identify the sub-group of patients who will fail tube thoracostomy and require surgical intervention. This is likely due, in part, to the fact that ultrasonographic features have not been shown to reliably differentiate CPPE from UPPE [34, 49].

Biochemical

As previously mentioned, initial studies evaluating the biochemical profile of PPE identified pleural pH as the most powerful indicator for tube thoracostomy [8, 66]. In addition, very low pleural fluid glucose levels (<40 mg/dL) and elevated LDH levels (>1000 IU/L) were shown to predict need for tube thoracostomy. In a recent study evaluating PPE in children, a combination of pleural fluid glucose and LDH was used to identify those at risk for a prolonged hospital course [67]. However, biochemical studies cannot reliably predict which patients will fail medical therapy or have increased mortality [60]. Additionally, while the aspiration of frank pus has been traditionally associated with poor outcomes, the recent study by Rahman et al. suggests improved outcomes [60, 61].

Management

Management of PPE and empyema requires risk stratification and a stepwise approach considering patients' co-morbidities and preferences into consideration.

General Principles

Patient presenting with pneumonia with or without parapneumonic effusion or empyema should be initiated on appropriate antibiotics in a timely manner. Important aspects of care include adequate fluid resuscitation, risk stratification for poor outcomes [clinical, ultrasonographic, and biochemical], venous thromboembolism prophylaxis, nutrition and early surgical consultation for multi-disciplinary discussion in patients with poor prognostic factors [1]. Treatment options include thoracentesis, chest tube drainage with or without intrapleural fibrinolytic/ mucolytic therapy, and surgical drainage of the pleural space. While the published guidelines provide guidance to the clinicians, individualized care relies on patient-centered approach and multi-disciplinary team discussions.

Thoracentesis

Once a likely PPE is identified a thoracentesis is performed to sample the fluid. Most often a therapeutic thoracentesis is recommended. Prior to widespread use of small-bore chest tubes, repeated drainage had been the standard of care for management of PPEs [58]. Several single center studies indicated success with this treatment plan with upwards of 80-90% cure rate without need for alternative therapies [12, 68]. In symptomatic patients without evidence of loculations, septations, or pleural acidosis, a thoracentesis may be all that is needed for drainage of the pleural space. Conversely, the need for repeated thoracentesis suggests the need for a more definitive drainage. A recent meta-analysis by ACCP comparing serial thoracentesis to other management options for PPEs, found that mortality was highest in thoracentesis alone group; about 10% compared to 8% for tube thoracostomy and 4% for fibrinolytic therapy and surgical intervention group. Additionally, >50% of patients on average required repeat intervention in the thoracentesis studies compared to 20% in fibrinolytic or surgical studies [4].

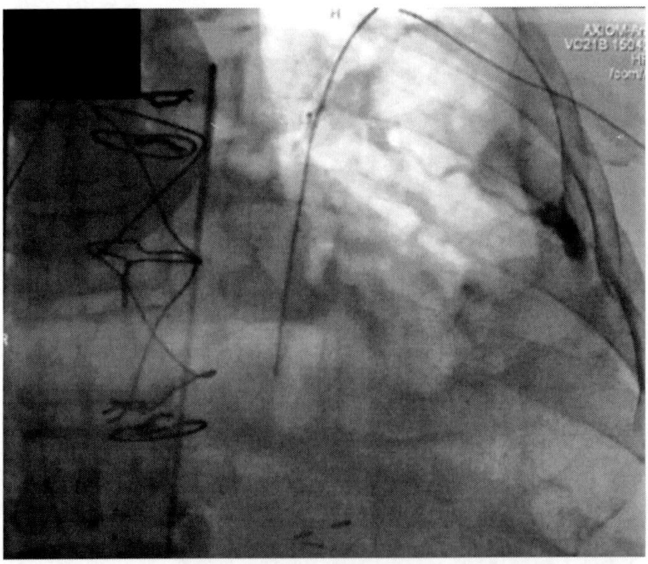

Figure 6. Intercostal artery (ICA) angiogram demonstrating “contrast blush” at the site of laceration. This patient underwent thoracentesis with a 5 French catheter and straw colored fluid was aspirated. The patient was successfully stabilized with volume resuscitation, tube thoracostomy, and ICA embolization.

Due to the evolving nature of PPEs and their tendency to septate/loculate, thoracentesis may inadequately drain the entire pleural space. While ultrasound guided thoracentesis may aid in the selection of repeat drainage sites and increase efficacy of the procedure, this approach exposes the patient to the increased risk of multiple procedures. The most recent expert consensus guidelines from the American Association of Thoracic Surgery (AATS) published in 2017, provide a class III recommendation for this treatment modality, meaning there is no benefit and serial thoracentesis is not recommended [69].

Thoracentesis, though a simple procedure, is not without associated risk of complications. Albeit uncommon, reported complications include pneumothorax, intercostal artery laceration and resultant hemorrhage, and rarely re-expansion pulmonary edema [70]. Complications occur despite all the precautions and one must be able to identify it and be prepared to manage these, as illustrated in Figure 6.

Tube Thoracostomy

As thoracentesis alone is unlikely to provide definitive treatment for PPEs and empyema especially in patients with complex pleural space, tube thoracostomy has become the preferred approach for ongoing drainage [69]. Percutaneous image-guided, ultrasound or CT, small-bore chest tube is recommended as an initial step for management of PPEs and empyema as they cause significantly less pain and similar clinical outcomes compared with large-bore tubes [71]. There are several aspects of tube thoracostomy that must be considered in patients with PPEs and empyema.

Traditionally, tube thoracostomy for PPEs, especially complicated ones or empyema, have used large-bore (>14 French) tubes via an open approach. These tubes have an apparent advantage of being able to traverse complicated septations or drain thick pus without clogging. However, this has not borne out in recent studies. One such study, looked retrospectively at 405 patients whose pleural infections were treated with chest tube drainage and intrapleural fibrinolytics. Compared to patients with chest tubes larger than 14 French, the smaller tube cohort had similar intervention rates, at about 35% and identical mortality rates and length of stay [71]. Similar results have been shown in other studies as well [72, 73], with a success rate of 80%; a rate that is comparable to historical studies where only large-bore chest tubes were used [74].

There are several features of these studies, however, that are important to keep in mind when making a decision on the utility of small-bore chest tubes for drainage of empyema. First, since none of these studies were randomized, it is difficult to ascertain which patients were selected to receive small-bore chest tube versus those that were excluded from the study and either referred for open tube drainage or direct to surgical management. Additionally, all small-bore chest tube placements were performed with image-guidance thereby providing additional advantage not observed in large-bore tube series. Finally, many studies using small-bore chest tubes also include use of intrapleural fibrinolytics which may overcome the deficit in size and propensity to clog. Despite these potential concerns, image-guided, small-bore chest tubes is recommended as an appropriate primary therapy for management of PPEs and empyemas [69].

Image-guided placement, especially of small-bore chest tubes, has become standard of care. The two primary modalities used for chest tube placement are ultrasound and CT guidance, each with its advantages and disadvantages. Ultrasound has the advantage of being portable, cheap, and relatively easy to use. It has limitations in its ability to visualize through bone though most loculated effusions can be accessed under ultrasound guidance. CT on the other hand has the advantage of accurately localizing the needle entry for effusions that are medial, subscapular, and fissural. At most institutions, the practitioner level of comfort with point-of-care ultrasound has continued to improve as a result of it being part of curriculum in training programs. Therefore, some predict that ultrasound will be shown to be as accurate as CT in identifying complex lesions [75]. Additionally, ultrasound use resulted in lowering of re-intervention rates and eliminated the need for additional or advanced imaging all of which resulted in lowering of hospital costs [76, 77]. Importantly, use of point-of-care ultrasound is associated with lower rates of procedure related complications [76, 78]. For these reasons, it has been the practice at our institution to consider ultrasound-guidance as preferred imaging modality for placement of chest tubes in patients with PPEs and empyema. CT guidance is performed for difficult anatomy or loculations that are unable to be identified using point-of-care ultrasound.

In order to optimally treat PPEs, complete drainage and full lung expansion is essential [79]. Despite routine use of image-guided chest tube drainage, inadequate resolution of PPEs and empyemas frequently occurs. Failure rate with chest tube drainage remain as high as 40% and delayed definitive treatment is associated with increased morbidity and mortality [4]. Frequent causes of failed chest tube therapy include: undrained collection, non-functional tube, and persistent inflammatory pleural peel or entrapment [80]. While chest tube drainage remains one of the most important treatment modalities for management of PPEs and empyema, incidence of high failure rate requires adjunctive and alternate therapies including intrapleural fibrinolytics and/or consideration for surgical drainage.

Management of Chest Tubes

The chest tubes, either small- or large-bore, can easily migrate during routine cares and nursing. As such the authors recommend securing the tube with 0 silk or prolene suture, for its tensile strength and inert characteristics. These physiognomies are important because of the amount of time the patient may have the tube. In general, a dry dressing without petroleum gauze is used. The addition of a 2-way or 3-way stop cock placed between the chest tube and pleurovac drainage line tubing allows for ease of fluid and medication instillation including fibrinolytic and mucolytic into the pleural space. This is demonstrated in Figure 7. Instillation is as simple as cleaning the hub, securing a leur-lock syringe with prescribed saline or medication, instilling it, then turning the stop-cock to the off position for a dwell time, if indicated. The reported blockage rates of chest tubes range from 11-30% and can be prevented by routine flushing [69]. This needs to be done under sterile pre-cautions. Daily evaluation of chest tubes is mandatory both to assess tube migration and any signs of local infection.

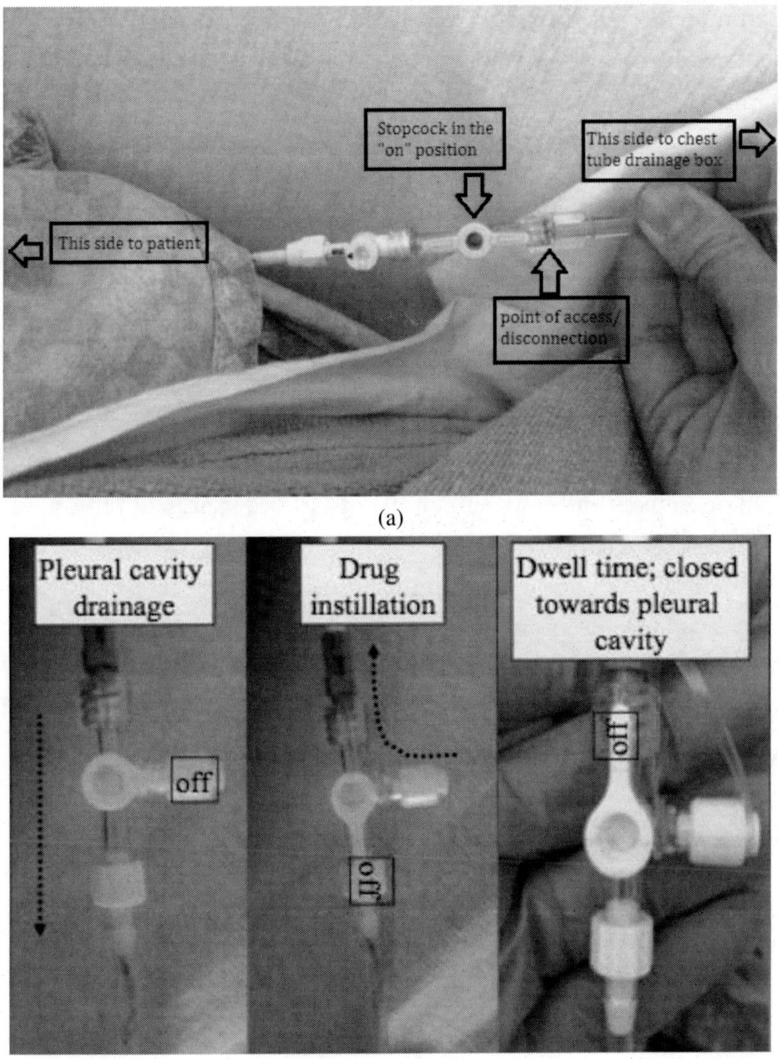

(b)

Figure 7. (a) An image of 2-way "stop-cock" interface with chest tube. (b) Similar set up but with a 3-way "stop-cock."

Intrapleural Fibrinolytics

The tendency of PPEs and empyemas to form loculations and to progress to fibrinous effusion has been the primary limitation of successful chest tube drainage management alone. Especially true for effusions in the fibrinopurulent stage, chest tube placement may only access one specific pocket of pleural infection or may become clogged prior to completely draining the space. Given the extensive fibrin deposition in advanced phase, many physicians over the past half a century have experimented with the use of fibrinolytic. Some of the earliest studies in the 1950s found that instillation of streptokinase had a tendency to promote drainage [81, 82]. However, fibrinolysis by means of streptokinase remained challenging due to development of antibodies and delayed hypersensitivity reaction [83]. Interest grew again in the later part of 20th century with the introduction of alternative fibrinolytics, including urokinase and tissue plasminogen activator (t-PA) and their use in several small studies that demonstrated radiologic and symptomatic improvement [84-86]. A large scale double-armed, randomized controlled trial of over 400 patients on the use of streptokinase in loculated PPEs did not find any improvement in mortality, rate of surgery or length of stay, the study also identified increased rate of complications with the use of streptokinase [72].

The subsequent MIST 2 trial added deoxyribonuclease (DNase) with the hypothesis that decreased viscosity would result in improved pleural drainage. Pleural drainage, as measured by chest radiographs, was improved in the arm that received both t-PA and DNase [87]. Improvement in secondary endpoints such as surgical referral and length of stay were also noted. Since the MIST2 trial, intrapleural fibrinolytic therapy has become a widely used adjunct to the chest tube drainage of PPEs, especially in the presence of complex loculations [88].

Intrapleural fibrinolytics are generally well tolerated but not without risks. Chest pain is the most common side effect occurring in approximately 20% of patients, which can be well managed and limits therapy in less than 5% of patients [88]. Intrapleural hemorrhage requiring intervention has been reported to be as high as 2-5% in a few large studies [87, 88]. Other rare complications including air embolism [89] and diffuse alveolar hemorrhage [90] have been reported as well. While it is clear t-PA/DNase has clinical utility, the optimal timing and dosing has yet to be established. One must be cautious to adopt this strategy in routine management of PPEs.

Surgical Management

Despite a timely and appropriate chest tube drainage of PPEs and empyema with or without fibrinolytic/mucolytic therapy, the failure rate of these approaches is not insignificant. In such cases, surgery remains an important treatment modality for definitive management, with options ranging from less invasive video assisted thoracoscopic surgery (VATS) to thoracotomy and complete decortication.

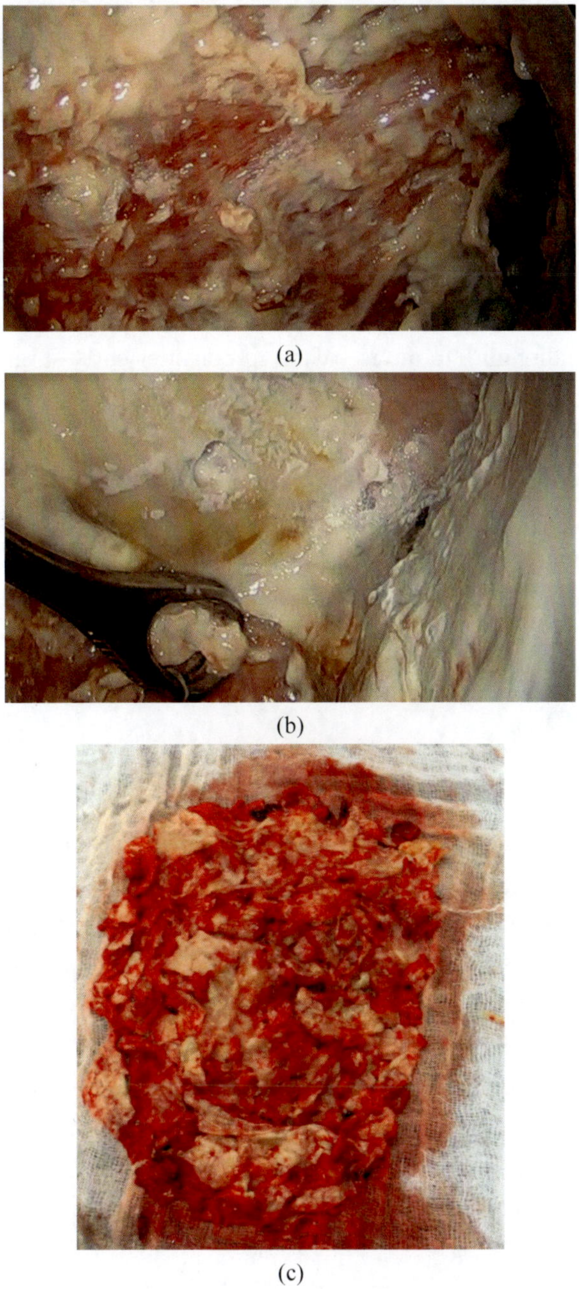

Figure 8. (a) Fibrinopurulent visceral peel. (b) Visceral pleural peel removed at pulmonary decortication. (c) Complete pulmonary decortication.

The most common indications for surgical intervention are incompletely drained PPEs and failure to achieve adequate response with medical therapy, including chest tube drainage, alone [9]. Several studies have shown that VATS is extremely successful in both breaking up the pleural loculations and completely draining infected fluid [91, 92]. Interestingly, a meta-analysis by the ACCP working group found that patients undergoing surgery had the lowest rate of additional intervention and lowest mortality rate at <4%, compared to 10% for primary tube thoracostomy [4]. If VATS is precluded because of inability to tolerate single lung ventilation or low likelihood of success, then conversion to open thoracotomy is needed. Reported conversion rates vary widely, ranging from 0-41%, and likely relate to preferences at individual centers, and the selection of patients taken to the operating room [69]. One recent study found that chronicity of infection and pleural thickness on CT imaging were significant predictors of necessity for conversion to an open procedure [93]. Figure 8 below illustrates the thick visceral pleural peel/rind found at VATS that required open thoracotomy and complete pulmonary decortication.

It still remains challenging to advise when to consider early surgical intervention. A recently published meta-analysis of 8 randomized controlled trials that included 391 patients, attempted to answer the question of surgical versus non-surgical management of empyema [94]. While there was no difference in mortality across all age groups, it did find a tendency towards shorter hospital length of stays in the groups that received surgery up front. Also, the procedure complication rates were similar between the tube thoracostomy and VATS groups, further promoting the idea that early surgical intervention may not only be effective but also safe.

Conclusion

Patients with parapneumonic effusions and empyema have higher morbidity and mortality. Prompt identification and management of these conditions is therefore critical. Point-of-care ultrasound evaluation is easy to perform and provides meaningful information to risk-stratify patients in addition to clinical scoring and biochemical parameters. Additionally, it has shown to decrease complications associated with performing thoracentesis and chest tube drainage. Along with fibrinolytic and mucolytic therapy, small-bore chest tubes have decreased the need for surgical intervention. Even so, the rate of treatment failure with these therapies is not inconsequential and many patients require surgical intervention. Early surgical referral along with a stepwise and multi-disciplinary team approach is recommended. This is likely to improve patient outcomes and decrease healthcare costs.

References

[1] Feller-Kopman, D. and R. Light. Pleural Disease. *N Engl J Med* 2018; 378 (18):1754. 10.1056/NEJMc1803858.

[2] Adams, F. The genuine works of Hippocrates. . *London: C. and J. Adlard Printers* 1848.

[3] Burgos, J., V. Falco, and A. Pahissa. The increasing incidence of empyema. *Curr Opin Pulm Med* 2013*;* 19 (4):350-6. 10.1097/MCP.0b013e3283606ab5.

[4] Colice, G. L., et al. Medical and surgical treatment of parapneumonic effusions: an evidence based guideline. *Chest* 2000*;* 118 (4):1158-71.

[5] Ahmed, R. A., T .J. Marrie, and J. Q. Huang. Thoracic empyema in patients with community acquired pneumonia. *Am J Med* 2006*;* 119 (10):877-83. 10.1016/j.amjmed.2006.03.042.

[6] Mandal, A. K., et al. Outcome of primary empyema thoracis: therapeutic and microbiologic aspects. *Ann Thorac Surg* 1998*;* 66 (5):1782-6.

[7] Halm, E. A. and A. S. Teirstein. Clinical practice. Management of community-acquired pneumonia. *N Engl J Med* 2002*;* 347 (25):2039-45. 10.1056/NEJMcp020499.

[8] Light, R. W., et al. Parapneumonic effusions. *Am J Med* 1980*;* 69 (4):507-12.

[9] Davies, H. E., et al. Management of pleural infection in adults: British Thoracic Society Pleural Disease Guideline 2010. *Thorax* 2010*;* 65 Suppl 2:ii41-53. 10.1136/thx.2010.137000.

[10] Goodnight, W. H. and D. E. Soper. Pneumonia in pregnancy. *Crit Care Med* 2005*;* 33 (10Suppl):S390-7.

[11] Chalmers, J. D., et al. Risk factors for complicated parapneumonic effusion and empyema on presentation to hospital with community-acquired pneumonia. *Thorax* 2009*;* 64 (7):592-7. 10.1136/thx.2008.105080.

[12] Ferguson, A. D., et al. The clinical course and management of thoracic empyema. *QJM* 1996*;* 89 (4):285-9.

[13] Finland, M. and M. W. Barnes. Changing ecology of acute bacterial empyema: occurrence and mortality at Boston City Hospital during 12 selected years from 1935 to 1972. *J Infect Dis* 1978*;* 137 (3):274-91.

[14] Weese, W. C., et al. Empyema of the thorax then and now. A study of 122 cases over four decades. *Arch Intern Med* 1973*;* 131 (4):516-20.

[15] Grijalva, C. G., et al. Emergence of parapneumonic empyema in the USA. *Thorax* 2011*;* 66 (8):663-8. 10.1136/thx.2010.156406.

[16] Farjah, F., et al. Management of pleural space infections: a population-based analysis. *J Thorac Cardiovasc Surg* 2007*;* 133 (2):346-51. 10.1016/j.jtcvs.2006.09.038.

[17] Munoz-Almagro, C., L. Selva, and R. Pallares. Influence of pneumococcal vaccine on the incidence of empyema. *Curr Opin Pulm Med* 2010*;* 16 (4):394-8. 10.1097/MCP.0b013e328338c19f.

[18] Hasley, P. B., et al. Do pulmonary radiographic findings at presentation predict mortality in patients with community-acquired pneumonia? *Arch Intern Med* 1996*;* 156 (19):2206-12.

[19] Menendez, R., et al. Risk factors of treatment failure in community acquired pneumonia: implications for disease outcome. *Thorax* 2004; 59 (11):960-5. 10.1136/thx.2003.017756.

[20] Maskell, N. A., et al. The bacteriology of pleural infection by genetic and standard methods and its mortality significance. *Am J Respir Crit Care Med* 2006; 174 (7):817-23.10.1164/rccm.200601-074OC.

[21] Ashbaugh, D. G. Empyema thoracis. Factors influencing morbidity and mortality. *Chest* 1991; 99 (5):1162-5.

[22] Bender, J. M., et al. Parapneumonic empyema deaths during past century, Utah. *Emerg Infect Dis* 2009; 15 (1):44-8. 10.3201/eid1501.080618.

[23] Popowicz, N. D., et al. Human pleural fluid is a potent growth medium for Streptococcus pneumoniae. *PLoS One* 2017; 12 (11):e0188833. 10.1371/journal.pone.0188833.

[24] Brook, I. and E. H. Frazier. Aerobic and anaerobic microbiology of empyema. A retrospective review in two military hospitals. *Chest* 1993; 103 (5):1502-7.

[25] Chen, K. Y., et al. A 10-year experience with bacteriology of acute thoracic empyema: emphasis on Klebsiella pneumoniae in patients with diabetes mellitus. *Chest* 2000; 117 (6):16859.

[26] Pinnola, A., et al. Bacteriology and Comorbidities in Patients Requiring Surgical Management of Empyema. *Am Surg* 2018; 84 (4):599-603.

[27] Vorster, M. J., et al. Tuberculous pleural effusions: advances and controversies. *J Thorac Dis* 2015; 7 (6):981-91. 10.3978/j.issn.2072-1439.2015.02.18.

[28] Gopi, A., et al. Diagnosis and treatment of tuberculous pleural effusion in 2006. *Chest* 2007;131 (3):880-889. 10.1378/chest.06-2063.

[29] El Solh, A. A., et al. A comparative study of community- and nursing home-acquired empyema thoracis. *J Am Geriatr Soc* 2007; 55 (11):1847-52. 10.1111/j.1532-5415.2007.01392.x.

[30] Community-acquired pneumonia in adults in British hospitals in 1982-1983: a survey of aetiology, mortality, prognostic factors and outcome. The British Thoracic Society and the Public Health Laboratory Service. *Q J Med* 1987; 62 (239):195-220.

[31] Goodman, L. R., R. A. Goren, and S. K. Teplick. The radiographic evaluation of pulmonary infection. *Med Clin North Am* 1980; 64 (3):553-74.

[32] Svigals, P. Z., et al. The accuracy of pleural ultrasonography in diagnosing complicated parapneumonic pleural effusions. *Thorax* 2017; 72 (1):94-95. 10.1136/thoraxjnl-2016-208904.

[33] Brixey, A. G., et al. The efficacy of chest radiographs in detecting parapneumonic effusions. *Respirology* 2011; 16 (6):1000-4. 10.1111/j.1440-1843.2011.02006.x.

[34] Porcel, J. M. Chest imaging for the diagnosis of complicated parapneumonic effusions. *Curr Opin Pulm Med* 2018; 24 (4):398-402. 10.1097/MCP.0000000000000485.

[35] Woodring, J. H. Recognition of pleural effusion on supine radiographs: how much fluid is required? *AJR Am J Roentgenol* 1984; 142 (1):59-64. 10.2214/ajr.142.1.59.

[36] Blackmore, C. C., et al. Pleural fluid volume estimation: a chest radiograph prediction rule. *Acad Radiol* 1996; 3 (2):103-9.

[37] Mandell, L. A., et al. Infectious Diseases Society of America/American Thoracic Society consensus guidelines on the management of community-acquired pneumonia in adults. *Clin Infect Dis* 2007; 44 Suppl 2:S27-72. 10.1086/511159.

[38] Moffett, B. K., et al. Comparing posteroanterior with lateral and anteroposterior chest radiography in the initial detection of parapneumonic effusions. *Am J Emerg Med* 2016; 34 (12):2402-2407. 10.1016/j.ajem.2016.09.021.

[39] Metersky, M. L. Is the lateral decubitus radiograph necessary for the management of a parapneumonic pleural effusion? *Chest* 2003; 124 (3):1129-32.

[40] Stark, D. D., et al. Differentiating lung abscess and empyema: radiography and computed tomography. *AJR Am J Roentgenol* 1983; 141 (1):163-7. 10.2214/ajr.141.1.163.

[41] Baber, C. E., et al. Differentiating empyemas and peripheral pulmonary abscesses: the value of computed tomography. *Radiology* 1980; 135 (3):755-8. 10.1148/radiology.135.3.7384467.

[42] Tsujimoto, N., et al. A Simple Method for Differentiating Complicated Parapneumonic Effusion/Empyema from Parapneumonic Effusion Using the Split Pleura Sign and the Amount of Pleural Effusion on Thoracic CT. *PLoS One* 2015; 10 (6):e0130141. 10.1371/journal.pone.0130141.

[43] Waite, R. J., et al. Parietal pleural changes in empyema: appearances at CT. *Radiology* 1990; 175 (1):145-50. 10.1148/radiology.175.1.2315473.

[44] Himelman, R.B. and P.W. Callen. The prognostic value of loculations in parapneumonic pleural effusions. *Chest* 1986; 90 (6):852-6.

[45] Doust, B. D., et al. Ultrasonic evaluation of pleural opacities. *Radiology* 1975; 114 (1):135 40. 10.1148/114.1.135.

[46] McLoud, T. C. and C. D. Flower. Imaging the pleura: sonography, CT, and MR imaging. *AJR Am J Roentgenol* 1991; 156 (6):1145-53. 10.2214/ajr.156.6.2028857.

[47] Yang, P. C., et al. Value of sonography in determining the nature of pleural effusion: analysis of 320 cases. *AJR Am J Roentgenol* 1992; 159 (1):29-33. 10.2214/ajr.159.1.1609716.

[48] Lomas, D. J., S. G. Padley, and C. D. Flower. The sonographic appearances of pleural fluid. *Br J Radiol* 1993; 66 (787):619-24. 10.1259/0007-1285-66-787-619.

[49] Kearney, S. E., et al. Computed tomography and ultrasound in parapneumonic effusions and empyema. *Clin Radiol* 2000; 55 (7):542-7. 10.1053/crad.1999.0480.

[50] Light, R. W., et al. Pleural effusions: the diagnostic separation of transudates and exudates. *Ann Intern Med* 1972; 77 (4):507-13.

[51] Roth, B. J., T. F. O'Meara, and W. H. Cragun. The serum-effusion albumin gradient in the evaluation of pleural effusions. *Chest* 1990; 98 (3):546-9.

[52] Joseph, J., et al. Is the pleural fluid transudate or exudate? A revisit of the diagnostic criteria. *Thorax* 2001; 56 (11):867-70.

[53] Sahn, S. A. Diagnosis and management of parapneumonic effusions and empyema. *Clin Infect Dis* 2007; 45 (11):1480-6. 10.1086/522996.

[54] Heffner, J. E., et al. Pleural fluid chemical analysis in parapneumonic effusions. A meta-analysis. *Am J Respir Crit Care Med* 1995; 151 (6):1700-8. 10.1164/ajrccm.151.6.7767510.

[55] Manuel Porcel, J., et al. Usefulness of the British Thoracic Society and the American College of Chest Physicians guidelines in predicting pleural drainage of non-purulent parapneumonic effusions. *Respir Med* 2006; 100 (5):933-7. 10.1016/j.rmed.2005.06.017.

[56] Wilkosz, S., et al. Characterization of a new mouse model of empyema and the mechanisms of pleural invasion by Streptococcus pneumoniae. *Am J Respir Cell Mol Biol* 2012; 46 (2):180-7. 10.1165/rcmb.2011-0182OC.

[57] Aleman, C., et al. Association between inflammatory mediators and the fibrinolysis system in infectious pleural effusions. *Clin Sci (Lond)* 2003; 105 (5):601-7. 10.1042/CS20030115.

[58] Andrews, N. C. Management of nontuberculous empyema: A statement of the subcommittee on surgery. *Am Rev Respir Dis* 1962; 85:935.

[59] Heffner, J. E., J. S. Klein, and C. Hampson. Interventional management of pleural infections. *Chest* 2009; 136 (4):1148-1159. 10.1378/chest.08-2956.

[60] Davies, C. W., et al. Predictors of outcome and long-term survival in patients with pleural infection. *Am J Respir Crit Care Med* 1999; 160 (5 Pt 1):1682-7. 10.1164/ajrccm.160.5.9903002.

[61] Rahman, N. M., et al. A clinical score (RAPID) to identify those at risk for poor outcome at presentation in patients with pleural infection. *Chest* 2014; 145 (4):848-855. 10.1378/chest.13 1558.

[62] White, H. D., et al. Predicting Long-Term Outcomes in Pleural Infections. RAPID Score for Risk Stratification. *Ann Am Thorac Soc* 2015; 12 (9):1310-6. 10.1513/AnnalsATS.201505 272OC.

[63] Touray, S., et al. Risk Stratification in Patients with Complicated Parapneumonic Effusions and Empyema Using the RAPID Score. *Lung* 2018. 10.1007/s00408-018-0146-2.

[64] Chen, K. Y., et al. Sonographic septation: a useful prognostic indicator of acute thoracic empyema. *J Ultrasound Med* 2000; 19 (12):837-43.

[65] Chen, C. H., et al. Transthoracic ultrasonography in predicting the outcome of small-bore catheter drainage in empyemas or complicated parapneumonic effusions. *Ultrasound Med Biol* 2009; 35 (9):1468-74. 10.1016/j.ultrasmedbio.2009.04.021.

[66] Light, R. W., et al. Diagnostic significance of pleural fluid pH and PCO2. *Chest* 1973; 64 (5):591-6.

[67] Breuer, O., et al. Predictors of Prolonged Hospitalizations in Pediatric Complicated Pneumonia. *Chest* 2018; 153 (1):172-180. 10.1016/j.chest.2017.09.021.

[68] Simmers, T. A., C. Jie, and B. Sie. Minimally invasive treatment of thoracic empyema. *Thorac Cardiovasc Surg* 1999; 47 (2):77-81. 10.1055/s-2007-1013115.

[69] Shen, K. R., et al. The American Association for Thoracic Surgery consensus guidelines for the management of empyema. *J Thorac Cardiovasc Surg* 2017; 153 (6):e129-e146. 10.1016/j.jtcvs.2017.01.030.

[70] Sachdeva, A., R. W. Shepherd, and H. J. Lee. Thoracentesis and thoracic ultrasound: state of the art in 2013. *Clin Chest Med* 2013; 34 (1):1-9. 10.1016/j.ccm.2012.11.005.

[71] Rahman, N. M., et al. The relationship between chest tube size and clinical outcome in pleural infection. *Chest* 2010; 137 (3):536-43. 10.1378/chest.09-1044.

[72] Maskell, N. A., et al. U.K. Controlled trial of intrapleural streptokinase for pleural infection. *N Engl J Med* 2005; 352 (9):865-74. 10.1056/NEJMoa042473.

[73] Westcott, J. L. Percutaneous catheter drainage of pleural effusion and empyema. *AJR Am J Roentgenol* 1985; 144 (6):1189-93. 10.2214/ajr.144.6.1189.

[74] Ali, I. and H. Unruh. Management of empyema thoracis. *Ann Thorac Surg* 1990; 50 (3):3559.

[75] Volpicelli, G., et al. International evidence-based recommendations for point-of-care lung ultrasound. *Intensive Care Med* 2012; 38 (4):577-91. 10.1007/s00134-012-2513-4.

[76] Patel, P. A., F. R. Ernst, and C. L. Gunnarsson. Ultrasonography guidance reduces complications and costs associated with thoracentesis procedures. *J Clin Ultrasound* 2012; 40 (3):135-41. 10.1002/jcu.20884.

[77] Peris, A., et al. The use of point-of-care bedside lung ultrasound significantly reduces the number of radiographs and computed tomography scans in critically ill patients. *Anesth Analg* 2010; 111 (3):687-92. 10.1213/ANE.0b013e3181e7cc42.

[78] Daniels, C. E. and J. H. Ryu. Improving the safety of thoracentesis. *Curr Opin Pulm Med* 2011; 17 (4):232-6. 10.1097/MCP.0b013e328345160b.

[79] Athanassiadi, K., M. Gerazounis, and N. Kalantzi. Treatment of post-pneumonic empyema thoracis. *Thorac Cardiovasc Surg* 2003; 51 (6):338-41. 10.1055/s-2003-45421.

[80] Silverman, S. G., et al. Thoracic empyema: management with image-guided catheter drainage. *Radiology* 1988; 169 (1):5-9. 10.1148/radiology.169.1.3047789.

[81] Tillett, W. S., S. Sherry, and C. T. Read. The use of streptokinase-streptodornase in the treatment of postneumonic empyema. *J Thorac Surg* 1951; 21 (3):275-97.

[82] Tillett, W. S., S. Sherry, and C. T. Read. The use of streptokinase-streptodornase in the treatment of chronic empyema; with an interpretive discussion of enzymatic actions in the field of intrathoracic diseases. *J Thorac Surg* 1951; 21 (4):325-41.

[83] Laisaar, T. and T. Pullerits. Effect of intrapleural streptokinase administration on antistreptokinase antibody level in patients with loculated pleural effusions. *Chest* 2003; 123 (2):432-5.

[84] Bouros, D., et al. Intrapleural streptokinase versus urokinase in the treatment of complicated parapneumonic effusions: a prospective, double-blind study. *Am J Respir Crit Care Med* 1997; 155 (1):291-5. 10.1164/ajrccm.155.1.9001327.

[85] Bouros, D., et al. Intrapleural urokinase versus normal saline in the treatment of complicated parapneumonic effusions and empyema. A randomized, double-blind study. *Am J Respir Crit Care Med* 1999; 159 (1):37-42. 10.1164/ajrccm.159.1.9803094.

[86] Skeete, D. A., et al. Intrapleural tissue plasminogen activator for complicated pleural effusions. *J Trauma* 2004; 57 (6):1178-83.

[87] Rahman, N. M., et al. Intrapleural use of tissue plasminogen activator and DNase in pleural infection. *N Engl J Med* 2011; 365 (6):518-26. 10.1056/NEJMoa1012740.

[88] Piccolo, F., et al. Intrapleural tissue plasminogen activator and deoxyribonuclease for pleural infection. An effective and safe alternative to surgery. *Ann Am Thorac Soc* 2014; 11 (9):1419-25. 10.1513/AnnalsATS.201407-329OC.

[89] Menendez-Gonzalez, M., P. Oliva-Nacarino, and A. Alvarez-Cofino. Cerebral gas embolism caused by pleural fibrinolytic treatment. *Stroke* 2007; 38 (9):2602-4. 10.1161/STROKEAHA.106.477752.

[90] Shah, R. M., et al. Diffuse Alveolar Hemorrhage as a Complication of Intrapleural Fibrinolytic Therapy. *J Bronchology Interv Pulmonol* 2017; 24 (4):e54-e56. 10.1097/LBR.0000000000000400.

[91] Angelillo-Mackinlay, T., et al. Surgical treatment of postpneumonic empyema. *World J Surg* 1999; 23 (11):1110-3.

[92] Wait, M. A., et al. A randomized trial of empyema therapy. *Chest* 1997; 111 (6):1548-51.

[93] Stefani, A., et al. Preoperative predictors of successful surgical treatment in the management of parapneumonic empyema. *Ann Thorac Surg* 2013; 96 (5):1812-9. 10.1016/j.athoracsur.2013.06.013.

[94] Redden, M. D., T. Y. Chin, and M. L. van Driel. Surgical versus non-surgical management for pleural empyema. *Cochrane Database Syst Rev* 2017; 3:CD010651. 10.1002/14651858.CD010651.pub2.

In: Pleural Effusions: Causes, Types and Treatment
Editor: Rahul Khosla
ISBN: 978-1-53614-683-7

Chapter 5

MALIGNANT PLEURAL EFFUSIONS

Amrik S. Ray, MD, Van K. Holden, MD, Or Kalchiem-Dekel, MD, Edward M. Pickering, MD and Ashutosh Sachdeva*, MBBS
Section of Interventional Pulmonology, Division of Pulmonary,
Critical Care, and Sleep Medicine, Department of Medicine,
University of Maryland School of Medicine, Baltimore, MD, US

ABSTRACT

Malignant pleural effusions (MPEs) are frequently encountered in patients with both intra- or extra-thoracic neoplasms and often portend a poor prognosis. The pathophysiology of MPE is varied and poorly understood. It is important to distinguish malignant from paramalignant effusions given the impact on staging and treatment decisions. Although the clinical presentation may vary, patients typically present with dyspnea or easy fatigability resulting in poor performance status. Imaging studies, typically ultrasonography and chest computed tomography (CT), are valuable for evaluation of MPE. CT imaging with contrast is helpful in identifying co-existing or alternate diagnoses. Ultrasonography provides point-of-care information to guide procedures and is superior to CT imaging in identifying pleural implants and loculations. Thoracentesis offers fluid for cytologic examination, relieves symptoms, and provides critical information on lung expandability. Long-term treatment options include therapeutic thoracenteses, indwelling pleural catheter placement, chemical pleurodesis, or a combination of indwelling pleural catheter and chemical pleurodesis. As patients with MPE may have limited prognosis, treatment options should balance, invasiveness, cost-effectiveness, quality of life, and patients' preferences. Furthermore, a multidisciplinary team approach is likely to close quality gaps, enhance patient safety, and provide guideline consistent care. This chapter provides an overview of the diagnosis and management of MPEs, while emphasizing practical aspects of care.

* Corresponding Author Email: asachdeva@som.umaryland.edu.

Keywords: malignant pleural effusions, pleurodesis, medical thoracoscopy, tunneled pleural catheters

INTRODUCTION

Malignant pleural effusions (MPEs) are a common complication of neoplastic disease. They are a frequent cause of hospital admission and are associated with significant morbidity and mortality. Inpatient mortality after diagnosis is 11.6% [1, 2], and median survival is 4-7 months from the time of diagnosis [2, 3]. Curative options are limited in most cases; thus, palliative management has taken precedence. Methods of providing effective palliation have emerged which has shifted most management to the outpatient setting, particularly with tunneled pleural catheters (TPCs) and rapid pleurodesis protocols.

Incidence

More than 150,000 MPEs are diagnosed every year in the United States, resulting in more than 125,000 hospital admissions per year [1, 2, 4]. It is estimated that 15% of all malignancies are complicated by pleural effusions [5]. In addition, the rate of recurrence of MPEs is as high as 30% within 15 days [6]. A majority of MPEs are exudative (44 - 77%) and are the second most common cause of exudative effusions among hospitalized patients after parapneumonic effusions [2]. Autopsy studies suggest that 60% of malignancies involve the pleura [7, 8]. Table 1 lists common causes of MPEs among hospitalized patients in United States [2].

Table 1. Causes of malignant pleural effusions [2]

Primary Malignancy Type	Percentage of MPEs
Lung cancer	37.8%
Breast cancer	15.2%
Hematologic cancer	11.2%
Gastrointestinal tract cancer	11.0%
Gynecologic cancer	9.0%
Other	22.2%
Unknown primary malignancy	11.2%

Prognosis

Aside from malignant mesothelioma, the presence of a MPE indicates metastatic disease. As such, MPE indicates advanced disease and the accordingly, the overall prognosis of MPEs remains poor despite advances in therapy. As noted above, estimates of the median survival after diagnosis range from 4-7 months [2, 3]; however, an individual patient's life expectancy can vary greatly depending on the underlying tumor subtype. The LENT score (pleural fluid lactate dehydrogenase [LDH] level, Eastern Cooperative Oncology [ECOG] performance status, neutrophil-lymphocyte ratio in the serum, and tumor type) has gained popularity in recent years in estimating the prognosis in patients with MPEs [9]. This may help guide patients with determining treatment options. Table 2 provides information on calculation of the LENT score. An aggregate LENT score of 0 - 1 is considered low risk, and patients with this score have a median survival of 319 days. A score of 2-4 (moderate risk) suggests a median survival of 130 days; a score of 5 or higher (high risk), a median survival of 44 days [9].

Table 2. LENT score calculation [9]

Category	Value	Score
Pleural LDH level	< 1500 IU per liter	0
	≥ 1500 IU per liter	1
ECOG Score	0 – Asymptomatic	0
	1 – Symptomatic but ambulatory	1
	2 – Symptomatic but in bed < 50% of the day	2
	3,4 – Symptomatic and in bed > 50% of the day or bedbound	3
Serum Neutrophil to Lymphocyte Ratio	< 9	0
	≥ 9	1
Tumor Type	Mesothelioma or hematologic malignancy	0
	Breast, gynecologic, or renal cell malignancy	1
	Lung or any other malignancy	2

PATHOPHYSIOLOGY

The pleural space typically contains 10-20mL of pleural fluid which is drained by stoma on the parietal pleura into the lymphatic system [10]. Fundamentally, fluid can develop in the setting of malignancy either by the introduction of malignant cells into the space, defining MPE, or from the accumulation of fluid via adjunctive methods resulting in a paramalignant pleural effusion. Paramalignant pleural effusions may arise from a variety of mechanisms, including obstruction of lymphatics, including the thoracic duct, bronchial obstruction leading to collapse and accumulation of reactive ipsilateral pleural fluid, trapped lung, chemotherapy or radiation-associated inflammation, post-obstructive pneumonia causing parapneumonic effusion, or pulmonary emboli causing effusions [7, 11, 12]. It is critical to ascertain whether an effusion is malignant or paramalignant as this will affect staging of malignancies, and thus treatment recommendations.

Malignancies can cause pleural effusions by a variety of mechanisms. First, neoplastic cells can directly invade the pleural space. This is most commonly seen in lung or breast neoplasms and is usually unilateral. Secondly, hematogenous spread of tumor cells to the pleura can occur, even in the absence of mediastinal lymph node involvement [5]. Breast cancer, when spread hematogenously, will often involve the liver and present with bilateral MPEs [13]. The development of MPEs occurs from any combination of increased fluid production due to fluid extravasation from parietal and visceral pleura, stomal obstruction, or obstruction of downstream lymphatics impairing drainage [14]. MPEs secondary to lymphoproliferative disease can be caused by either direct pleural invasion, as is more commonly seen in non-Hodgkin's lymphoma, or via hematogenous spread, which is more commonly seen in Hodgkin's lymphoma [15]. Of note, while lymphomas can present with chylothoraces due to lymphatic or thoracic duct obstruction, the incidence of this phenomenon is quite low [16].

CLINICAL PRESENTATION

A patient's clinical presentation can range from minimal or no symptoms to respiratory distress. Many factors including volume of fluid, rate of fluid accumulation, patient's weight, and underlying cardiopulmonary comorbidities play into the severity of any individual patient's symptoms [17]. The most common presenting symptom is dyspnea, likely from reduced lung volumes and impaired diaphragmatic excursion. Pain and cough are the next most common symptoms. Patients with MPEs may present with pleuritic chest pain. However, patients with mesothelioma often have dull chest pain unless there is chest wall or nerve invasion, which may result in severe pain. Patients may have early satiety as a result of impaired stomach expansion due to downward displacement of diaphragm and typically report improved appetite after pleural fluid drainage. Physical exams typically demonstrate dullness to percussion and diminished breath sounds on auscultation at the base of the side with pleural effusion [18].

IMAGING CHARACTERISTICS

Chest Radiography

Chest radiography is typically the most common test that patients with dyspnea undergo on evaluation. It can at times be helpful in identifying loculated effusions [Figure 1]. Among patients with symptomatic MPE who undergo chest radiography, 80% demonstrate with moderate to large sized effusions [Figure 2], 10% demonstrate massive effusions, and 10% demonstrate small effusions of < 500mL [19, 20]. However, about one-half of small and one-third of moderate-sized effusions can be misdiagnosed as parenchymal opacities or not identified at all on chest x-rays [21].

Thoracic Ultrasonography

Bedside or formal thoracic ultrasonography has a higher sensitivity in detecting pleural effusions compared to chest radiography [22, 23]. Effusions can appear anechoic in comparison to surrounding structures as demonstrated in Figure 3. Highly cellular, sanguineous, or proteinaceous fluid may appear cloudy and hyperechogenic when compared to benign pleural fluid. Pleural thickening may suggest a MPE. Pleural-based metastases are often visible on ultrasound and appear as either hyperechogenic nodules or larger more complex cystic structures. These can be found on either the visceral or parietal pleura [22-24]. In addition, ultrasonography is sensitive in identifying a complex pleural space, including septations or adhesion bands as demonstrated in Figure 4a. These patients may require earlier and more invasive therapeutic approaches.

Chest Computerized Tomography

CT chest with or without contrast is useful in evaluating pleural effusions. Use of intravenous contrast is preferable when possible as it can further delineate pleural structures [25]. CT findings that are characteristic of MPE include the presence of pleural nodules, pleural thickening, ipsilateral lung nodules or masses, distant metastasis (particularly in the liver), and medial or interlobar fissure pleural thickening [25-27] [Figure 5 - 7]. If possible, obtaining CT imaging after pleural fluid drainage provides optimal evaluation, especially that of an underlying parenchymal process.

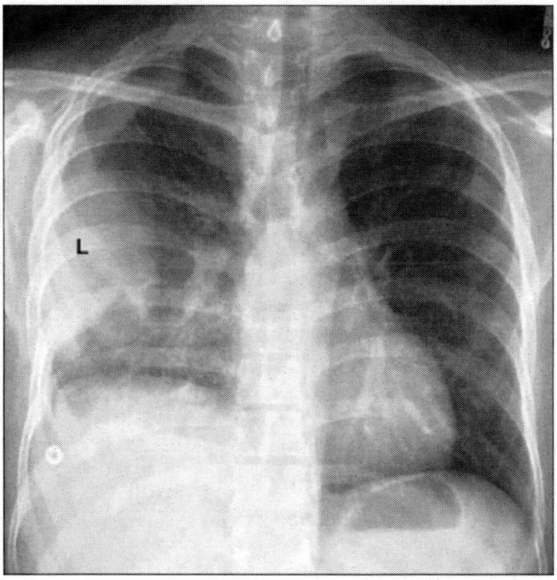

Figure 1. Chest radiograph demonstrated a loculated right-sided pleural effusion (L) in a patient with history of breast cancer who presented with pleuritic chest pain.

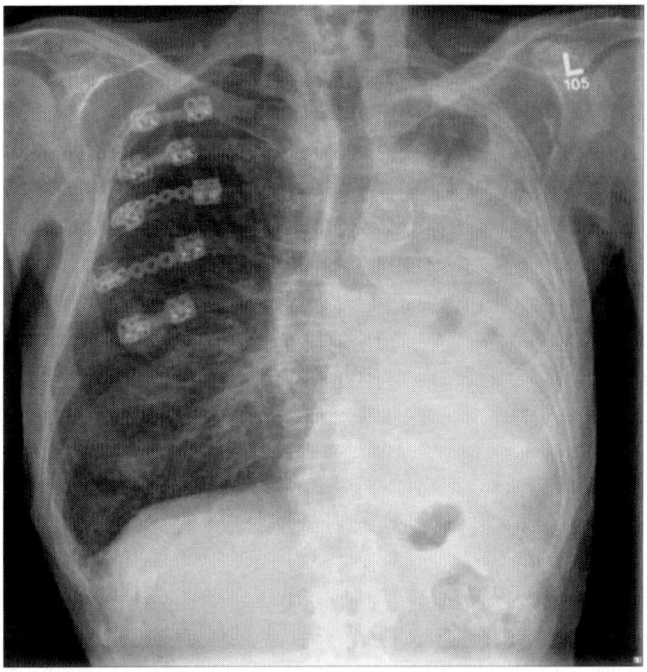

Figure 2. Chest radiograph showing a large left-sided pleural effusion with ipsilateral mediastinal shift as result of co-existing central airway obstruction. The patient presented with symptoms of cough and shortness of breath and had a prior history of non-small cell lung cancer.

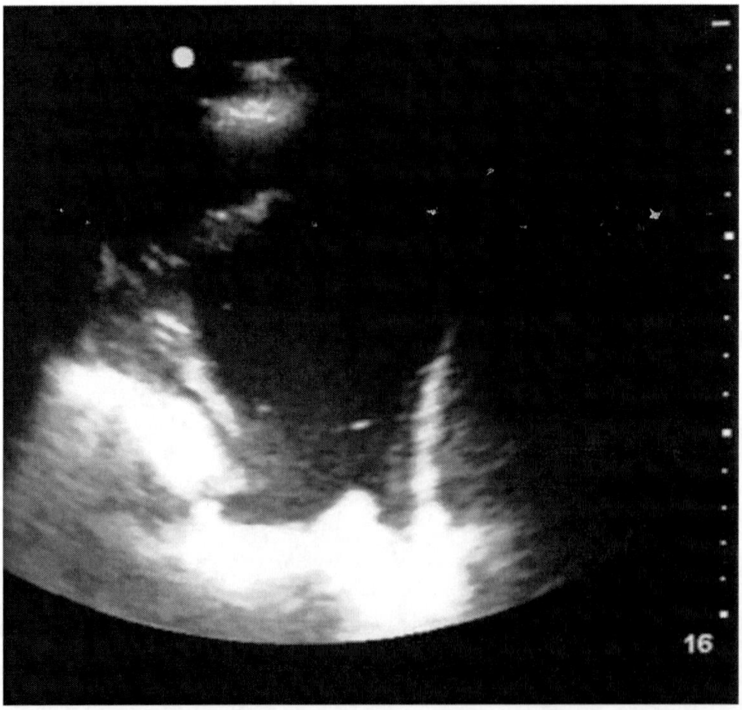

Figure 3. Transthoracic ultrasound demonstrating a large anechoic pleural effusion in a patient with metastatic breast cancer.

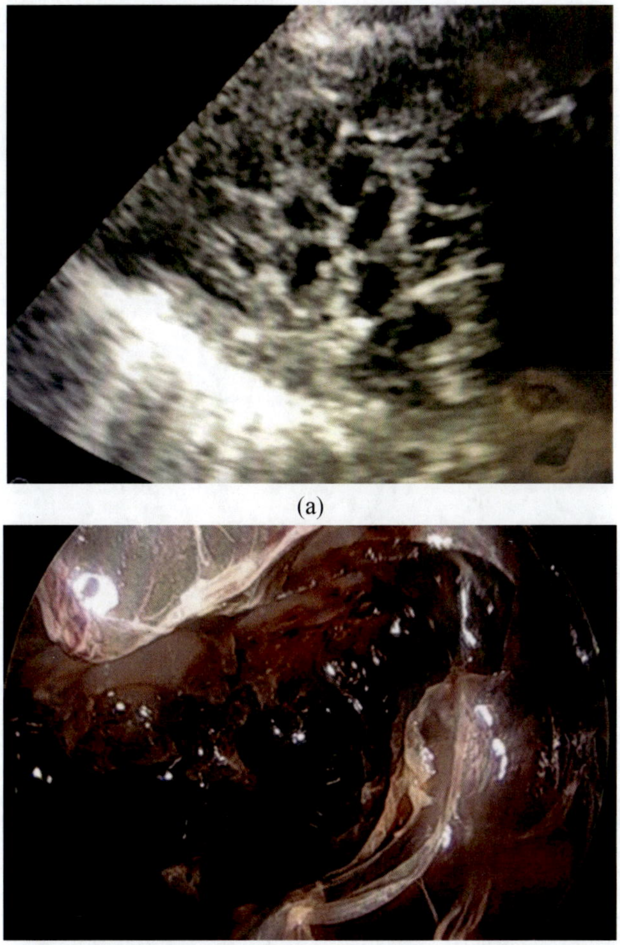

(a)

(b)

Figure 4 (a-b). A patient with a history of non-small cell lung cancer who presented with shortness of breath and pleuritic chest pain. Figure 4a. Transthoracic ultrasonographic image demonstrating this complex effusion. Figure 4b. Thoracoscopic image of the same patient during video-assisted partial decortication and placement of tunneled catheter.

PET-CT

PET-CT imaging utilizing fluorodeoxyglucose (FDG) uptake is a routine imaging study used to radiographically stage malignancies; however, it has a high false-positive rate as areas of infection or inflammation will also demonstrate FDG-avidity [28]. If there is low suspicion for infection or inflammation, PET-CT performs adequately [Figure 8] with a reported sensitivity of 81% and specificity of 74% [29]. On the other hand, concerns over the false-positive rate limit its utility in the diagnosis of MPEs without some other method of verification. One area of utility is in differentiating areas of mesothelioma from benign asbestos-related pleural effusions [29]. Areas with mesothelioma will often have higher FDG uptake than the surrounding benign effusion. Additionally, PET-CT is helpful in identifying targetable sites for biopsy and optimal tissue acquisition.

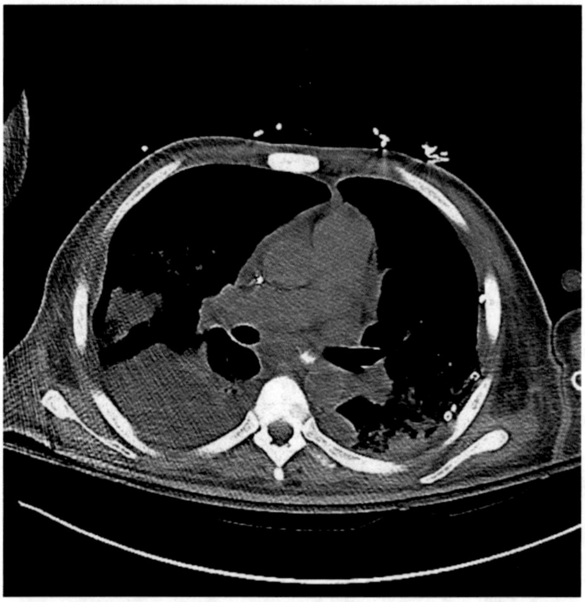

Figure 5. Axial CT images of the chest without intravenous contrast demonstrating a loculated malignant right-sided pleural effusion and ipsilateral lung mass.

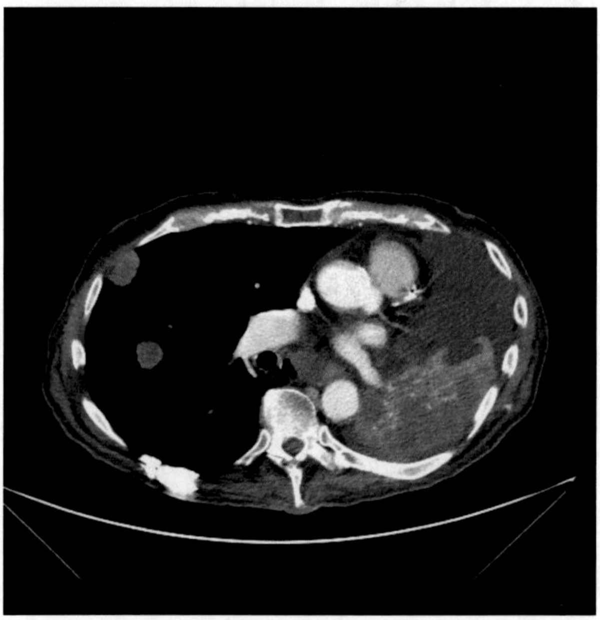

Figure 6. Axial CT image of the chest with intravenous contrast-enhancement with a loculated malignant left-sided pleural effusion with two contralateral lung nodules and contrast enhancement of the ipsilateral atelectatic lung.

Diagnosis

Pleural Fluid Cytology

The most common method of diagnosing MPE is via cytologic analysis. This is most commonly obtained by ultrasound-guided thoracentesis but can be obtained during insertion of a chest tube or during thoracoscopy as well. Sixty to one hundred mL fluid are sufficient to obtain a diagnosis of malignancy, but additional fluid should be sent if it is obtained [28, 30]. The reported diagnostic rate is 60% for one cytology specimen [28, 31-33]. The utility of a second sample has been questioned, but one study reported a combined diagnostic rate of 87% for two cytology specimens. Additional samples do not increase the diagnostic yield [32]. Tumor type and burden of disease can influence the diagnostic rate for one pleural fluid specimen with the highest reported yield in adenocarcinoma and the lowest in mesothelioma [34-36].

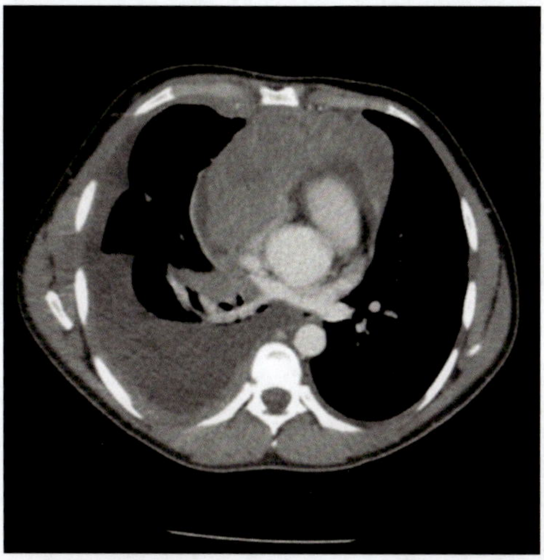

(a)

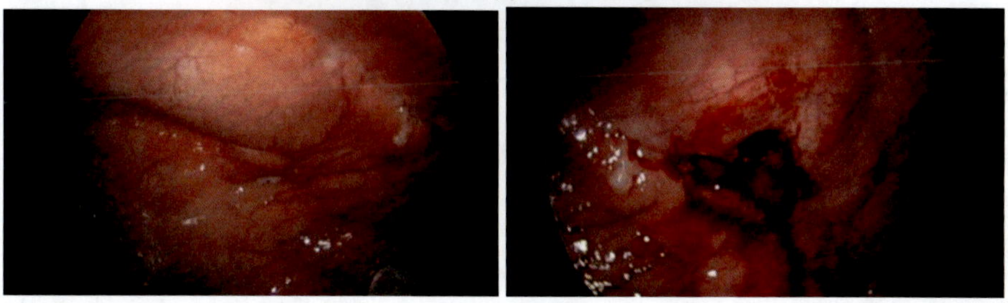

(b)

Figure 7. (a-b). A patient presenting with a large right sided malignant pleural effusion and mediastinal mass caused by T-cell lymphoma. Figure 7a. Axial CT of the chest demonstrating contrast enhancement of the right pleura and a large right sided pleural effusion. Figure 7b. Video assisted thoracoscopic pleural biopsy, images showing pre and post biopsy.

Pleural fluid cytology can be processed typically either as a smear or in a cell block. Smear processing includes placing a small sample of fluid on to a slide, allowing it to dry, and staining it accordingly. A cell block is prepared by centrifuging a larger volume of fluid, fixating the pelleted cellular material, sectioning the material, and finally staining it accordingly. Multiple studies have shown increased diagnostic yield in body fluids evaluated using a cell block as compared to a smear [37, 38].

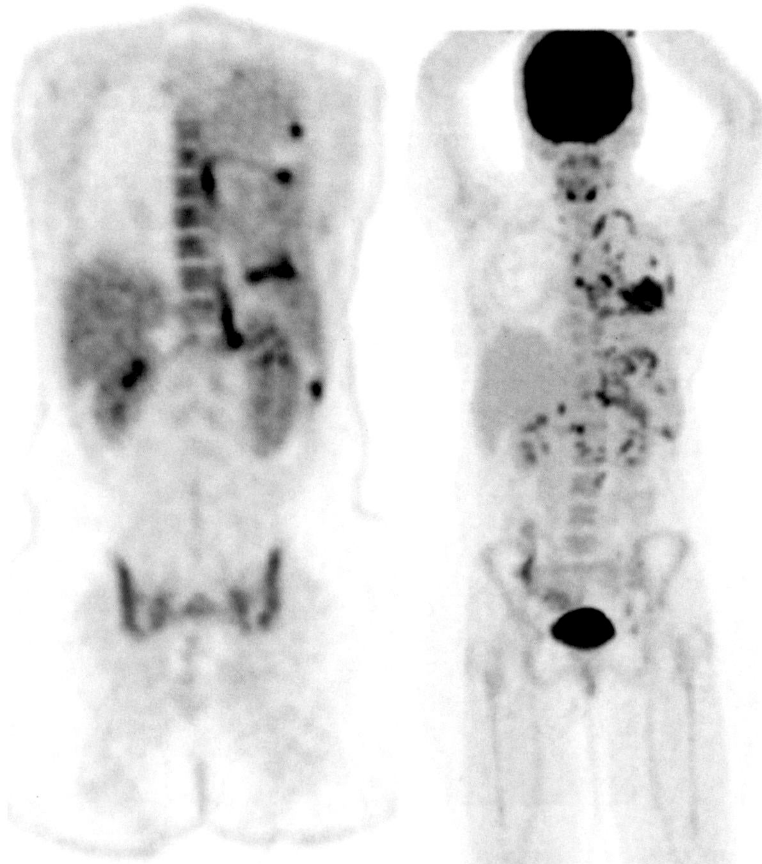

(a) (b)

Figure 8. (a-b). PET imaging of a 50-year-old woman, never smoker, who presented with symptoms of cough and progressive dyspnea. Figure 8a. PET imaging demonstrating multiple areas of FDG avidity; Figure 8b. A localizing PET-CT fusion image demonstrating intense FDG avidity with a SUV = 9.9 in the left pleura consistent with metastatic disease.

Pleural fluid can be successfully tested for next-generation driver mutations. One study reports a 86.7% concordance rate comparing thoracic biopsy to pleural cytology testing for EGFR, KRAS, and ALK mutations [39]. Larger volumes of fluid (> 100mL) did not increase the yield of sequencing for EGFR, KRAS, BRAF, ALK, and ROS1 mutations [40]. While pleural fluid PDL-1 immunohistochemistry testing is being performed at multiple centers, it has not been validated in the literature.

Pleural Biopsy

If standard pleural fluid cytology is non-diagnostic, the next step is a pleural biopsy. There are 3 general methods for obtaining pleural tissue: closed, image-guided, and thoracoscopic pleural biopsy. Closed or "blind" pleural biopsy is performed worldwide as it is relatively straightforward to perform, requires minimal equipment, and is inexpensive [41]. However, it does have significant limitations. It has lower sensitivity for malignancy than medical thoracoscopy [18] with an overall sensitivity of 50% [42], and the complication rate has been reported to be 14.4% in total with a 9.4% incidence of pneumothoraces [43]. We do not recommend performing a closed pleural biopsy unless imaging guidance or thoracoscopy is not available or feasible.

Image-guided pleural biopsy can be performed under CT or ultrasound guidance. Typically, patients require either pleural-based nodules or pleural thickening to target. The sensitivity of CT-guided pleural biopsies for pleural thickening ranges from 76 - 88%, and the specificity approaches 100%. Specifically, the sensitivity for mesothelioma is 83 - 86%, which is much higher than that of blind closed pleural biopsy [44-47]. The sensitivity of ultrasound-guided pleural biopsies is 70 - 94%, again higher than that of blind closed pleural biopsy [44-46, 48, 49]. If there is a suspicion for mesothelioma, pleural thickening alone is sufficient to biopsy, and imaging guidance has been shown to be superior to closed pleural biopsy [50].

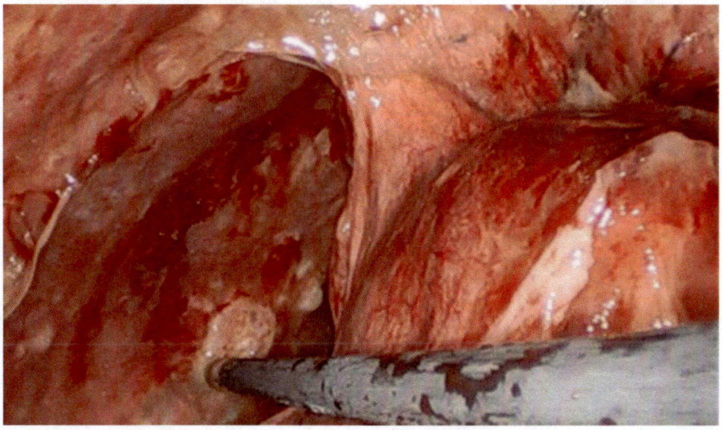

Figure 9. Thoracoscopic pleural biopsy in a patient with metastatic non-small cell lung cancer.

Lastly, thoracoscopic pleural biopsy is becoming more utilized in the diagnostic algorithm for exudative effusions. It also allows for management of the effusion with placement of a TPC and performing talc poudrage during the same procedure. This can be via medical thoracoscopy (MT) or video-assisted thoracoscopic surgery (VATS). MT differs from VATS in that it is typically done in an endoscopy or procedural suite, utilizes a single port system via a rigid or flexible-rigid pleuroscope, and is usually performed under monitored anesthesia care. This enables direct visualization of the pleura [Figure 4b, 7b] to perform biopsies, using either forceps or cryoprobe [Figure 9]. The advantages of MT compared to VATS are one small incision, avoidance of general anesthesia, and lower costs. However, there is limited to no ability to decorticate or perform parenchymal biopsies via MT.

The reported sensitivity of MT for MPE is 91 - 94% [51]. Ultrasonography is typically used to identify the access site immediately pre-procedurally [52, 53]. The overall complication rate of MT is quite low at 1.8%, and the procedure attributable mortality is 0.34% [51, 54]. Of note, a number of the complications is attributed to the concurrent administration of a pleurodesis agent during the procedure rather than to the MT itself [51]. Potential complications include infection, hemorrhage, port site or tract metastasis (most commonly seen in mesothelioma, though this is possible in any carcinoma), alveolar-pleural fistula, pneumothorax, and death [51, 54]. One consideration to minimize the occurrence of port site tract seeding in mesothelioma is to perform port site radiation post-procedurally [55] though recent studies have not shown benefit in prophylactic radiotherapy prior to pleural interventions [56, 57].

Summary of Diagnostic Methods

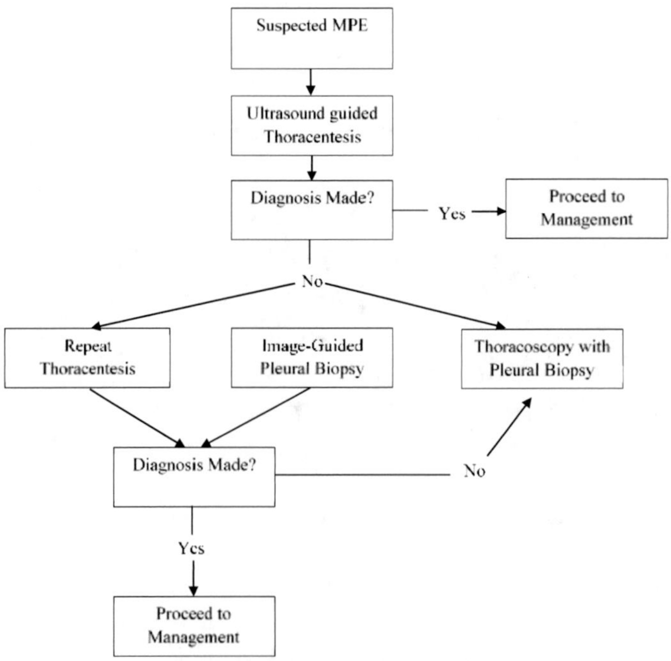

Figure 10. Suspected malignant pleural effusion.

Thoracentesis is the first choice in determining the etiology of a pleural effusion as it is safe, quick, inexpensive, and provides immediate therapeutic relief. One can also gather information regarding lung re-expansion via pleural manometry or chest X-ray, which influences future management. If the first thoracentesis is non-diagnostic, repeat thoracentesis is reasonable, especially if the patient has a poor performance status or poor prognosis (≤ 4 weeks, LENT score ≥ 5). If the patient has a good performance status and favorable prognosis (> 4 weeks, LENT score ≤ 4), then thoracoscopic pleural biopsy is indicated. If thoracoscopy is not available or if there is a pleural-based nodule or implant, then image-guided pleural biopsy is indicated. Closed pleural biopsy is not recommended unless there are no alternatives available. A suggested diagnostic algorithm for suspected MPE is shown in Figure 10.

MANAGEMENT

Overall, the management of MPE must be tailored to the patient. The goal of therapy for MPE is to palliate symptoms. If a patient is asymptomatic, no treatment may be necessary. This contrasts with a patient who has limited survival, in which case minimal therapy is reasonable. The majority of patients fall between these two extremes, and additional therapies are appropriate.

Therapeutic Thoracentesis

Therapeutic thoracentesis under ultrasound guidance is typically the initial procedure performed during the evaluation of pleural effusion. It is quick, inexpensive, safe, and can be performed with minimal analgesia [18]. If a patient is in distress from a rapidly accumulating pleural effusion, a thoracentesis can usually be performed with minimal preparatory time. It is useful in determining the etiology of pleural effusions through pleural fluid analyses and in ascertaining how much of a patient's dyspnea is attributable to it. It is also helpful in evaluating whether a patient has an expandable lung using pleural manometry [58] or a post-procedure chest x-ray. If a lung is thought to be non-expandable, then care should be taken during drainage to minimize patient discomfort related to an ex-vacuo pneumothorax. In patients with limited prognosis, repeated thoracenteses may be the only clinically appropriate procedure, though this must be balanced against the risk of repeated procedures.

Tunneled Pleural Catheters

In a patient with recurring symptomatic pleural effusion, the next step in management can be either TPC placement or pleurodesis, assuming the patient has a reasonable life expectancy. TPCs attempt to control symptoms by draining effusions on an outpatient basis as needed. TPC placement is a relatively inexpensive, outpatient procedure, which can be performed using local anesthesia with or without sedation. Typically, a tunneled silicone catheter is placed in the lower anterolateral chest with the site of entry into the pleural cavity localized by ultrasound. TPC placement is usually well-tolerated, and post-procedural pain can be alleviated by oral analgesics.

After placement, pleural effusions are drained via the TPC at home by the patient alone or with assistance from family members or home health aides. TPC drainage can be done safely via family members [59] and has been shown to be as safe and effective as drainage by nurses [60].

Recommendations for drainage are variable, symptom-based, but are usually performed three to four times per week. TPC placement can lead to spontaneous pleurodesis over time, with an overall rate of 45.6% and average time to pleurodesis of 52 days [61]. This potentially allows for eventual removal of the TPC. The ASAP trial showed that daily drainage has a higher rate of (47% vs 24%) and earlier auto-pleurodesis (54 vs 90 days) as compared to three times weekly drainage; however, there was a significant number of patients, especially in the standard arm, who did not complete the trial [62]. This likely resulted in a substantially lower auto-pleurodesis rate in the 3 times weekly drainage arm than previous studies [61].

Almost all patients (95.6%) have symptomatic improvement [61] with TPC drainage. In a large meta-analysis of 1,370 patients undergoing TPC placement, the overall complication rate for TPCs was 12.5%. Complications included empyema (2.8%), cellulitis (3.4%), obstruction (3.7%), pneumothorax requiring chest tube placement (5.9%), and catheter malfunction (9.1%) [61]. Fifty-four percent of pleural infections were successfully treated without removing the TPCs in one study [63]. They can also be left in when treating with antibiotics for cellulitis with close monitoring for response to therapy. Fibrinolytic instillation is efficacious in resolving catheter obstruction [64]. Importantly, TPCs can be safely placed and used in patients who are immunosuppressed due to antineoplastic therapy patients with a similar rate of infectious complications as patients without immune-suppression [65].

Pleurodesis

Pleurodesis involves obliteration of the pleural space via fusion of the visceral and parietal pleura. Patients with an expandable lung and longer life expectancy are considered good candidates for pleurodesis. Patients typically withstand pleurodesis well, and prior pulmonary function testing studies showed minimal long-term restrictive ventilatory deficits [66]. The 2010 British Thoracic Society guidelines suggest pleurodesis as first-line therapy for MPE with TPC placement only after pleurodesis failure [67].

Pleurodesis can be performed mechanically via a surgical procedure or chemically via introduction of a pleurodesis agent into the pleural cavity. There has been little data to support mechanical pleurodesis over chemical pleurodesis via a chest drain [68, 69]. There is some evidence to suggest that patients have better survival with pleurodesis over TPC placement. However, this could be confounded as patients with more advanced disease, entrapped lung, and poor performance status typically can only undergo TPC placement [70] and not pleurodesis. Mechanical pleurodesis is performed via VATS, often at the same time as the diagnostic procedure. Mechanical trauma is intentionally done to the visceral pleura with concurrent administration of a chemical pleurodesis agent, most commonly talc. Chemical pleurodesis can be performed via a chest tube or at the same time as thoracoscopic surgery or medical thoracoscopy. Chest tube pleurodesis requires admission for pain control and chest tube drainage, which increases initial costs [71]. Two studies demonstrated a higher but not statistically significant pleurodesis failure with small bore (12Fr) vs. large bore (24Fr) chest tube placement, but a higher pain score was documented in patients with large bore chest tubes as compared to patient's with small bore tubes [72, 73].

The most commonly used and best studied pleurodesis agent is talc, which can be administered via poudrage or slurry. Talc poudrage is an aerosolized sterile talcum powder that must be given either via VATS or MT. Talc slurry is a liquid suspension of talcum that can be introduced via a chest tube or TPC. Although a recent Cochrane analysis suggests that talc poudrage is a highly efficacious pleurodesis method, additional studies are needed to evaluate superiority to talc slurry [74], which may not be as evenly distributed throughout the pleural cavity [75]. There have been a variety of other agents used, such as, bleomycin [76, 77], doxycycline [78, 79], povidone-iodine [80, 81], mepacrine [77], and viscum [78, 82]. However, there are reports of various reactions to each of these agents. Povidone-iodine has been used more frequently in Asia given its performance profile, low risk of side effects, and low cost. Talc remains the agent of choice in most of North America and Europe. Pain is the most common side effect of pleurodesis, though other major side effects have been reported. Bleomycin has a higher risk of major side effects and should be avoided unless necessary [74].

Rapid Pleurodesis

The original study of a rapid pleurodesis protocol involved MT with talc poudrage and placement of a TPC. Mean duration of hospitalization was 3.2 days, and the TPC was removed around day 17 from the procedure. The pleurodesis rate was high at 92% at 6 months [83]. These early studies investigated TPC placement at the same time as MT with talc poudrage [84, 85]. In recent years, rapid pleurodesis via TPC placement has emerged as a viable alternative to standard chest tube or thoracoscopic chemical pleurodesis. The advantage of pleurodesis via TPC is that it can be done as an outpatient with associated cost savings [86]. Typically, a TPC is placed in a patient with a known MPE, and a pleurodesis agent is administered immediately thereafter. A recent study evaluated outpatient talc slurry administration via TPC and demonstrated a pleurodesis rate of 43% at day 35 [87]. Rates of pleurodesis have ranged from 47 - 80%. Evaluation of silver impregnation of TPCs in animal models has demonstrated rapid pleurodesis [88]. An in-human trial of the silver nitrate-coated TPC demonstrated an 89% pleurodesis rate after a median of 4 days in 9 patients [89].

Summary of Therapeutic Methods

MPEs are an important clinical problem in patients with intra- and extra-thoracic malignancies and portend a poor prognosis. Once diagnosed, management is tailored to patient's comfort, and in asymptomatic patients no specific pleural intervention may be needed. If the patient derives symptomatic relief with thoracentesis, then drainage by methods described or an attempt at pleurodesis is appropriate. If the patient has a poor prognosis (≤ 4 weeks, LENT score ≥ 5), then repeated thoracenteses is recommended. If the patient has an expandable lung and a favorable prognosis (> 4 weeks, LENT score ≤ 4), then chemical pleurodesis via either MT, TPC alone, or a rapid pleurodesis protocol may be appropriate. If the patient does not have an expandable lung and a favorable prognosis, then TPC placement alone is indicated. If MT is utilized, talc poudrage is the preferred agent for chemical pleurodesis. A patient-centered approach is recommended with palliation of symptoms the main goal of therapy. However, care must be taken to advance patients to more definitive therapies as opposed to needlessly repeating thoracenteses as often happens. One study found that in patients who had recurrent MPE who should have been advanced to a more definitive management option such as TPC or pleurodesis, only 24% of patients actually received a definitive management option [90]. A suggested management algorithm is shown in Figure 11.

Summary

Malignant pleural effusions are a frequent cause of morbidity and hospitalizations and are associated with a poor prognosis. Many malignancies are associated with malignant pleural effusions, but lung cancers, breast cancers, and lymphoma are the most common causes. Patients usually present with symptoms of cough or shortness of breath and have typical findings on imaging studies. The diagnosis of malignant pleural effusion is confirmed via cytologic analysis of pleural fluid, most commonly obtained via thoracentesis, or via image-guided or thoracoscopic pleural biopsy. Management plan should be patient-centered, minimally invasive, and include multi-disciplinary team discussion. As treatment options that may impact survival expand for patients with malignant diseases, one could anticipate change in management strategies and future research for unanswered questions.

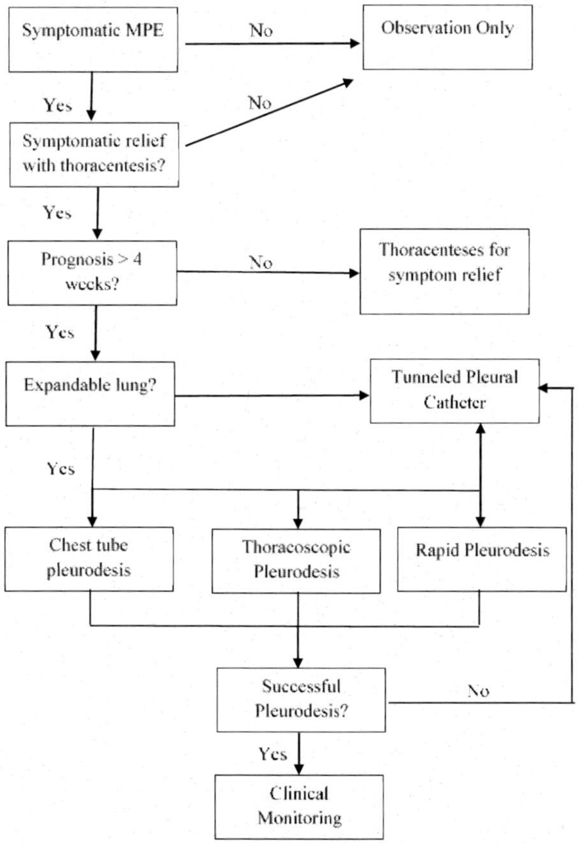

Figure 11. Management algorithm.

REFERENCES

[1] Feller-Kopman, D; Light, RW. Pleural Disease. *New England Journal of Medicine*, 2018, 378(8), 740-751. 10.1056/NEJMra1 403503.

[2] Taghizadeh, N; Fortin, M; Tremblay, A. US Hospitalizations for Malignant Pleural Effusions: Data From the 2012 National Inpatient Sample. *Chest*, 2017, 151 (4), 845-854. 10.1016/j.chest.2016.11.010.

[3] Porcel, JM; et al. Clinical features and survival of lung cancer patients with pleural effusions. *Respirology*, 2015, 20 (4), 654-9. 10.1111/resp.12496.

[4] Desai, NR; Lee, HJ. Diagnosis and management of malignant pleural effusions: state of the art in 2017. *Journal of Thoracic Disease*, 2017, 9 (Supplement 10), S1111-S1122.

[5] Rodriguez-Pandero, F; Borderas Naranjo, F; Lopez Mejias, J. Pleural Metastatic Tumours and Effusions. Frequency and Pathogenic Mechanisms in a Post-Mortem Series. *European Respiratory Journal*, 1989, 2 (4), 366-369.

[6] Grosu, HB; et al. Risk factors for pleural effusion recurrence in patients with malignancy. *Respirology*, 2018, 10.1111/resp.13362.

[7] Thomas, JM; Musani, AI. Malignant Pleural Effusions: A Review. *Clinics in Chest Medicine*, 2013, 34 (3), 459-471. 10.1016/j.ccm. 2013.05.004.

[8] Light, RW; Hamm, H. Malignant Pleural Effusion: Would the Real Cause Please Stand Up? *European Respiratory Journal*, 1997, 10 (8), 1701-1702.

[9] Clive, AO; et al. Predicting survival in malignant pleural effusion: development and validation of the LENT prognostic score. *Thorax*, 2014, 69 (12), 1098-1104. 10.1136/thoraxjnl-2014-205285.

[10] Chernow, B; Sahn, SA; Chernow, B; Shahn, SA. Carcinomatous involvement of the pleura. *American Journal of Medicine*, 1977, 63 (5), 695-702. 10.1016/0002-9343(77)90154-1.

[11] Hsia, D; Musani, AI. Management of Malignant Pleural Effusions. *Current Pulmonology Reports*, 2012, 1, 73-81. DOI 10.1007/s13665-012-0012-2.

[12] Fentiman, IS; Rubens, RD; Hayward, JL. Control of pleural effusions in patients with breast cancer. A randomized trial. *Cancer*, 1983, 52 (4), 737-9.

[13] Stathopoulos, GT; Kalomenidis, I. Malignant pleural effusion: tumor-host interactions unleashed. *Am J Respir Crit Care Med*, 2012, 186 (6), 487-92. 10.1164/rccm.201203-0465PP.

[14] Tremblay, A; Michaud, G. Single-center experience with 250 tunnelled pleural catheter insertions for malignant pleural effusion. *Chest*, 2006, 129 (2), 362-8. 10.1378/chest.129.2.362.

[15] Doerr, CH; et al. Etiology of chylothorax in 203 patients. *Mayo Clin Proc*, 2005, 80 (7), 867-70. 10.4065/80.7.867.

[16] Doelken, P; et al. Effect of thoracentesis on respiratory mechanics and gas exchange in the patient receiving mechanical ventilation. *Chest*, 2006, 130 (5), 1354-61. 10.1378/chest.130.5.1354.

[17] American Thoracic Society, A. Management of malignant pleural effusions. *American Journal of Respiratory & Critical Care Medicine*, 2000, 162 (5), 1987-2001. 10.1164/ajrccm.162.5.ats8-00.

[18] Chernow, B; Sahn, SA. Carcinomatous involvement of the pleura. *The American Journal of Medicine*, 1977, 63 (5), 695-702. 10.1016/ 0002-9343(77)90154-1.

[76] Ibrahim, IM; et al. Povidone-iodine pleurodesis versus talc pleurodesis in preventing recurrence of malignant pleural effusion. *Journal of Cardiothoracic Surgery* 2015, 10, 64. 10.1186/s13019-015-0270-5.

[77] Agarwal, R; et al. Efficacy & safety of iodopovidone pleurodesis: a systematic review & meta analysis. *The Indian Journal of Medical Research*, 2012, 135 (3), 297-304.

[78] Cho, JS; et al. Chemical Pleurodesis Using Mistletoe Extraction (ABNOVA-viscum(®) Injection) for Malignant Pleural Effusion. *Annals of Thoracic and Cardiovascular Surgery*, 2016, 22 (1), 20-26. 10.5761/atcs.oa.15-00230.

[79] Reddy, C; et al. Rapid pleurodesis for malignant pleural effusions: a pilot study. *Chest*, 2011, 139(6), 1419-1423. 10.1378/chest.10-1868.

[80] Boujaoude, Z; et al. Pleuroscopic Pleurodesis Combined With Tunneled Pleural Catheter for Management of Malignant Pleural Effusion: A Prospective Observational Study. *J Bronchology Interv Pulmonol*, 2015, 22 (3), 237-43. 10.1097/lbr.0000000000000186.

[81] Krochmal, R; et al. Patient evaluation for rapid pleurodesis of malignant pleural effusions. *J Thorac Dis*, 2016, 8 (9), 2538-2543. 10.21037/jtd.2016.08.55.

[82] Fysh, ETH; et al. Indwelling pleural catheters reduce inpatient days over pleurodesis for malignant pleural effusion. *Chest*, 2012, 142 (2), 394-400. 10.1378/chest.11-2657.

[83] Bhatnagar, R; et al. Outpatient Talc Administration by Indwelling Pleural Catheter for Malignant Effusion. *New England Journal of Medicine*, 2018, 378 (14), 1313-1322. 10.1056/NEJMoa 1716883.

[84] Tremblay, A; et al. Local and systemic effects of a silver nitrate coated indwelling pleural catheter in an animal model of pleurodesis. *Experimental Lung Research*, 2017, 43 (9-10), 388-394. 10.1080/ 01902148.2017.1384865.

[85] Bhatnagar, R; et al. A Novel Drug-Eluting Indwelling Pleural Catheter for the Management of Malignant Effusions. *Am J Respir Crit Care Med*, 2018, 197 (1), 136-138. 10.1164/rccm.201701-0097L E.

In: Pleural Effusions: Causes, Types and Treatment
Editor: Rahul Khosla
ISBN: 978-1-53614-683-7

Chapter 6

HEMOTHORAX, CHYLOTHORAX, AND PSEUDOCHYLOTHORAX

Katie R. Jeans, MD, Stephen Bujarski, MD, Venkata Bandi, MD and Donald R. Lazarus, MD**[*]**

Pulmonary, Critical Care, and Sleep Section,
Baylor College of Medicine and the Michael E. DeBakey
VA Medical Center, Houston, TX, US

ABSTRACT

Hemothorax, chylothorax, and pseudochylothorax are types of pleural effusion that differ in appearance, prognosis, and management from most other pleural effusions. Hemothorax, defined as blood in the pleural space, is most often the result of thoracic trauma. The mainstay of treatment is placement of a chest tube with close observation. Surgery is sometimes needed when hemorrhage continues or retained clot is unable to be evacuated by chest tube alone. Chylothorax results from the accumulation of chyle in the pleural space, usually because the thoracic duct is damaged or obstructed. Common associated conditions are trauma and lymphoma. The pleural fluid in chylothorax is milky in appearance and diagnosis is confirmed by pleural fluid triglyceride levels > 110 ml/dL and the presence of chylomicrons in the pleural fluid. Chylothorax may resolve spontaneously with time and treatment of the underlying cause. Some cases of chylothorax may require surgical treatment. Palliation with pleurodesis, pleural drainage, and a low-fat diet supplemented with medium-chain fatty acids are also frequently helpful. Pseudochylothorax is also a milky, turbid effusion. It results from the presence of a longstanding pleural effusion, most commonly related to rheumatoid arthritis or tuberculosis. The pleura is usually thickened and often calcified in pseudochylothorax. It is differentiated from chylothorax by pleural fluid cholesterol levels above 200 mg/dL, normal pleural fluid triglyceride levels, and the absence of chylomicrons in pleural fluid.

[*] Corresponding Author Email: Donald.Lazarus@bcm.edu.

Management includes determining and treating the underlying cause. Therapeutic thoracentesis and surgical decortication are also sometimes required.

Keywords: hemothorax, chylothorax, pseudochylothorax, chyliform effusion, pleural effusion

Introduction

Hemothorax, chylothorax, and pseudochylothorax are types of pleural effusions uncommonly encountered in clinical practice. Hemothorax, defined as blood in the pleural space, is most frequently associated with trauma [1, 2]. Chylothorax is defined as the accumulation of chyle within the pleural space and is typically caused by damage to or obstruction of the thoracic duct by trauma or malignancy [3]. Pseudochylothorax consists of non-chylous cholesterol-rich fluid which usually evolves from a longstanding inflammatory effusion [4]. The pathophysiology and management of each differs from that of the more common types of pleural effusion and will be reviewed in this chapter.

Hemothorax

Hemothorax is defined as the presence of blood in the pleural space [1, 2]. Because hemothorax is most frequently associated with thoracic trauma, it should be suspected in any patient with a new pleural effusion who has a history of such trauma or an invasive thoracic procedure. While imaging and an appropriate clinical scenario can suggest the presence of hemothorax, thoracentesis with pleural fluid analysis is required for diagnosis. Because pleural fluid may appear grossly bloody with as little as 5% hematocrit relative to that of the patient's blood, it is critical to measure the pleural fluid hematocrit in order to distinguish a true hemothorax from a hemorrhagic or bloody pleural effusion [1, 2]. Pleural fluid with a fluid hematocrit > 50% of the hematocrit of the patient's blood is considered diagnostic of hemithorax [1]. Since pleural fluid hematocrit may be falsely low due to dilution if not analyzed within the first few days, some authors have proposed changing the definition to include those effusions with a hematocrit > 25% of the blood's hematocrit [1, 2].

In addition to ensuring hemodynamic stability, the evaluation of patients with suspected hemothorax should include imaging studies to guide diagnostic and therapeutic interventions. Chest x-ray has long been the standard imaging modality used in the evaluation of chest trauma. If an upright film can be obtained hemothorax may be indicated when there is any evidence of pleural effusion such as blunted costophrenic angles or opacification of a hemithorax. Unfortunately most trauma patients are not able to have upright chest x-rays done, and the more commonly used supine film is much less sensitive for pleural effusions [2]. Computed tomography (CT) of the chest is now commonly a part of the initial emergency room evaluation of trauma patients, and is much more sensitive than chest x-ray for detecting pleural effusions. Any new pleural effusion after chest trauma should be presumed to be blood until proven otherwise. In patients with chronic pleural effusions the CT measurement of Hounsfield units (HU) may help determine if there is a concomitant hemothorax [Figure 1] [2]. In a retrospective study, hemothorax was successfully differentiated from pleural effusion by CT using HU of 15.6 as the cut off value [5]. More recently point of care ultrasonography is being utilized in emergency rooms as part of standard care in the evaluation of trauma patients. It is both sensitive and specific in identifying pleural effusion and at times can help distinguish potential pleural fluid characteristics such as blood based on its ultrasound appearance [2, 6].

Etiology of Hemothorax

Hemothorax is generally classified by etiology and divided primarily into traumatic or spontaneous hemothorax [1, 2]. The causes of hemothorax are summarized in Table 1. Traumatic hemothorax can be related to any injury to the vasculature in the chest. Both open and closed chest trauma, as well as thoracic procedures such as central venous catheter placement, thoracentesis, chest tube placement, and lung or pleural biopsy can result in bleeding into the pleural space [1, 2]. Hemothorax is a common complication of chest trauma. Chest trauma is present in up to 60% of multi-trauma patients and such injuries are responsible for 20 - 25% of trauma-related mortality [2]. A study of 1359 consecutive patients with chest trauma by Kulshrestha and colleagues demonstrated that the majority of chest injuries were related to blunt trauma, and the mortality due to traumatic chest injury was 9.4% [7]. Liman et al. demonstrated that the incidence of hemothorax increases with the number of rib fractures after a chest trauma. Only 6.7% of patients without rib fractures developed hemothorax, but 24.9% of those with 1-2 rib fractures and > 80% of patients with > 2 rib fractures had a hemothorax at presentation [8]. Hemothorax is a rare complication of central line placement as well as thoracentesis with rates of 0.4 - 0.6% and 0.18 - 2% respectively [9]. Interestingly, known coagulopathy (INR > 3) or thrombocytopenia do not appear to confer increased risk of hemothorax during those procedures [10, 11].

Spontaneous hemothorax is defined as bleeding into the pleural space occurring in the absence of chest trauma or intervention. Spontaneous hemothorax is rare and so much of what we know about it is derived from case reports and series, and its management is generally extrapolated from studies of the management of traumatic hemothorax [2]. Spontaneous hemothorax can occur in conjunction with a pneumothorax (hemopneumothorax) or may be related to vascular changes in the chest, costal exostoses, endometriosis, neoplasia, or coagulopathy.

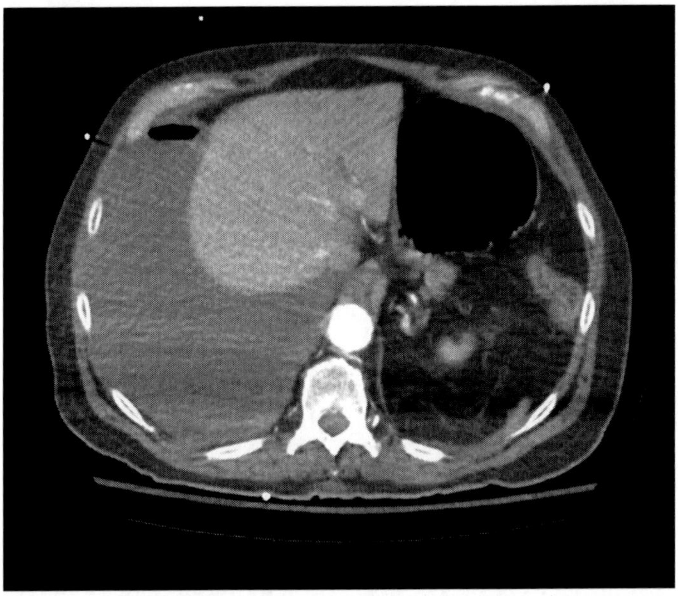

Figure 1. Computed tomogram of the chest showing right hemothorax. The dependent areas of lighter density are blood.

Table 1. Causes of hemothorax

Trauma	Spontaneous
• Penetrating chest trauma • Blunt chest trauma Iatrogenic • Central venous catheterization • Thoracentesis • Chest tube placement • Lung biopsy • Pleural biopsy	• Spontaneous hemopneumothorax • Aortic dissection • Pulmonary arteriovenous malformations • Ehlers-Danlos syndrome type IV • Neurofibromatosis • Costal exostoses • Pleural endometriosis (catamenial) • Neoplasm • Coagulopathy • Pulmonary infarction • Idiopathic

Hemothorax is a relatively common complication of spontaneous pneumothorax. Incidence rates are reported to be between 3 - 7%. It typically occurs more frequently in young patients and the size of hemothorax is variable [1]. Spontaneous hemopneumothoraces range in size from a few hundred milliliters (mL) to as much as 1.5 liters (L). The presentation of spontaneous hemopneumothorax varies from asymptomatic pleural effusion to hemorrhagic shock [12]. Multiple mechanisms have been proposed as the etiology of bleeding. The most common etiology is a torn vascularized adhesion between the parietal and visceral pleura [2, 13]. This is usually bleeding from a small vessel on the parietal pleura. A second mechanism is bleeding from the rupture of vascularized bullae. The last proposed mechanism is bleeding from congenitally aberrant vessels between the parietal pleural and bullae [14]. The lung is less able to tamponade the bleeding vessel in the setting of concomitant pneumothorax, allowing more blood to enter the pleural space [2]. If the hemothorax is massive, it is more likely to be related to the rupture of a branch of a systemic artery. The higher pressures present in the systemic circulation lead to increased bleeding, further compounding the inability of the collapsed lung to offer effective tamponade to the source of hemorrhage [1].

Multiple vascular abnormalities, both acquired and inherited, can lead to hemothorax. The most common vascular condition leading to spontaneous hemothorax is probably aortic dissection or rupture. Aortic dissection or rupture is usually apparent from history and physical examination. The patient will typically present with tearing chest pain and a CT scan with contrast can confirm the diagnosis [2]. In this situation, hemothorax generally occurs on the left side [1]. Pulmonary arteriovenous malformations (PAVMs), which are abnormal connections between the pulmonary arterial and venous circulation, can also lead to hemothorax. PAVMs are rare and can occur spontaneously or as a manifestation of another systemic disease such as hereditary hemorrhagic telangiectasia (HHT, or Osler-Weber-Rendu syndrome) [2, 15]. PAVMs are suspected when an echo with bubble study demonstrates the delayed appearance of bubbles in the left heart. They can occur within the lung parenchyma or in subpleural locations. Intraparenchymal PAVMs are most common and often present with hemoptysis. Subpleural PAVMs leading to hemothorax are rarer and have been reported in approximately 4% of PAVMs [2, 15, 16]. Of the reported cases of hemothorax due to PAVMs, about half were in patients with documented HHT and between 30% and 50% occurred in women who were pregnant. It has been proposed that the increased incidence of rupture during pregnancy is related to the physiologic increased blood volume and cardiac output of the gravid state [2, 17, 18]. Some physicians recommend screening all women with HHT for PAVMs prior to their becoming pregnant [1, 18].

Another hereditary etiology of vascular hemothorax is Ehlers-Danlos syndrome type IV (vascular-type), which is a defect of type III collagen. This leads to thin-walled, ectatic vessels which are more likely to develop aneurysms and rupture [1, 19]. Arterial tears are the most serious reported complication. Hemothorax has been linked to rupture of the internal mammary artery, pulmonary arteries, ruptured bullae, or pneumothorax in this condition [1, 20, 21]. Neurofibromatosis (von Recklinghausens disease) can lead to hemothorax as well. Two distinct mechanisms are proposed. In the first, large vessels (aorta, subclavian artery, internal mammary artery) develop stenotic or aneurysmal changes which lead to dissection and rupture. The second proposed mechanism is related to arterial dysplasia of smaller vessels which also makes them prone to bleed [1, 22-25].

Costal exostoses are bony outgrowths from the ribs, and they are a rare cause of hemothorax and hemopneumothorax. The growths are sometimes associated with hereditary multiple exostoses syndrome, but can also occur alone. The method in which these growths lead to hemothorax is not understood, but it is hypothesized that it is related to injury of the pleura by direct contact with the bony outgrowth. Another hypothesis is that bleeding is related to repetitive irritation of the pleura and rupture of underlying dilated vessels [1, 2, 26]. Whatever the mechanism, there have been many case reports of exostoses leading to hemothorax, mostly in younger patients [1, 27-29].

Endometriosis can lead to catamenial hemothorax when endometrial tissue migrates across fenestrations in the diaphragm and implants on the pleural surface. This tissue continues to respond to hormonal cycles in menstruating women, and can lead to recurrent spontaneous hemithorax [1, 30]. Hemothorax is a relatively common presentation of thoracic endometriosis, with rates as high as 14% reported [1, 31]. It is generally unilateral, occurs on the right side more than 80% of the time, and is always associated with pelvic endometriosis [1, 31, 32]. Patients may present with symptoms and radiographic changes that recur with menses [30]. Catamenial hemothorax most commonly occurs in young, nulliparous, black women [1, 33]. Diagnosis is often delayed. Pleural fluid cytology usually does not reveal endometrial cells, and may only demonstrate hemosiderin-laden histiocytes which are a nonspecific finding. Confident diagnosis may even require thoracoscopy with direct visualization and biopsy of endometrial pleural implants [1].

Many types of neoplasia can lead to hemothorax. The most common neoplasms resulting in hemothorax are schwannomas of the pleura associated with neurofibromatosis and soft tissue tumors such as sarcomas that have metastasized to the lung and pleura [1, 34, 35]. Hemothorax in the setting of sarcoma is an especially poor prognostic sign, with 6-8 month mortality greater than 80% [1, 36]. Others include hepatocellular carcinoma and mediastinal tumors which invade the pleural space directly [1, 37, 38]. Interestingly lung cancer is rarely the etiology of hemothorax, even when associated with pleural extension or metastasis [1, 2]. Diagnosis of tumor-related hemothorax can be difficult. Thoracentesis with pleural fluid cytology may yield tumor cells, but the large amount of blood seen makes cytologic diagnosis more difficult. Immunohistochemical markers can increase the cytological yield but pleural fluid cytology is often not sufficient to make the diagnosis alone. Thoracoscopy with biopsy is frequently required [2].

Coagulopathy can predispose to both spontaneous and traumatic hemothorax. Coagulopathy may be hereditary, such as hemophilia, or acquired, such as systemic anticoagulation [2]. There are numerous well-documented reports of spontaneous hemothorax in the setting of systemic anticoagulation. Most cases involved heparin and warfarin, but one case was associated with enoxaparin. The level of anticoagulation was supratherapeutic in only 30% of the reported patients [1, 39]. Most of the cases of spontaneous hemothorax occurring in anticoagulated patients took place in patients with venous thromboembolic disease who were being treated with anticoagulation [1, 40]. When hemothorax related to pulmonary embolism (PE) develops it is most likely to occur during the first week of anticoagulation therapy and generally takes place on the same side as the PE [1, 40]. There is high morbidity and mortality in hemothorax associated with coagulopathy with reported mortality of 20% [1, 41]. There have also been reported cases of hemothorax in the setting of anticoagulation not associated with thromboembolic disease: one for mechanical heart valve, another after angioplasty, and 2 reports of spontaneous hemothorax related to the direct thrombin inhibitor dabigatran given for nonvalvular atrial fibrillation [1, 42-44].

Management of Hemothorax

Most evidence regarding the management of hemothorax has been in the trauma setting. In addition to resuscitation and stabilization, the initial management of hemothorax is tube thoracostomy in most cases [2, 7]. When possible, the tube should be inserted at the mid-axillary line and placed posteriorly to aid in drainage while the patient is supine. Although the optimal size of the chest tube is still debated, large bore chest tubes are generally favored [45, 46]. Among surgical chest tubes, tubes of 28-32 Fr diameter have been shown to be as effective for hemothorax in trauma patients as those of 36 - 40 Fr diameter [46]. Prophylactic antibiotics given along with chest tube placement for traumatic hemothorax have been shown to reduce the incidence of pneumonia but not empyema [47].

Surgical intervention for traumatic hemothorax can sometimes be necessary in a subset of patients, especially those with evidence of ongoing bleeding. Patients with chest tubes draining more than 200 mL per hour for 4 hours, with initial drainage of more than 1500 mL of blood, and who are hemodynamically unstable warrant early surgical intervention [2]. The standard surgical approach for hemothorax is an anterior thoracotomy which allows access to many of the great vessels, pericardium, and lung [2]. The incision may be extended across the sternum for a clamshell approach, which gives better visualization of the mediastinum. Posterolateral thoracotomy is preferred for injuries to the esophagus or airway but should only be performed in stable patients as patient positioning may be difficult to achieve in those who are unstable. If superior intrathoracic vessels are thought to be contributing to bleeding a cervical or supraclavicular incision may be added. Median sternotomy is a superior approach for injuries to the heart, but it takes longer to perform and has a higher post-op complication rate than other thoracotomy in this setting. Complications include sternal nonunion and osteomyelitis [2]. In patients with acute thoracic trauma the use of video-assisted thoracic surgery (VATS) is controversial since visualization with VATS is more difficult than with thoracotomy during severe active bleeding. VATS may be considered in selected cases to control minor bleeding, evacuate the hemothorax, or explore the pleural space of a stable patient [2]. Thoracic arterial angiography can be both diagnostic and therapeutic, although there is a small risk of embolization of the anterior spinal artery [48].

The general management of spontaneous hemothorax is extrapolated from that of traumatic pneumothorax given the paucity of evidence specific to its management. There are some nuances to the management of spontaneous hemothorax that vary with the underlying cause, and we will review these below. Spontaneous hemopneumothorax is generally treated with tube thoracostomy initially. If the lung is unable to expand with chest tube placement and thereby tamponade the source of bleeding then surgical intervention may be required. Several retrospective series have suggested that early surgical intervention with VATS or open thoracotomy may be a superior approach to conservative treatment in this setting [1, 49]. Another advantage of surgical intervention for hemopneumothorax is that it also allows the etiology of the pneumothorax to be addressed simultaneously [50].

The treatment of vascular-related hemothorax includes drainage of the pleural space with tube thoracostomy but often surgical intervention via VATS or open thoracotomy with attempts at hemostasis with coagulation or ligation of the bleeding vessel is needed. If patients are hemodynamically stable, vascular localization with angiogram and attempt at embolization may be considered [1]. Embolization is not without risk, and complications including respiratory distress, cerebral ischemia, brain abscess, hemoptysis, and seizure have been reported during vascular embolization procedures. These are believed to be due to collateral or accessory vessels, recanalization of previously embolized vessels, or residual PAVMs [51]. Embolization has been shown to be effective in reducing right to left shunt, improving arterial hypoxemia, and increasing exercise capacity. Embolization of the bleeding PAVM can stop ongoing bleeding, but patients remain at risk for development of re-bleeding from collateral vessels or subsequent recanalization. Unstable patients should be surgically managed with immediate thoracotomy or VATS to stop bleeding [2].

Hemothorax from costal exostoses is initially managed with tube thoracostomy. Definitive treatment is surgical resection of the exostoses, generally with VATS or thoracotomy [1, 2]. After initial stabilization with chest tube placement and resuscitation the treatment of catamenial hemothorax is primarily with hormonal therapy to decrease estrogen secretion and promote amenorrhea [1, 32, 52, 53]. Surgical resection of implants may be required when hormonal agents are inadequate for management. In some cases surgeons are also able to repair diaphragmatic fenestrations at the time of resection of endometrial pleural implants [32, 53]. The treatment of neoplasia-related hemothorax is not well described. Most reported treatments consist of tube thoracostomy, arterial embolization, and conservative management and are only described in case reports. However, hemothorax in these situations is a very poor prognostic indicator with survival typically being just a few to several months [1, 37, 38]. The treatment of coagulopathy-related hemothorax should begin with reversing the coagulopathy, which is usually sufficient to halt the accumulation. Tube thoracotomy is also necessary to drain the hemothorax and if pulmonary infarction is the etiology, a thoracic surgeon should be consulted for consideration of definitive surgical management [1, 2].

Retained Hemothorax

Retained hemothorax occurs when blood in the pleural space becomes clotted or loculated and cannot be drained via chest tube. The diagnosis and management of retained hemothorax are controversial [2, 54, 55]. The incidence of retained hemothorax ranges from 5 - 30% of patients with hemothorax [1, 56]. It is often suspected when persistent radiographic pleural effusion remains for more than 2-3 days after tube thoracostomy [1, 54]. When blood enters the pleural space, it is constantly agitated by the movement of the heart and lung and rapidly defibrinates. This leads to fibrin clot formation along the pleura and eventually to trapped lung. By the 7th day after hemorrhage the pleural membrane becomes thickened and organized, making it more difficult to treat. Therefore, retained hemothorax should be evacuated within 7-10 days to prevent the need for decortication [1, 57]. Retained hemothorax puts patients at risk for complications including empyema, fibrothorax, lung entrapment, and restrictive lung disease [1]. In the AAST study, the incidence of empyema was 26.8%, and nearly all of these patients required additional interventions. Rib fractures and injury severity score >25 are both risk factors for developing empyema and subsequent longer hospital stays [55].

If the retained hemothorax is small, observation alone may be sufficient [2, 54, 58]. Most experts believe that drainage is necessary if the volume of retained blood is larger than 200-300ml to prevent further complications [1]. Although thoracotomy has long been the standard surgical approach for retained hemothorax, it has significant associated morbidity and has fallen somewhat out of favor for this indication [2, 54]. In the current era VATS is now used more frequently than thoracotomy for retained hemothorax. The effectiveness of VATS for retained hemothorax has been reported to be as high as 70 - 80% with less associated morbidity than thoracotomy [1, 59]. It allows for inspection of the pleura, evacuation of any retained blood and new thoracostomy tubes can be placed simultaneously [2, 54, 59, 60]. In addition, early intervention with VATS appears to be superior to late intervention in some studies [2, 60, 61]. Placement of a second thoracostomy tube is another option for treatment of retained hemothorax, but it is less effective than surgery because of the presence of loculations and clots [2, 62]. Meyer et al. compared placing an additional chest tube versus thoracoscopy for retained hemothorax. The thoracoscopy arm had a shorter chest tube duration, shorter hospital stay, and reduced total hospital costs compared to the chest tube group [62]. In the Dubose study, 64% of the patients who were treated with additional chest tube placement required additional interventions [54]. Intrapleural fibrinolytic therapy can also be used in conjunction with chest tube placement for retained hemothorax, but many of the studies describing this are retrospective and have small sample sizes [2, 56, 63, 64]. In one representative retrospective study VATS demonstrated a shorter hospital stay and decreased need for thoracotomy when compared to intrapleural streptokinase in retained hemothorax [56]. In another multicenter study of patients with loculated effusions including 18 patients with hemothorax, fibrinolysis was successful 92% of the time [65]. One small study by Kimbrell at al demonstrated that 6 days of intrapleural streptokinase or urokinase achieved resolution of hemothorax in 90% of their patients without bleeding complications [64]. Intrapleural fibrinolytic therapy should be used with caution for retained hemothorax because of bleeding risk. It should be avoided in those cases of hemothorax caused by coagulopathy or vascular lesions so as to avoid re-bleeding [1].

CHYLOTHORAX

The accumulation of chyle in the pleural space defines chylothorax [3]. Chyle is a noninflammatory, bacteriostatic, milky fluid originating in the small intestine during digestion that is transported to the circulation by the lymphatic drainage system [Figure 2]. It is characterized by variable protein and fat concentrations (2.2 - 6.0 g/dl and 0.4 - 6 g/dl respectively), high triglycerides (TG) (> 110 mg/dl), lower than serum cholesterol levels (65 - 220 mg/dl), and a T-lymphocytic predominance (usually > 80%). It is also made up of fat-soluble vitamins, water, and other solutes. Some of the variability, especially in fat and triglyceride content, depends on dietary consumption. These concentrations are especially lowered in fasting states.

Chylomicrons are lipoproteins that assist in "packaging" and transporting a substantial proportion of consumed triglycerides to the blood by way of the lymphatic drainage system. These chylomicrons form from the breakdown of long-chain triglycerides from dietary fat in the intestine and transport them to lymph vessels to introduce them into the circulatory system. Unlike medium chain triglycerides which can be directly absorbed into the portal vein, these long-chain triglycerides normally constitute 95% of consumed triglyceride [3, 4, 66, 67].

Lymph vessels serve as the major "railway" for chyle. Almost all the lymph, and therefore dietary fat including triglycerides, eventually passes into the thorax via the thoracic duct or smaller lymphatics prior to entering the vascular system. The thoracic duct transports between 2 and 4 L of fluid per day [68]. It ranges in length from 36-45 cm and measures 2-5 mm in diameter. Although significant anatomic variability exists, lymph vessels traditionally coalesce at the posterior aspect of the abdominal aorta anterior to the second lumbar vertebrae, forming the origin of the thoracic duct called the cisterna chyli. After following the abdominal aorta, the thoracic duct enters the chest through the aortic hiatus of the diaphragm and ascends in the posterior mediastinum along the right side of the vertebral column. The thoracic duct then crosses over to the left side of the body around the level of the carina or third to fifth thoracic vertebrae. From here, it continues cephalad posterior to the esophagus. It then exits the mediastinum and finally terminates after arching above the clavicle into the neck at the junction of the left internal jugular vein and left subclavian vein. Although variations are seen in up to 50% of the population, this common route helps explain why injuries to the thoracic duct below the third to fifth thoracic vertebrae typically result in right sided chylothorax and injuries above this location often result in left sided chylothorax [3, 4, 66, 67, 69].

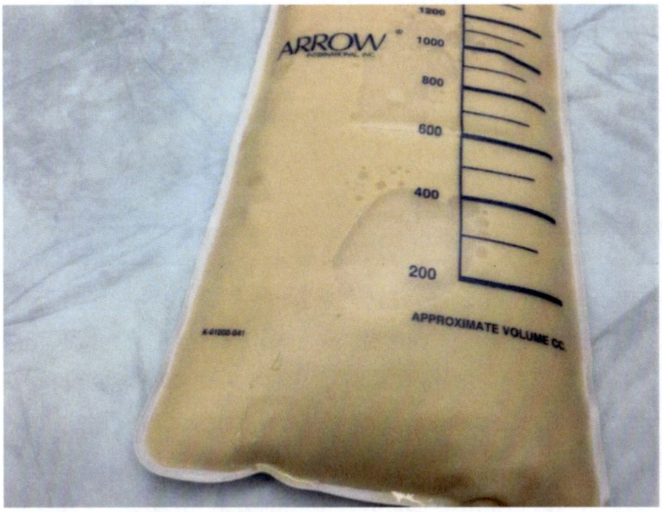

Figure 2. Fluid from chylothorax after drainage by thoracentesis.

The presentation of chylothorax differs depending on its exact etiology. Although bilateral chylothoraces can develop, nearly 80% present as unilateral pleural effusions. Of these, two-thirds are right sided [70]. Post-surgical chylothorax related to direct damage to the thoracic duct may present with rapid-onset high-volume accumulation of chylous fluid in the pleural space. If the smaller lymphatics are damaged the presentation may be more gradual and insidious. Chylothorax secondary to medical etiologies usually results in a gradual and progressive worsening of shortness of breath caused by the accumulating the pleural effusion. Pleurisy is unusual in chylothorax, but cough is common. As many as one-third of chylothoraces due to medical etiologies will result in minimal or no symptoms and are discovered only after incidental imaging studies reveal a new pleural effusion [71].

Chylothorax is often not suspected until thoracentesis of a new pleural effusion reveals milky fluid. The gold standard for confirmation of the diagnosis of suspected chylothorax is the detection of chylomicrons in the pleural fluid. Traditionally chylous fluid is described as milky white and turbid (See Figure 2). Diagnostic studies will often demonstrate a lymphocytic predominant exudate with low LDH levels and TG levels > 110 ml/dL. However, less than half of chylothoraces will have the classic "milky" appearance and a significant percentage will not have the typical pleural fluid characteristics. Although it is extremely rare to find a chylothorax with TG < 50mg/dl, many chylothoraces will have TG levels between 50-110 ml/dl, especially in those individuals who are in a fasting state or are malnourished. Patients with conditions resulting in transudative effusions such as cirrhosis, heart failure, and nephropathic associated pleural effusions can also develop a transudative chylothorax [72]. Therefore, a high index of suspicion should be maintained when assessing pleural effusions in individuals with risk factors for chylothorax. These include recent thoracic interventions, malignancy, and cirrhosis. In addition, if a chylothorax is detected but pleural fluid analysis does not demonstrate the traditional exudate with low LDH pattern, the clinician should strongly consider evaluation for an additional contributing mechanism for the pleural effusion since this may strongly influence initial and subsequent management options.

Etiology of Chylothorax

Accumulation of chyle in the pleural space is usually the result of fluid leakage due to thoracic duct or lymphatic disruption or to limited re-absorption due to lymphatic obstruction another location. Etiologies of chylothorax are summarized in Table 2 and can be categorized as iatrogenic trauma, non-iatrogenic trauma, including blunt and penetrating injuries, and secondary to other medical etiologies.

Iatrogenic causes of chylothorax include surgical and other invasive diagnostic and therapeutic procedures primarily of the chest. This accounts for as many as 30 - 50% of all chylothoraces seen in clinical practice. Cardiothoracic surgeries account for the large majority of cases in large part due to the variable unpredictable course of the thoracic duct and its various collaterals within the chest. Although chylothorax is rare even in cardiothoracic surgery, those procedures that are complicated by chylothorax have significantly worse outcomes including increased mortality [73]. The most common cardiothoracic surgeries to be result in chylothorax are esophageal procedures such as resections and reconstructions. Chylothorax has been reported to occur in 2 - 8% of esophagectomies [4]. Its incidence has declined in recent years with this change influenced by changes in the chosen procedure and technique. When chylothorax occurs after esophageal surgery it is usually as a result of disruption to main thoracic duct leading to immediate high volume chylothorax. When smaller lymphatics are damaged instead patients may present with a more delayed and gradual onset of symptoms [74]. Post-surgical chylothorax can occur (albeit less frequently) in a number of other cardiothoracic surgical procedures. Less than 2% of pulmonary resections, mediastinal lymph node dissections, congenital heart surgeries, coronary artery bypass graft surgeries, and radical neck dissections are complicated by chylothorax [71, 74-77]. Even less common causes of chylothorax are direct injury to the thoracic duct from non-surgical procedures such as central vein catheterization or indirect injury from potential catheter associated venous obstruction from indwelling vascular access [71].

Table 2. Causes of Chylothorax

Iatrogenic	Medical
• Cardiothoracic surgery • Neck surgery • Central venous catheter placement • Venous obstruction from indwelling vascular access devices Trauma • Penetrating chest wound • Blunt chest trauma • Spinal fracture • Childbirth • Retching • Weight lifting	• Malignancy (especially lymphoma) • Sarcoidosis • Fungal infection • Tuberculosis • Lymphangioleiyomyomatosis • Yellow nail syndrome • Heart failure • Post radiotherapy • Central venous thrombosis or stenosis • Idiopathic

The most common non-iatrogenic traumatic causes of chylothorax include penetrating chest injuries such as gunshot and knife wounds as well as high impact closed chest blunt trauma. These cause chylothorax by disrupting the thoracic duct or other lymphatics. Other less common minor traumatic injuries such as hyperextension or fractures of the spine, childbirth, severe emesis or coughing, and weight lifting have been rarely reported to cause chylothorax as well. Overall, these etiologies likely account for 2% or less of all chylothorax cases but may be seen more frequently in trauma centers [71].

Medical etiologies of chylothorax can be further divided into cancer related, miscellaneous causes, and idiopathic and account for up to 40% of cases. Most of these are related to lymphatic obstruction by enlarged lymph nodes or tumors [3, 4, 71]. Of the medical cause of chylothorax malignancy accounts for the majority with lymphoma the most common, making up 75% of malignant etiologies of chylothorax. Overall, malignant etiologies are thought to represent nearly one-third of all cases of chylothorax [4]. Chylothorax secondary to lymphatic obstruction due to non-malignant enlargement of mediastinal lymph nodes can be seen in medical conditions such as sarcoidosis, tuberculosis, and histoplasmosis among others [3]. Other rare parenchymal and chest related diseases that involve the lymphatics, such as lymphangioleiyomyomatosis (LAM) and the yellow nail syndrome can also be complicated by chylothorax. Although the pathophysiology of chylothorax in these conditions is not certain, they are hypothesized to result in chylothorax due to direct chyle leak from proximal lymphatic obstruction, general oozing from lymphatic vessels, and/or transdiaphragmatic flow of chylous ascites [3]. At times chylothorax is secondary to a non-thoracic etiology as can be seen in cases of chylous ascites from cirrhosis or other intra-abdominal pathologic processes such as pancreatic or gynecological tumors [3]. A number of other miscellaneous causes of chylothorax have been reported to include heart failure, post thoracic or mediastinal radiation, multiple myeloma, Kaposi sarcoma, and central venous thrombosis or obstruction [68]. In around 5% of cases no attributable cause can be found for a chylothorax, and these cases are labeled idiopathic [68].

Management of Chylothorax

Management strategies for chylothorax include conservative, surgical, and other interventional approaches. The type of intervention selected depends on several factors including the underlying etiology of the chylothorax, patient characteristics including surgical risk, and institutional experience and available resources [78]. In most cases, an initial conservative approach is appropriate with escalation to more aggressive strategies for cases that do not resolve or that recur despite conservative management. Overall, traumatic chylothorax is generally more responsive to conservative management than chylothorax due to non-traumatic etiologies. Up to 50% of traumatic chylothoraces will respond to initial conservative strategies alone and most of the other half will respond well to invasive therapies [68, 78]. Unfortunately patients who have chylothorax due to medical causes have worse outcomes. Less than one-third of these patients are able to be successfully managed conservatively [68]. Even when more aggressive interventions such as surgery, pleurodesis, or embolization are attempted as many as one in three patients with non-traumatic chylothorax will experience recurrent disease. In such cases less-traditional long-term palliative interventions such as tunneled indwelling pleural catheters (TIPC) should be considered [78]. In addition to the direct management of the chylothorax, treating clinicians must be cognizant of the potential long-term consequences of chyle leak including nutritional losses, volume depletion, and potential immunosuppression due to loss of lymphocytes.

Conservative management of chylothorax includes one or more of the following strategies: treatment of the underlying medical issue, dietary modification, intermittent thoracentesis, chest tube drainage, and use of octreotide [78]. Treatment of the underlying medical condition is often the most useful approach to management of non-traumatic chylothorax. Chylothorax secondary to malignant etiologies including lymphoma may respond to treatment of the cancer with chemotherapy and radiation. Chylothorax caused by non-malignant causes of mediastinal lymphadenopathy such as sarcoidosis or endemic fungal infections may respond to treatment of the underlying disease as well. When chylothorax is caused by venous obstruction targeted interventions such as stenting to relieve the obstruction may be attempted. Aggressive management of chronic disease states such as heart failure, cirrhosis, or renal failure which may contribute to the persistence of chylothorax is also recommended [3, 4, 68, 78]. Another important component of conservative management of chylothorax is dietary modification. The production of chyle is a direct consequence of dietary intake of long-chain fatty acids. By reducing intake of long-chain fatty acids and overall dietary fat the production of chyle may also be reduced, limiting the output from the damaged thoracic duct and potentially allowing for healing of the leaking area. As overall dietary fat and long-chain fatty acids are reduced they are replaced with medium-chain triglycerides (MCT). MCT are able to be directly absorbed from the gut into the portal circulation, bypassing the lymphatic system and providing necessary dietary lipid while reducing chyle formation. In some cases transient fasting with utilization of parenteral nutrition can aid in this strategy [3, 4, 78]. The somatostatin analogue octreotide has also been used to treat chylothorax. Octreotide inhibits production of chyle, intestinal absorption of fat, and decreases in splanchnic blood flow. Most reports utilize doses of 50 micrograms every 8 hours in combination with dietary modification for 1-2 weeks with the largest impact on chyle flow occurring in the first week [4, 79]. Intermittent therapeutic thoracentesis is also indicated for symptom control when symptomatic chylothorax does not respond to treatment targeted at optimizing the underlying medical condition. Thoracentesis is primarily targeted at symptom relief. In patients who have rapid symptomatic re-accumulation of chylothorax chest tube placement is occasionally required. Chest drainage allows for quantification of chyle output which may be used to select patients who may benefit from earlier aggressive treatment. In patients who have chyle output of more than 1100 mL/24 hours for two consecutive days or who have continued output lasting for more than 9 days early surgery or other invasive techniques are recommended [73, 76].

Various invasive surgical or interventional techniques for managing chylothorax exist. A multidisciplinary approach is frequently helpful for these complex patients. Traditional operative approaches employed by cardiothoracic surgeons include thoracic duct ligation (TDL), repair of the injured thoracic duct, and mechanical or chemical pleurodesis [76, 78]. Both open thoracotomy and VATS are used for surgical palliation of chylothorax. Minimally invasive techniques such as VATS should be utilized preferentially for TDL and pleurodesis if feasible as they are less invasive than thoracotomy. The chosen approach and technique depend on available resources, institutional expertise, and individual patient characteristics. Often surgeons use pre-operative intake of a high fat diet with or without a coloring agent to help visualize and localize the leak during the procedure. This can allow for potential direct repair of injury to the thoracic duct or more commonly distal ligation of the duct. Mechanical and chemical pleurodesis can be accomplished at time of surgical intervention but chemical pleurodesis can also be considered via chest tube instillation, especially in patients who are poor surgical candidates and do not respond to conservative management [76, 78].

In patients who are not surgical candidates interventional radiologists play a vital role in the management of chylothorax [80]. Localization attempts with percutaneous lymphangiography as well as therapeutic interventions with thoracic duct embolization (TDE) have been described. These procedures, although appealing given their less invasive nature, are often very technically challenging and therefore have highly variable rates of success. Reported rates of successful treatment of chylothorax with TDE are typically between 30 - 50% [3, 68, 80]. Much of the technical challenge of TDE stems from frequent anatomic variation among individuals and difficulty to successfully catheterizing the thoracic duct from a suitable abdominal lymph vessel. In addition, not all institutions have personnel with experience in these modalities and some sources of chyle leak may not be amenable to such interventions.

Additional interventions for chylothorax that are less commonly used include pleuroperitoneal shunts and tunneled indwelling pleural catheters (TIPC). Pleuroperitoneal shunts allow chylous pleural fluid to be transported from the thorax to the abdomen through a subcutaneous shunt. They are indicated for patients with recurrent chylothorax refractory to conservative management, most often caused by central venous thrombosis or stenosis. Recently, tunneled indwelling pleural catheters have been utilized more frequently in the management of recurrent non-malignant pleural effusions. Traditionally, there was a concern recurrent and prolonged drainage of chylothorax could and would result in nutritional and immune depletion. However, recent studies support the safe and efficacious use of TIPC for malignant, non-malignant, and traumatic recurrent chylothorax. Although limited data exists, reported results demonstrate a high rate of symptom relief and spontaneous pleurodesis without evidence of clinically significant volume, nutritional, or immune depletion [81, 82]. Additional advantages of TIPC include very low rates of other complications and the ability to manage recurrent effusions in the outpatient setting. Early placement of TIPC may also obviate the need for subsequent additional invasive procedures. TIPC has also been used for long-term drainage of post-operative chylothorax refractory to other attempted treatment modalities [76].

PSEUDOCHYLOTHORAX

Pseudochylothorax (PCT), also known as a cholesterol or chyliform effusion, was first described by Weems in 1918 as a cholesterol-rich effusion not related to thoracic duct disruption. It is a lipid rich pleural fluid with cholesterol levels > 200 mg/dL and also often containing cholesterol crystals [4]. It is generally described as being milky in appearance, but may also be cloudy, opaque, “oily yellow”, bloody, or serous [83]. It most commonly occurs in patients with chronic inflammation in the pleural space due to rheumatoid arthritis

[17] Kjeldsen, AD; Oxhoj, H; Andersen, PE; Green, A; Vase, P. "Prevalence of Pulmonary Arteriovenous Malformations (Pavms) and Occurrence of Neurological Symptoms in Patients with Hereditary Haemorrhagic Telangiectasia (Hht)." *J Intern Med*, 248, no. 3, (Sep 2000), 255-62.

[18] Bevelaqua, FA; Ordorica, SA; Lefleur, R; Young, B. "Osler-Weber-Rendu Disease. Diagnosis and Management of Spontaneous Hemothorax During Pregnancy." *N Y State J Med*, 92, no. 12, (Dec 1992), 551-2.

[19] Dowton, SB; Pincott, S; Demmer, L. "Respiratory Complications of Ehlers-Danlos Syndrome Type Iv." *Clin Genet*, 50, no. 6, (Dec 1996), 510-4.

[20] Phan, TG; Sakulsaengprapha, A; Wilson, M; Wing, R. "Ruptured Internal Mammary Artery Aneurysm Presenting as Massive Spontaneous Haemothorax in a Patient with Ehlers-Danlos Syndrome." *Aust N Z J Med*, 28, no. 2, (Apr 1998), 210-1.

[21] Hasan, RI; Krysiak, P; Deiranyia, AK; Hooper, T. "Spontaneous Rupture of the Internal Mammary Artery in Ehlers-Danlos Syndrome." *J Thorac Cardiovasc Surg*, 106, no. 1, (Jul 1993), 184-5.

[22] Yoshida, K; Tobe, S. "Dissection and Rupture of the Left Subclavian Artery Presenting as Hemothorax in a Patient with Von Recklinghausen's Disease." *Jpn J Thorac Cardiovasc Surg*, 53, no. 2, (Feb 2005), 117-9.

[23] Tatebe, S; Asami, F; Shinohara, H; Okamoto, T; Kuraoka, S. "Ruptured Aneurysm of the Subclavian Artery in a Patient with Von Recklinghausen's Disease." *Circ J*, 69, no. 4, (Apr 2005), 503-6.

[24] Kim, SJ; Kim, CW; Kim, S; Lee, TH; Kim, KI; Moon, TY; Chung, SW. "Endovascular Treatment of a Ruptured Internal Thoracic Artery Pseudoaneurysm Presenting as a Massive Hemothorax in a Patient with Type I Neurofibromatosis." *Cardiovasc Intervent Radiol*, 28, no. 6, (Nov-Dec 2005), 818-21.

[25] Butchart, EG; Grotte, GJ; Barnsley, WC. "Spotaneous Rupture of an Intercostal Artery in a Patient with Neurofibromatosis and Scoliosis." *J Thorac Cardiovasc Surg*, 69, no. 6, (Jun 1975), 919-21.

[26] Uchida, K; Kurihara, Y; Sekiguchi, S; Doi, Y; Matsuda, K; Miyanaga, M; Ikeda, Y. "Spontaneous Haemothorax Caused by Costal Exostosis." *Eur Respir J*, 10, no. 3, (Mar 1997), 735-6.

[27] Martino, A; Fabrizzi, G; Costarelli, L; Ilari, M; de Benedictis, FM. "Haemothorax Caused by Isolated Costal Exostosis." *Eur J Pediatr Surg*, 17, no. 2, (Apr 2007), 129-31.

[28] Huang, HR; Lin, TY; Wong, KS. "Costal Exostosis Presenting with Hemothorax: Report of One Case." *Eur J Pediatr*, 165, no. 5, (May 2006), 342-3.

[29] Hayes, D. Jr. "Chest Pain. Hemothorax." *Clin Pediatr (Phila)*, 46, no. 8, (Oct 2007), 746-7.

[30] Johnson, MM. "Catamenial Pneumothorax and Other Thoracic Manifestations of Endometriosis." *Clin Chest Med*, 25, no. 2, (Jun 2004), 311-9.

[31] Dhanaworavibul, K; Hanprasertpong, J; Cheewadhanaraks, S; Buhachat, R. "Bilateral Pleural Endometriosis." *J Obstet Gynaecol Res*, 32, no. 1, (Feb 2006), 86-9.

[32] Joseph, J; Sahn, SA. "Thoracic Endometriosis Syndrome: New Observations from an Analysis of 110 Cases." *Am J Med*, 100, no. 2, (Feb 1996), 164-70.

[33] Bhojawala, J; Heller, DS; Cracchiolo, B; Sama, J. "Endometriosis Presenting as Bloody Pleural Effusion and Ascites-Report of a Case and Review of the Literature." *Arch Gynecol Obstet*, 264, no. 1, (Jul 2000), 39-41.

[34] Liu, SF; Wu, CC; Lai, YF; Hsieh, MJ. "Massive Hemoptysis and Hemothorax Caused by Pleuropulmonary Angiosarcoma." *Am J Emerg Med*, 20, no. 4, (Jul 2002), 374-5.

[35] Alexiou, C; Clelland, CA; Robinson, D; Morgan, WE. "Primary Angiosarcomas of the Chest Wall and Pleura." *Eur J Cardiothorac Surg*, 14, no. 5, (Nov 1998), 523-6.

[36] Moriya, Y; Sugawara, T; Arai, M; Tsuda, Y; Uchida, K; Noguchi, T; Arai, T; Takahashi, H. "Bilateral Massive Bloody Pleurisy Complicated by Angiosarcoma." *Intern Med*, 46, no. 3, (2007), 125-8.

[37] Nakashima, T; Okuda, K; Kojiro, M; Jimi, A; Yamaguchi, R; Sakamoto, K; Ikari, T. "Pathology of Hepatocellular Carcinoma in Japan. 232 Consecutive Cases Autopsied in Ten Years." *Cancer*, 51, no. 5, (Mar 1, 1983), 863-77.

[38] Sohara, N; Takagi, H; Yamada, T; Abe, T; Mori, M. "Hepatocellular Carcinoma Complicated by Hemothorax." *J Gastroenterol*, 35, no. 3, (2000), 240-4.

[39] Mrug, M; Mishra, PV; Lusane, HC; Cunningham, JM; Alpert, MA. "Hemothorax and Retroperitoneal Hematoma after Anticoagulation with Enoxaparin." *South Med J*, 95, no. 8, (Aug 2002), 936-8.

[40] Rostand, RA; Feldman, RL; Block, ER. "Massive Hemothorax Complicating Heparin Anticoagulation for Pulmonary Embolus." *South Med J*, 70, no. 9, (Sep 1977), 1128-30.

[41] Simon, HB; Daggett, WM; DeSanctis, RW. "Hemothorax as a Complication of Anticoagulant Therapy in the Presence of Pulmonary Infarction." *JAMA*, 208, no. 10, (Jun 9, 1969), 1830-4.

[42] Robinson, NM; Thomas, MR; Jewitt, DE. "Spontaneous Haemothorax as a Complication of Anti-Coagulation Following Coronary Angioplasty." *Respir Med*, 89, no. 9, (Oct 1995), 629-30.

[43] Akgedik, R; Gunaydin, Z; Bektas, O; Karagoz, A; Ozturk, H. "Spontaneous Hemothorax Due to Dabigatran Use in a Patient with Atrial Fibrillation." *Clin Respir J*, 11, no. 3, (May 2017), 394-96.

[44] Huang, J; Lin, W; Lv, D; Yu, L; Wu, L; Jin, H; Deng, Z; Ding, Q. "Dabigatran-Induced Massive Spontaneous Hemothorax." *Drug Saf Case Rep*, 4, no. 1, (Sep 22, 2017), 12.

[45] Kortbeek, JB; Al Turki, SA; Ali, J; Antoine, JA; Bouillon, B; Brasel, K; Brenneman, F; et al. "Advanced Trauma Life Support, 8th Edition, the Evidence for Change." *J Trauma*, 64, no. 6, (Jun 2008), 1638-50.

[46] Inaba, K; Lustenberger, T; Recinos, G; Georgiou, C; Velmahos, GC; Brown, C; Salim, A; Demetriades, D; Rhee, P. "Does Size Matter? A Prospective Analysis of 28-32 Versus 36-40 French Chest Tube Size in Trauma." *J Trauma Acute Care Surg*, 72, no. 2, (Feb 2012), 422-7.

[47] Luchette, FA; Barrie, PS; Oswanski, MF; Spain, DA; Mullins, CD; Palumbo, F; Pasquale, MD. "Practice Management Guidelines for Prophylactic Antibiotic Use in Tube Thoracostomy for Traumatic Hemopneumothorax: The East Practice Management Guidelines Work Group. Eastern Association for Trauma." *J Trauma*, 48, no. 4, (Apr 2000), 753-7.

[48] Santamarina, MG; Beddings, I; Lermanda Holmgren, GV; Opazo Sanchez, H; Volpacchio, MM. "Multidetector Ct for Evaluation of the Extrapleural Space." *Radiographics*, 37, no. 5, (Sep-Oct 2017), 1352-70.

[49] Chang, YT; Dai, ZK; Kao, EL; Chuang, HY; Cheng, YJ; Chou, SH; Huang, MF. "Early Video-Assisted Thoracic Surgery for Primary Spontaneous Hemopneumothorax." *World J Surg*, 31, no. 1, (Jan 2007), 19-25.

[50] Kakaris, S; Athanassiadi, K; Vassilikos, K; Skottis, I. "Spontaneous Hemopneumothorax: A Rare but Life-Threatening Entity." *Eur J Cardiothorac Surg*, 25, no. 5, (May 2004), 856-8.

[51] Pollak, JS; Saluja, S; Thabet, A; Henderson, KJ; Denbow, N; White, RI. Jr. "Clinical and Anatomic Outcomes after Embolotherapy of Pulmonary Arteriovenous Malformations." *J Vasc Interv Radiol*, 17, no. 1, (Jan 2006), 35-44, quiz 45.

[52] Olive, DL; Pritts, EA. "Treatment of Endometriosis." *N Engl J Med*, 345, no. 4, (Jul26 2001), 266-75.

[53] Bagan, P; Le Pimpec Barthes, F; Assouad, J; Souilamas, R; Riquet, M. "Catamenial Pneumothorax: Retrospective Study of Surgical Treatment." *Ann Thorac Surg*, 75, no. 2, (Feb 2003), 378-81, discusssion 81.

[54] DuBose, J; Inaba, K; Demetriades, D; Scalea, TM; O'Connor, J; Menaker, J; Morales, C; et al. "Management of Post-Traumatic Retained Hemothorax: A Prospective, Observational, Multicenter Aast Study." *J Trauma Acute Care Surg*, 72, no. 1, (Jan 2012), 11-22, discussion 22-4, quiz 316.

[55] DuBose, J; Inaba, K; Okoye, O; Demetriades, D; Scalea, T; O'Connor, J; Menaker, J; et al. "Development of Posttraumatic Empyema in Patients with Retained Hemothorax: Results of a Prospective, Observational Aast Study." *J Trauma Acute Care Surg*, 73, no. 3, (Sep 2012), 752-7.

[56] Oguzkaya, F; Akcali, Y; Bilgin, M. "Videothoracoscopy Versus Intrapleural Streptokinase for Management of Post Traumatic Retained Haemothorax: A Retrospective Study of 65 Cases." *Injury*, 36, no. 4, (Apr 2005), 526-9.

[57] Burford, TH; Parker, EF; Samson, PC. "Early Pulmonary Decortication in the Treatment of Posttraumatic Empyema." *Ann Surg*, 122, no. 2, (Aug 1945), 163-90.

[58] Bilello, JF; Davis, JW; Lemaster, DM. "Occult Traumatic Hemothorax: When Can Sleeping Dogs Lie?". *Am J Surg*, 190, no. 6, (Dec 2005), 841-4.

[59] Navsaria, PH; Vogel, RJ; Nicol, AJ. "Thoracoscopic Evacuation of Retained Posttraumatic Hemothorax." *Ann Thorac Surg*, 78, no. 1, (Jul 2004), 282-5, discussion 85-6.

[60] Velmahos, GC; Demetriades, D. "Early Thoracoscopy for the Evacuation of Undrained Haemothorax." *Eur J Surg*, 165, no. 10, (Oct 1999), 924-9.

[61] Morales Uribe, CH; Villegas Lanau, MI; Petro Sanchez, RD. "Best Timing for Thoracoscopic Evacuation of Retained Post-Traumatic Hemothorax." *Surg Endosc*, 22, no. 1, (Jan 2008), 91-5.

[62] Meyer, DM; Jessen, ME; Wait, MA; Estrera, AS. "Early Evacuation of Traumatic Retained Hemothoraces Using Thoracoscopy: A Prospective, Randomized Trial." *Ann Thorac Surg*, 64, no. 5, (Nov 1997), 1396-400, discussion 400-1.

[63] Hunt, I; Thakar, C; Southon, R; Bedard, EL. "Establishing a Role for Intra-Pleural Fibrinolysis in Managing Traumatic Haemothoraces." *Interact Cardiovasc Thorac Surg*, 8, no. 1, (Jan 2009), 129-33.

[64] Kimbrell, BJ; Yamzon, J; Petrone, P; Asensio, JA; Velmahos, GC. "Intrapleural Thrombolysis for the Management of Undrained Traumatic Hemothorax: A Prospective Observational Study." *J Trauma*, 62, no. 5, (May 2007), 1175-8, discussion 78-9.

[65] Jerjes-Sanchez, C; Ramirez-Rivera, A; Elizalde, JJ; Delgado, R; Cicero, R; Ibarra Perez, C; Arroliga, AC; et al. "Intrapleural Fibrinolysis with Streptokinase as an Adjunctive Treatment in Hemothorax and Empyema: A Multicenter Trial." *Chest*, 109, no. 6, (Jun 1996), 1514-9.

[66] Skouras, V; Kalomenidis, I. "Chylothorax: Diagnostic Approach." *Curr Opin Pulm Med*, 16, no. 4, (Jul 2010), 387-93.

[67] Staats, BA; Ellefson, RD; Budahn, LL; Dines, DE; Prakash, UB; Offord, K. "TheLipoprotein Profile of Chylous and Nonchylous Pleural Effusions." *Mayo Clin Proc*, 55, no. 11, (Nov 1980), 700-4.

[68] Schild, HH; Strassburg, CP; Welz, A; Kalff, J. "Treatment Options in Patients with Chylothorax." *Dtsch Arztebl Int*, 110, no. 48, (Nov 29, 2013), 819-26.

[69] Johnson, OW; Chick, JF; Chauhan, NR; Fairchild, AH; Fan, CM; Stecker, MS; Killoran, TP; Suzuki-Han, A. "The Thoracic Duct: Clinical Importance, Anatomic Variation, Imaging, and Embolization." *Eur Radiol*, 26, no. 8, (Aug 2016), 2482-93.

[70] Maldonado, F; Hawkins, FJ; Daniels, CE; Doerr, CH; Decker, PA; Ryu, JH. "Pleural Fluid Characteristics of Chylothorax." *Mayo Clin Proc*, 84, no. 2, (Feb 2009), 129-33.

[71] Doerr, CH; Allen, MS; Nichols, FC; 3rd. Ryu, JH. "Etiology of Chylothorax in 203 Patients." *Mayo Clin Proc*, 80, no. 7, (Jul 2005), 867-70.

[72] Agrawal, V; Doelken, P; Sahn, SA. "Pleural Fluid Analysis in Chylous Pleural Effusion." *Chest*, 133, no. 6, (Jun 2008), 1436-41.

[73] Shah, RD; Luketich, JD; Schuchert, MJ; Christie, NA; Pennathur, A; Landreneau, RJ; Nason, KS. "Postesophagectomy Chylothorax: Incidence, Risk Factors, and Outcomes." *Ann Thorac Surg*, 93, no. 3, (Mar 2012), 897-903, discussion 03-4.

[74] Bryant, AS; Minnich, DJ; Wei, B; Cerfolio, RJ. "The Incidence and Management of Postoperative Chylothorax after Pulmonary Resection and Thoracic Mediastinal Lymph Node Dissection." *Ann Thorac Surg*, 98, no. 1, (Jul 2014), 232-5, discussion 35-7.

[75] Ziarnik, E; Grogan, EL. "Postlobectomy Early Complications." *Thorac Surg Clin*, 25, no. 3, (Aug 2015), 355-64.

[76] Reisenauer, JS; Puig, CA; Reisenauer, CJ; Allen, MS; Bendel, E; Cassivi, SD; Nichols, FC; et al. "Treatment of Postsurgical Chylothorax." *Ann Thorac Surg*, 105, no. 1, (Jan 2018), 254-62.

[77] Cerfolio, RJ; Allen, MS; Deschamps, C; Trastek, VF; Pairolero, PC. "Postoperative Chylothorax." *J Thorac Cardiovasc Surg*, 112, no. 5, (Nov 1996), 1361-5, discussion 65-6.

[78] Maldonado, F; Cartin-Ceba, R; Hawkins, FJ; Ryu, JH. "Medical and Surgical Management of Chylothorax and Associated Outcomes." *Am J Med Sci*, 339, no. 4, (Apr 2010), 314-8.

[79] Kalomenidis, I. "Octreotide and Chylothorax." *Curr Opin Pulm Med*, 12, no. 4, (Jul 2006), 264-7.

[80] Toliyat, M; Singh, K; Sibley, RC; Chamarthy, M; Kalva, SP; Pillai, AK. "Interventional Radiology in the Management of Thoracic Duct Injuries: Anatomy, Techniques and Results." *Clin Imaging*, 42, (Mar - Apr 2017), 183-92.

[81] Jimenez, CA; Mhatre, AD; Martinez, CH; Eapen, GA; Onn, A; Morice, RC. "Use of an Indwelling Pleural Catheter for the Management of Recurrent Chylothorax in Patients with Cancer." *Chest*, 132, no. 5, (Nov 2007), 1584-90.

[82] DePew, ZS; Iqbal, S; Mullon, JJ; Nichols, FC; Maldonado, F. "The Role for Tunneled Indwelling Pleural Catheters in Patients with Persistent Benign Chylothorax." *Am J Med Sci*, 346, no. 5, (Nov 2013), 349-52.

[83] Lama, A; Ferreiro, L; Toubes, ME; Golpe, A; Gude, F; Alvarez-Dobano, JM; Gonzalez-Barcala, FJ; et al. "Characteristics of Patients with Pseudochylothorax-a Systematic Review." *J Thorac Dis*, 8, no. 8, (Aug 2016), 2093-101.

[84] Sassoon, CS; Light, RW. "Chylothorax and Pseudochylothorax." *Clin Chest Med*, 6, no. 1, (Mar 1985), 163-71.

[85] Coe, JE; Aikawa, JK. "Cholesterol Pleural Effusion. Report of 2 Cases Studied with Isotopic Techniques and Review of the World Literature." *Arch Intern Med*, 108, (Nov 1961), 763-74.

[86] Garcia-Zamalloa, A; Ruiz-Irastorza, G; Aguayo, FJ; Gurrutxaga, N. "Pseudochylothorax. Report of 2 Cases and Review of the Literature." *Medicine (Baltimore)*, 78, no. 3, (May 1999), 200-7.

[87] Hillerdal, G. "Chyliform (Cholesterol) Pleural Effusion." *Chest*, 88, no. 3, (Sep 1985), 426-8.

[88] Hillerdal, G. "Chylothorax and Pseudochylothorax." *Eur Respir J*, 10, no. 5, (May 1997), 1157-62.

[89] Hamm, H; Pfalzer, B; Fabel, H. "Lipoprotein Analysis in a Chyliform Pleural Effusion: Implications for Pathogenesis and Diagnosis." *Respiration*, 58, no. 5-6, (1991), 294-300.

[90] Wrightson, JM; Stanton, AE; Maskell, NA; Davies, RJO; Lee, YCG. "Pseudochylothorax without Pleural Thickening: Time to Reconsider Pathogenesis?". *Chest*, 136, no. 4, (Oct 2009), 1144-47.

[91] Priya, MP; Dharmic, S; Kar, A; Suryanarayana, V. "An Unusual Case of Pseudochylothorax." *J Pharm Bioallied Sci*, 7, no. Suppl 1, (Apr 2015), S80-2.

[92] Balbir-Gurman, A; Yigla, M; Nahir, AM; Braun-Moscovici, Y. "Rheumatoid Pleural Effusion." *Semin Arthritis Rheum*, 35, no. 6, (Jun 2006), 368-78.

[93] Shaw, M; Collins, BF; Ho, LA; Raghu, G. "Rheumatoid Arthritis-Associated Lung Disease." *Eur Respir Rev*, 24, no. 135, (Mar 2015), 1-16.

[94] Ryu, JH; Tomassetti, S; Maldonado, F. "Update on Uncommon Pleural Effusions." *Respirology*, 16, no. 2, (Feb 2011), 238-43.

In: Pleural Effusions: Causes, Types and Treatment ISBN: 978-1-53614-683-7
Editor: Rahul Khosla

Chapter 7

TUBERCULOUS AND FUNGAL PLEURAL EFFUSION

Ramasubramanian Balachandran[1*], MD and Janaki Deepak[2], MD
[1]Division of Pulmonary and Critical Care,
University Of Maryland School of Medicine, Baltimore, MD, US
[2]Pulmonary and CCM Section, Veterans Affairs Medical Center, Baltimore, MD, US

ABSTRACT

This chapter will elaborate on tuberculous and fungal pleural effusion. While the former is the most common cause of pleural effusion worldwide, the incidence of the latter has been steadily increasing. The world of medicine has been battling mycobacterium tuberculosis, one of the deadliest communicable diseases, for many years. The emergence of Human immunodeficiency virus (HIV) infection led to the resurgence of this problem. Diagnosis of this disorder is challenging. Though the gold standard method of diagnosis is detection of the bacteria in pleural fluid and pleural biopsy, clinical suspicion and knowledge of biomarkers is required to tailor a diagnostic approach. The incidence of fungal infections is increasing due to the rising number of critically ill patients, use of intra-vascular devices, immunosuppressive medications, broad-spectrum antibiotics and incidence of cancer. Fungal empyema carries a high morbidity and mortality. Since many fungi are commensals in skin and are ubiquitous in the environment, diagnosis can be difficult. We shall review the risk factors, diagnosis, treatment and natural history of tubercular and fungal pleural infections in this chapter.

Keywords: fungal, tuberculosis, pleural effusion, adenosine deaminase

[*]Corresponding Author Email: rambaalachandran@umm.edu

INTRODUCTION

Mycobacterium Tuberculosis (MTB) is known to man since pre-historic times and is the most common cause of death due to an infectious organism. Over 1.6 million deaths were associated with MTB in 2016 [1]. Pleural TB is the second most common site of extra-pulmonary TB, after lymph nodes. One of the first case reports of this clinical entity was almost 65 years ago [27]. Very little progress has been made in the diagnosis and management because of its low incidence, difficulty in identification and delay in therapy.

TUBERCULAR PLEURAL EFFUSION

Epidemiology

Mycobacterium Tuberculosis (MTB) is known to man since pre-historic times and is the most common cause of death due to an infectious organism. Over 1.6 million deaths were associated with MTB in 2016 [1]. Pleural TB is the second most common site of extra-pulmonary TB, after lymph nodes. In developed countries, less than 1% of all exudative pleural effusions are due to tuberculous etiology and 3-5% of TB patients develop pleural effusions [2].

The emergence of human immunodeficiency viral infection (HIV) and multi-drug resistant (MDR) TB are changing the epidemiology of this disease. Recent studies reveal MDR-TB pleural effusions account for 19 and 9% of their country's MDR- TB burden in Iran [3] and Peru [4], respectively.

Pathogenesis

Pleural TB can occur in primary and post-primary or reactivated TB. The following mechanisms have been described [5].

1. *Delayed Hypersensitivity*: Mycobacterial antigen triggers a delayed hypersensitivity reaction in the pleural space.
2. *Contiguous spread:* Direct inoculation in the pleura from contiguous lung lesions or sub-diaphragmatic focus.
3. *Lymphatic spread.*
4. *Hematogenous spread.*

Clinical Presentation

Majority of the patients are symptomatic. It is rarely detected incidentally on chest radiograph. The most common symptoms are fever, chest pain and cough. Some patients present with non-specific symptoms like anorexia, weight loss, malaise, generalized weakness, fatigability and night sweats [6]. Dramatic presentation with symptoms is more common in immunocompetent individuals, while HIV patients are less symptomatic. Age also plays an important role in determining the duration of symptoms. Elderly patients have a longer symptomatic period prior to presentation [7].

Unilateral effusion is the rule with bilateral effusion limited to case reports and the volume of effusion is usually low. Rarely, it can track to the skin and present as chest wall swelling and empyema necessitans. Thus, to conclude, the symptoms and signs of a tubercular effusion vary and are nonspecific [5].

Diagnosis

Ultrasound

Ultrasound of the pleura is useful not only in diagnosis, but also to predict the sequelae of tuberculous effusion. The presence of complex septate pattern on sonography in lymphocyte rich effusions indicates tuberculous cause with a specificity, positive predictive value and positive likelihood ratio of 96%, 94% and 12 respectively [8]. In a prospective study, complex septate pleural effusion [Figure 1] in pleural TB proved to be a significant marker of residual pleural thickening (RPT) after 1 year. This is clinically relevant, since patients with RPT also had significantly lower forced vital capacity [9].

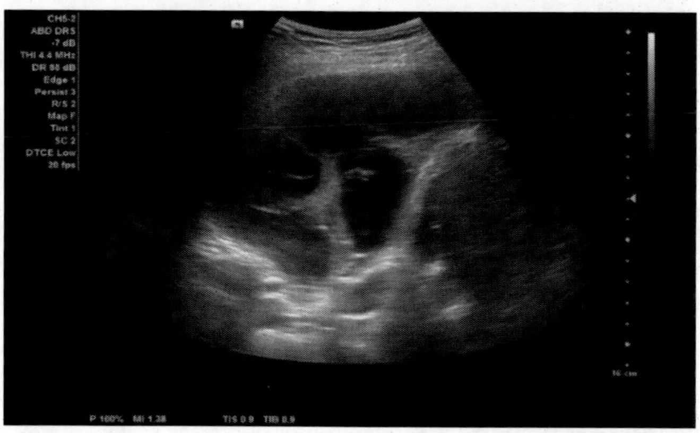

Figure 1. Complex septate pleural effusion: This shows a large right pleural effusion with multiple, thick septae. Tuberculous effusion is one of the commonest causes of this pattern. Despite the presence of multiple thick fibrous bands, the fluid appears relatively clear.

Other Imaging

Computed Tomography (CT) of the chest is not useful in volumetric assessment of pleural effusion but can reveal parenchymal lesions. Majority of the patients with tuberculous pleuritis have associated parenchymal lesions [10]. Magnetic Resonance Imaging of chest (MRI) is less useful, but can help in differentiating benign from malignant etiology [11].

Pleural Fluid Analysis

The following characteristics are commonly noted in pleural fluid analysis of pleural tuberculosis [7]:

- Exudative
- Pleural fluid pH between 7.3-7.4
- Pleural fluid glucose greater than 60 mg/dl
- Lymphocytic predominance
- Mean protein content above 5 g/dl
- 90–95% of the pleural fluid cells are T-lymphocytes

Neutrophilic predominance can also observed in pleural TB, though less commonly than lymphocytic predominance. Microbiological detection of MTB from pleural fluid and sputum is more frequent in the neutrophil-predominant group than the lymphocyte-predominant group [12].

Pleural Fluid Microbiology

Pleural TB is a paucibacillary process, thus making microbiological detection very difficult. Recent increase in the incidence of multi-drug resistant (MDR) TB makes isolation and drug sensitivity testing very important. The following samples can be used for detection with smear and/or culture:

1. *Sputum:* Induced sputum has a culture positive rate of 55%, including patients without evidence of parenchymal involvement in chest radiograph [13]. This also helps in identifying patients who are more infective.
2. *Broncho-alveolar lavage (BAL)*
3. *Pleural fluid:* The yield of pleural fluid microscopy is around 10%. The sensitivity of pleural fluid culture is also low, around 10-35% [13].

4. *Pleural biopsy:* This technique has a diagnostic yield of 76%. Tissue can be obtained by closed pleural biopsy, medical thoracoscopy, video-assisted thoracoscopy and open surgical biopsy. US guided pleural biopsy has a diagnostic yield of 90%, while pleural biopsies taken under direct visualization via thoracoscopy can achieve a sensitivity of up to 100% [14].

The following factors increase the microbiological yield:

1. *HIV* patients have higher rate of positive cultures. This is probably due to ineffective clearance of bacteria [15].
2. *Liquid culture* has higher sensitivity (30% to 70%) and faster time to positivity (2 weeks compared to 6 weeks) [16].
3. *Neutrophilic* predominant pleural effusions [12].

Combining different techniques for obtaining specimen can increase the yield. When pleural biopsy and thoracentesis are combined the diagnostic yield for MTB increases from 77.8% to 88.9% [17]. A higher sensitivity (93%) and specificity (100%) can be achieved by combining closed pleural biopsy with ADA of more than 50 IU/L, lymphocyte/neutrophil ratio more than 0.75 [14].

Table 1. Diagnostic tools for pleural TB

Diagnostic method	Sensitivity (%)	Specificity (%)
ADA >=50 U/L	95	89
Pleural fluid culture	7	100
Medical Thoracoscopy AFB stain and Histology Culture	100 76	100 100

Adenosine Deaminase (ADA)

ADA is an enzyme in the purine salvage pathway of De-oxyribonucleic acid (DNA) metabolism. It is significantly increased in granulomatous inflammation, thus being useful in diagnosis of MTB infection. ADA alone at a cut-off value of ≥40 IU/L attained 87% diagnostic accuracy and had a positive likelihood ratio (LR) of 6.6 and a negative LR of 0.2. It also performed better than other clinical prediction models [18]. Pleural fluid levels greater than equal to 41.5 U/L has good sensitivity (97.1%) and specificity (92.9%) in low-moderate incidence setting. In the same study conducted in France, the positive and negative predictive value were 86.8% and 98.5%, respectively [19]. Empyema and malignancy are important causes of false positive result. Thus, caution is needed while interpreting ADA levels in patients older than 50 years of age, with h/o malignancy and large or massive pleural effusion. The suggested algorithm for diagnosing pleural TB is shown below[Figure 3].

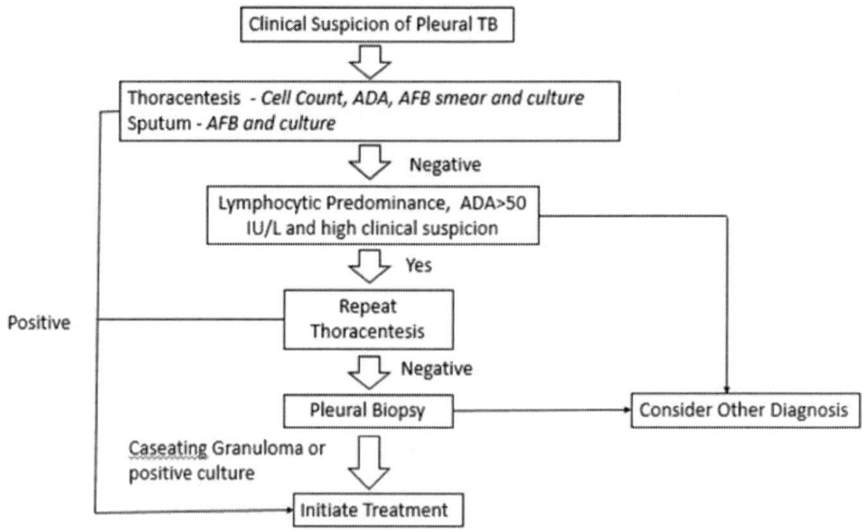

Figure 3. Suggested Algorithm for diagnosis of Pleural TB.

Treatment

The main goals of treatment are:

1. Prevent the development of active TB
2. Relief of symptoms
3. Prevent the development of complications like fibrothorax

Antibiotic therapy for pleural TB consists of 2 months of intensive therapy and 4 months of continuation therapy. The following regimens have been shown to be equally effective [5].

1. Isoniazid (H), Rifampin (R), Pyrazinamide (Z) and Ethambutol (E) for 2 months and maintenance therapy with Isoniazid (H) and Rifampin (R), for 4 months.
2. Since the disease is paucibacillary, six month treatment with Isoniazid (H) and Rifampin (R) was equally effective in a 130-patient trial [20].
3. *MDR-TB:* WHO recommends a 5- Drug regimen with add-on drugs it be used as necessary. The duration of treatment is also longer- 20 months.

4. *HIV:* In newly diagnosed HIV and TB, Anti-retroviral therapy should be initiated at least 8 weeks after initiation of anti-TB therapy. It can be started earlier if CD4 count is less than 50 cells/cu.mm [21].

At present, the use of steroids is not recommended for pleural TB [22, 23]. In loculated tuberculous pleural effusion, combining anti-tubercular therapy, chest tube drainage and fibrinolytic therapy is associated with faster clearance of pleural effusion, reduce the occurrence of RPT and accelerate pulmonary function recovery [24].

Table 2. Sequelae of pleural TB

Sequelae of Pleural TB	Incidence
Spontaneous resolution	90%
Active TB after 5 years without treatment	40-60%
Residual pleural thickening	50%
Fibrothorax	5%

Without treatment majority of tuberculous pleural effusions (90%) resolve spontaneously while 40-60% develop active TB, thus necessitating treatment. Residual pleural thickening (RPT) is a common sequelae and may occur in up to 50% of cases. The risk factors for development of RPT includes the lower pleural fluid glucose, pH, higher TNF-a levels [25] complex septate pattern on ultrasonography [9] and elevated TIMP-1 levels at the completion of anti-tuberculosis medications [26]. In a Cochrane review in 2017, it was concluded that the impact of pleural TB on long-term respiratory function is unknown [23]. Fibrothorax, defined as a pleural membrane of at least 5mm thickness occurs in 5% of the patients. Tubercular empyema almost invariably develop extensive calcified fibrothorax, that is, pleuritis caldaria [7]. The studies on recurrence of pleural effusion after treatment are limited. In a study from Sub Saharan Africa in patients with smear negative parenchymal and pleural TB (most of them who were HIV positive) after standard unsupervised treatment, it was noted that the recurrence rate for pleural TB was 10.8%. The mortality in isolated pleural TB was lower than that of parenchymal TB.

FUNGAL PLEURAL EFFUSION

Introduction

One of the first case reports of this clinical entity was almost 65 years ago [7]. Very little progress has been made in the diagnosis and management because of its low incidence, difficulty in identification and delay in therapy.

Epidemiology

The overall incidence of fungal pleural effusion is low. In a retrospective analysis of pleural infection, the incidence of fungal empyema thoracis (FET) was only 7% [28]. But the incidence has been increasing over the past years, especially of candida and aspergillus [29]. In a more recent retrospective study among cancer patients the incidence was 16% [30]. The reason for this is unclear. It could be due in the increase in number of immunocompromised patients being admitted to our hospitals and/or better fungal identification techniques. Airways and lung are common sites of fungal infection after blood stream and urinary tract.

This unusual infection is more common in males and the median age of diagnosis is 64 years [30]. Majority of the patients acquire the infection in health care setting, mostly acquired in ICU [31].

Risk Factors

Most patients with FET have underlying medical conditions. Immunosuppression and malignancy are the most important risk factors. Presence of conditions with compromised immunity like HIV, long term steroid use and organ transplantation are also predictors of mortality [31]. Abdominal and hematological malignancies are the more common culprits among the cancers. Solid malignancies are associated with candida pleural effusions more than aspergillus [30]. Use of broad spectrum antibiotics disrupts the normal gastrointestinal (GI) flora. This results in overgrowth of candida, which translocates to the blood stream resulting in invasive candidiasis [32].

Candida species commonly colonizes the skin, gastro-intestinal tract and airways. Thus, any disruption to the epithelial and mucosal barrier in these organs puts the patient at risk for developing fungal infections. In pleural infections due to other pathogens broncho-pulmonary infection and spread to pleura is the important pathogenic mechanism. On the other hand, many FET cases have a preceding acute or sub-acute abdominal disease, especially in those with candida pleural effusion. Isolation of Candida species in pleural fluid can be an important clue for suspecting gastrointestinal tract perforation, GI fistulae and GI malignancies [33]. Most patients with candida (especially candida albicans) pleural effusion have had abdominal or thoracic surgery within 30 days of index culture [30].

Candida species commonly colonizes the skin, gastro-intestinal tract and airways. Thus any disruption to the epithelial and mucosal barrier in these organs puts the patient at risk for developing fungal infections. In pleural infections due to other pathogens broncho-pulmonary infection and spread to pleura is the important pathogenic mechanism. On the other hand, many FET cases have a preceding acute or sub-acute abdominal disease, especially in those with candida pleural effusion. Isolation of Candida species in pleural fluid can be an important clue for suspecting gastrointestinal tract perforation, GI fistulae and GI malignancies [33]. Most patients with candida (especially candida albicans) pleural effusion have had abdominal or thoracic surgery within 30 days of index culture [30].

Pneumonia and lung abscess are important risk factors in FET due to aspergillus. Prior colonization of respiratory tract is an important risk factor for development in critically ill and post-surgical patients [34]. Rarely FET can occur after repeated thoracentesis and chest tube drainage due to aseptic techniques [35]. Any break in the skin barrier can predispose to invasive fungal infections. Thus, hyperalimentation, chest and abdominal surgery and invasive devices like central vascular catheters, urinary catheters, and chest tubes are important risk factors [35, 36].

Clinical Presentation

The most common complaints at presentation are fever and dyspnea [31]. Fever is less common among cancer patients [30]. Most patients have leukocytosis with white blood cell counts reaching greater than 20,000 per cc of blood. Neutropenia is seen in some patients, especially after chemotherapy. The pleural effusion can be simple or loculated. Abnormal parenchymal changes are more common in aspergillus infections. This is not surprising since Aspergillus is associated more with broncho-pulmonary infections, while Candida is associated abdominal disease. Exudative pleural effusion is the rule and transudative effusion is very rare. The Lactate dehydrogenase concentrations are usually high and glucose concentration is low. Eosinophilia has not been reported and neutrophilic predominance is common in pleural fluid.

Table 3. Risk factors for fungal pleural effusion

Most common
Immunosuppression
Malignancy
For Candida
Gastro-intestinal diseases
Abdominal and thoracic surgery
Use of broad-spectrum antibiotics
Invasive devices (central lines, urinary catheter)
For other Fungi
Alcoholism
Uremia
HIV
Steroid use
Organ transplantation
Hyperalimentation
Respiratory colonization

Table 4. Fungal isolates from pleural effusion

Fungal Isolates	No. (%)
Candida Species	47(64(
C.albicans	28(38)
C.tropicalis	12(18)
C.parapsilosis	2(3)
C.guilliermondii	2(3)
C.humicola	1(1)
C.famata	1(1)
Torulopsis glabrata	13(18)
Cryptococcus species	3(4)
Aspergillus psecies	9(12)
Rhizopus species	1(1)

Microbiology

Candida is the most common fungi isolated, candida albicans being the most frequent. Aspergillus is the second most common fungi seen. Pleural Cryptococcosis is associated with HIV infection [37] liver cirrhosis and Bruton's agammaglobulinemia. There are very few case reports of other filamentous fungi causing pleural effusion. Uncommon molds (e.g., penicillium) are usually contaminants and treatment is not required. In the study by Nigo et al. they were associated with very low mortality even without treatment. Endemic mycosis can also cause pleural effusion [38].

Concomitant bacterial infection is seen in in around a quarter of the patients. The bacteria usually isolated are vary widely. Nosocomial pathogens like Pseudomonas aeruginosa, coagulase negative staphylococci and staphylococcus aureus are more common. This is consistent with the fact that majority of the fungal empyema cases are nosocomial.

Pathophysioloy

The infection spreads to the pleura by 2 ways, hematogenous and contiguous spread. Hematogenous spread is seen with candida and is associated with poor outcome [39]. Candida empyema thoracis due to contiguous infection is more common than those due to noncontiguous infection. Contiguous spread is the rule is aspergillus infections, usually from rupture of lung abscess.

Diagnosis

It is important to recognize the importance of contamination while interpreting positive fungal cultures of pleural fluid. In the absence of risk factors, clinical features of infection, and exudative pleural fluid it is unlikely to be an infection. Isolation of uncommon molds is likely to represent a contamination of the pleural fluid [30]. There are some guidelines for establishing invasive fungal infections (IFI) but these criteria are not sensitive and may not apply for unusual sites like the pleura [40].

Treatment

Antifungal Therapy

Earlier studies report high mortality among patient who did not receive anti-fungal agents. The more recent studies report a lower mortality. This indicates the need for better criteria to differentiate between contamination and infection. Amphotericin B (for aspergillus) and fluconazole (for candida) are most commonly used antifungal agents. Dual antifungal therapy is more commonly employed with aspergillus infection, Amphotericin B and Voriconazole being the most popular combination therapy. When dual therapy is needed in candida infections – usually a combination of an azole and an echinocandin is used. Data on the concentration of antifungal agents in the pleural fluid is limited. Some studies suggest that voriconazole achieves therapeutic concentrations in the pleural space [41] whereas the concentration of echinocandins in the pleural fluid is marginal [42].

Irrigation

Irrigation with normal saline, fluconazole and amphotericin B is less popular. The use of intrapleural instillation of an antifungal has been sporadically reported as an effective adjunctive therapy for FET due to Mucorales, Aspergillus or Candida spp. [43].

Other Procedures

Chest tube drainage and fibrinolytic therapy is more commonly employed in candida infection and the response is variable. In complicated infections, not responding to above therapies surgical options like decortication and lung resection are considered. Aspergillus pleural effusions needs surgical treatment more often than candida. Data supporting one particular therapeutic strategy over the others is lacking and further studies are needed.

Natural History and Outcome

Fungal empyema is associated with prolonged hospital stay, increased morbidity and mortality the mortality approaches as high as 73% in some retrospective studies [31]. In a more recent study the mortality has decreased to 34% [30]. The mortality risk factors are:

- Lack of antifungal treatment
- Compromised immunity
- Respiratory Failure
- Isolation of multiple fungal strain

Conclusion

Pleural TB is the second most common extrapulmonary site after lymph nodes with varied pathogenesis. Most patients are symptomatic with fever chest pain and cough. Ultrasound is the preferred imaging technique and is helpful in predicting sequelae. Exudative, lymphocytic predominant pleural effusions with ADA > 50 IU/L have a high predictive value. Pleural TB is usually paucibacillary. Treatment includes 2 months of intensive therapy with 4 drug regimen followed by 4 months of two drug regimen. Most effusions spontaneously resolve, with 50% of cases showing residual pleural thickening and 5% develop Fibrothorax.

Fungal infections are less common, mostly nosocomial in an immunocompromised host. Fever and leukocytosis being the clinical presentation, with mostly exudative effusions with neutrophilic predominance and a low glucose. Candida and Aspergillus are the most common species isolated from the effusions. Medical therapy consists of dual antifungal therapy as a norm for aspergillus effusions. Candidial effusions usually respond to an Azole monotherapy but when dual therapy is required an Echinocandin is added. Other therapies like irrigation of the pleural space with antifungals, chest tube drainage etc. have mixed results. Surgical decortication is reserved for the severe cases.

References

[1] Bahrmand, A R, A Siadati, G Samar, and A Sanami. 1996. "[Report of drug resistance in strains of Mycobacterium tuberculosis isolated from patients in Iran]." *Revista cubana de medicina tropical* 48 (2). Cuba: 92–97.

[2] Baumann, Michael H, Rathel Nolan, Marcy Petrini, Y C Gary Lee, Richard W Light, and Eileen Schneider. 2007. "Pleural Tuberculosis in the United States: Incidence

and Drug Resistance." *Chest* 131 (4). United States: 1125–32. https://doi.org/10.1378/chest.06-2352.

[3] Bittner, R. C., and R. Felix. 1998. "Magnetic Resonance (MR) Imaging of the Chest: State-of-the-Art." *European Respiratory Journal* 11 (6): 1392–1404. https://doi.org/10.1183/09031936.98.11061392.

[4] Canete, C, I Galarza, A Granados, E Farrero, R Estopa, and F Manresa. 1994. "Tuberculous Pleural Effusion: Experience with Six Months of Treatment with Isoniazid and Rifampicin." *Thorax* 49 (11). England: 1160–61.

[5] Chan, C H, M Arnold, C Y Chan, T W Mak, and G B Hoheisel. 1991. "Clinical and Pathological Features of Tuberculous Pleural Effusion and Its Long-Term Consequences." *Respiration; International Review of Thoracic Diseases* 58 (3–4). Switzerland: 171–75. https://doi.org/10.1159/000195921.

[6] Chen, Hung-jen, Wu-huei Hsu, Chih-yen Tu, Yang-hao Yu, Kuo-liang Chiu, Liang-wen Hang, Te-chun Hsia, and Chuen-ming Shih. 2006. "Sonographic Septations in Lymphocyte Rich Exudative Pleural Effusions." *J Ultrasound Med 2006;* no. 25: 857–63.

[7] Choi, Hayoung, Hae Ri Chon, Kang Kim, Sukyeon Kim, Ki Jong Oh, Suk Hyeon Jeong, Woo Jin Jung, et al. 2016. "Clinical and Laboratory Differences between Lymphocyte- and Neutrophil-Predominant Pleural Tuberculosis." *PLoS ONE* 11 (10): 1–10. https://doi.org/10.1371/journal.pone.0165428.

[8] Chung, C. L., C. H. Chen, C. Y. Yeh, J. R. Sheu, and S. C. Chang. 2008. "Early Effective Drainage in the Treatment of Loculated Tuberculous Pleurisy." *European Respiratory Journal* 31 (6): 1261–67. https://doi.org/10.1183/09031936.00122207.

[9] Conde, Marcus B., Angela Chindamo Loivos, Valeria M. Rezende, Sergio L.M. Soares, Fernanda C.Q. Mello, Arthur L. Reingold, Charles L. Daley, and Afranio L. Kritski. 2003. "Yield of Sputum Induction in the Diagnosis of Pleural Tuberculosis." *American Journal of Respiratory and Critical Care Medicine* 167 (5): 723–25. https://doi.org/10.1164/rccm.2111019.

[10] Denkinger, Claudia M., Samuel G. Schumacher, Catharina C. Boehme, Nandini Dendukuri, Madhukar Pai, and Karen R. Steingart. 2014. "Xpert MTB/RIF Assay for the Diagnosis of Extrapulmonary Tuberculosis: A Systematic Review and Meta-Analysis." *European Respiratory Journal* 44 (2): 435–46. https://doi.org/10.1183/09031936.00007814.

[11] Diacon AH, Van de Wal BW, Wyser C, et al. 2003. "Diagnostic Tools in Tuberculous Pleurisy: A Direct Comparative Study." *European Respiratory Journal* 22 (4): 589–91. https://doi.org/10.1183/09031936.03.00017103.

[12] Engel, M E, P T Matchaba, and J Volmink. 2007. "Corticosteroids for Tuberculous Pleurisy." *The Cochrane Database of Systematic Reviews*, no. 4(October). England: CD001876. https://doi.org/10.1002/14651858.CD001876.pub2.

[13] Gopi, Arun, Sethu M. Madhavan, Surendra K. Sharma, and Steven A. Sahn. 2007. "Diagnosis and Treatment of Tuberculous Pleural Effusion in 2006." *Chest* 131 (3). The American College of Chest Physicians: 880–89. https://doi.org/10.1378/chest.06-2063.

[14] Hwang, Ki-Eun, Young-Jun Shon, Byong-Ki Cha, Mi-Jeong Park, Min-Su Chu, Young-Jun Kim, Eun-Taik Jeong, and Hak-Ryul Kim. 2015. "Tissue Inhibitor of Metalloproteinase-1 Is Responsible for Residual Pleural Thickening in Pleural Tuberculosis." *Tohoku Journal of Experimental Medicine* 235 (4): 327. https://doi.org/10.1620/tjem.235.327.Correspondence.

[15] Kawai, Vivian, Giselle Soto, Robert H Gilman, Christian T Bautista, Luz Caviedes, Luz Huaroto, Eduardo Ticona, et al. 2006. "Tuberculosis Mortality, Drug Resistance, and Infectiousness in Patients with and without HIV Infection in Peru." *The American Journal of Tropical Medicine and Hygiene* 75 (6). United States: 1027–33.

[16] Kim, Hee Joung, Hyun Ju Lee, Sung Youn Kwon, Ho Il Yoon, Hee Soon Chung, Choon Taek Lee, Sung Koo Han, Young Soo Shim, and Jae Joon Yim. 2006. "The Prevalence of Pulmonary Parenchymal Tuberculosis in Patients with Tuberculous Pleuritis." *Chest* 129 (5). The American College of Chest Physicians: 1253–58. https://doi.org/10.1378/chest.129.5.1253.

[17] Koegelenberg, Coenraad Frederik N., Elvis Malcom Irusen, Florian Von Groote-Bidlingmaier, Johannes Willem Bruwer, Enas Mansour A. Batubara, and Andreas Henri Diacon. 2015. "The Utility of Ultrasound-Guided Thoracentesis and Pleural Biopsy in Undiagnosed Pleural Exudates." *Thorax* 70 (10): 995–97. https://doi.org/10.1136/thoraxjnl-2014-206567.

[18] Lai, Y. F., M. C. Su, H. H. Weng, J. T. Wu, and C. T. Chiu. 2009. "Sonographic Septation: A Predictor of Sequelae of Tuberculous Pleurisy after Treatment." *Thorax* 64 (9): 806–9. https://doi.org/10.1136/thx.2008.110197.

[19] Maartens, G, and E D Bateman. 1991. "Tuberculous Pleural Effusions: Increased Culture Yield with Bedside Inoculation of Pleural Fluid and Poor Diagnostic Value of Adenosine Deaminase." *Thorax* 46 (2). BMJ Publishing Group Ltd: 96–99. https://doi.org/10.1136/thx.46.2.96.

[20] Michot, Jean Marie, Yoann Madec, Sophie Bulifon, Cécile Thorette-Tcherniak, Nicolas Fortineau, Nicolas Noël, Olivier Lambotte, et al. 2016. "Adenosine Deaminase Is a Useful Biomarker to Diagnose Pleural Tuberculosis in Low to Medium Prevalence Settings." *Diagnostic Microbiology and Infectious Disease* 84 (3). Elsevier Inc.: 215–20. https://doi.org/10.1016/j.diagmicrobio.2015.11.007.

[21] Pablo, Alicia De, Victoria Villena, José Echave-Sustaeta, and Angel López Encuentra. 1997. "Are Pleural Fluid Parameters Related to the Development of Residual Pleural Thickening in Tuberculosis?" *Chest* 112 (5): 1293–97. https://doi.org/10.1378/chest.112.5.1293.

[22] Pai, Madhukar, Laura L. Flores, Alan Hubbard, Lee W. Riley, and John M. Colford. 2004. "Nucleic Acid Amplification Tests in the Diagnosis of Tuberculous Pleuritis: A Systematic Review and Meta-Analysis." *BMC Infectious Diseases* 4: 1–14. https://doi.org/10.1186/1471-2334-4-6.

[23] Ryan, Hannah, Jinho Yoo, and Padmapriya Darsini. 2017. "Corticosteroids for Tuberculous Pleurisy." *The Cochrane Database of Systematic Reviews* 3 (March). England: CD001876. https://doi.org/10.1002/14651858.CD001876.pub3.

[24] Shaw, Jane A., Elvis M. Irusen, Andreas H. Diacon, and Coenraad F. Koegelenberg. 2018. "Pleural Tuberculosis: A Concise Clinical Review." *Clinical Respiratory Journal* 12 (5): 1779–86. https://doi.org/10.1111/crj.12900.

[25] Solari, Lely, Alonso Soto, and Patrick Van der Stuyft. 2017. "Performance of Clinical Prediction Rules for Diagnosis of Pleural Tuberculosis in a High-Incidence Setting." *Tropical Medicine and International Health* 22 (10): 1283–92. https://doi.org/10.1111/tmi.12932.

[26] Udwadia, Zarir F., and Tiyas Sen. 2010. "Pleural Tuberculosis: An Update." *Current Opinion in Pulmonary Medicine* 16 (4): 399–406. https://doi.org/10.1097/MCP.0b013e328339cf6e.

[27] WHO. 2017. "*Global Tuberculosis*." Geneva. http://www.who.int/tb/publications/global_report/en/.

[28] World Health Organization. 2017. *Guidelines for Treatment of Tuberculosis and Patient Care*. *Who*. Vol. 1. https://doi.org/10.1586/17476348.1.1.85.

[29] Alan, S Katz, Leonard Niesenbaum, and Burton Mass. 1989. "Pleural Effusion as the Initial Manifestation of Disseminated Cryptococcosis in Acquired Immune Deficiency Syndrome. Diagnosis by Pleural Biopsy." *Chest* 96 (August). Elsevier Inc.: 440–41. http://10.0.5.98/chest.96.2.440.

[30] Barlow D. 1954. "Aspergillosis Complicating Pulmonary Tuberculosis." *Proc R Soc Med 1954; 47(10):877.* 47 (10): 877.

[31] Bitar, Dounia, Olivier Lortholary, Yann Le Strat, Javier Nicolau, Bruno Coignard, Pierre Tattevin, Didier Che, and Françoise Dromer. 2014. "Population-Based Analysis of Invasive Fungal Infections." *Emerging Infectious Diseases* 20 (7): 1149–55. https://doi.org/10.3201/eid2007.140087.

[32] Crompton, J A, D Alexander, and T Somerville. 1900. "Lipid-Based Amphotericin in Pulmonary Zygomycosis : Safety and E⁄Cacy of High Exposure in a Renal Allograft Recipient." *Antimicrobial Agents and Chemotherapy.* United States 55 (5): 2478–80.

[33] Felton, Timothy, Peter F. Troke, and William W. Hope. 2014. "Tissue Penetration of Antifungal Agents." *Clinical Microbiology Reviews* 27 (1): 68–88. https://doi.org/10.1128/CMR.00046-13.

[34] Giamarellou, H, and A Antoniadou. 1996. "Epidemiology, Diagnosis, and Therapy of Fungal Infections in Surgery." *Infection Control and Hospital Epidemiology* 17

(8). Athens University School of Medicine, First Department of Propedeutic Medicine, Laiko General Hospital, Greece.: Cambridge University Press: 558–64.

[35] Ishiguro, Takashi, Noboru Takayanagi, Tomohiko Ikeya, Hiroaki Yoshioka, Tsutomu Yanagisawa, Eishin Hoshi, Toshiko Hoshi, Yutaka Sugita, and Yoshinori Kawabata. 2010. "Isolation of Candida Species Is an Important Clue for Suspecting Gastrointestinal Tract Perforation as a Cause of Empyema." *Internal Medicine (Tokyo, Japan)* 49 (18). Department of Respiratory Medicine, Saitama Cardio-vascular and Respiratory Center, Kumagaya. ishiguro.takashi@pref.saitama.lg.jp: Japanese Society of Internal Medicine: 1957–64.

[36] Jonathan, Meakins. 1994. *Surgical Infections : Diagnosis and Treatment.* New York : Scientific American, Inc., c1994.

[37] Ko, Shiann Chin, Kuan Yu Chen, Po Ren Hsueh, Kwen Tay Luh, and Pan Chyr Yang. 2000. "Fungal Empyema Thoracis: An Emerging Clinical Entity." *Chest* 117 (6): 1672–78. https://doi.org/10.1378/chest.117.6.1672.

[38] León, Cristóbal, Sergio Ruiz-Santana, Pedro Saavedra, Benito Almirante, Juan Nolla-Salas, Francisco Álvarez-Lerma, José Garnacho-Montero, and María Ángeles León. 2006. "A Bedside Scoring System ('Candida Score') for Early Antifungal Treatment in Non neutropenic Critically Ill Patients with Candida Colonization." *Critical Care Medicine* 34 (3): 730–37. https://doi.org/10.1097/01.CCM.0000202208.37364.7D.

[39] Lin, Kuo Hsi, Yuag Meng Liu, Po Chang Lin, Cheng Mao Ho, Chia Hui Chou, Jui Hsing Wang, Chih Yu Chi, Mao Wang Ho, and Jen Hsien Wang. 2014. "Report of a 63-Case Series of Candida Empyema Thoracis: 9-Year Experience of Two Medical Centers in Central Taiwan." *Journal of Microbiology, Immunology and Infection* 47 (1). Elsevier Taiwan LLC: 36–41. https://doi.org/10.1016/j.jmii.2012.08.010.

[40] Moriyama, Brad, Marisa Ditullio, Eleanor Wilson, Stacey A. Henning, Scott R. Penzak, Robert L. Danner, Gennethel Pennick, et al. 2011. "Pharmacokinetics of Anidulafungin in Pleural Fluid during the Treatment of a Patient with Candida Empyema." *Antimicrobial Agents and Chemotherapy* 55 (5): 2478–80. https://doi.org/10.1128/AAC.01560-10.

[41] Seero CB, Dall Bello AG, Oliveira Fde M, Guazzelli LS, Tregnago R, Haas M, Hochhegger B, Severo LC. etal, 2013. Pleural effusion an unusual feature of paracoccidioidomycosis: report of two new cases with a systematic review of the literature. *Mycopathologia.* 2013 Apr; 175 (3-4):323-30.

[42] Nigo, Masayuki, Macarena R. Vial, Jose M. Munita, Ying Jiang, Jeffrey Tarrand, Carlos A. Jimenez, and Dimitrios P. Kontoyiannis. 2016. "Fungal Empyema Thoracis in Cancer Patients." *Journal of Infection* 72 (5): 615–21. https://doi.org/10.1016/j.jinf.2016.02.014.

[43] Pauw, Ben De, Thomas J. Walsh, J. Peter Donnelly, David A. Stevens, John E. Edwards, Thierry Calandra, Peter G. Pappas, et al. 2008. "Revised Definitions of

Invasive Fungal Disease from the European Organization for Research and Treatment of Cancer/Invasive Fungal Infections Cooperative Group and the National Institute of Allergy and Infectious Diseases Mycoses Study Group (EORTC/MSG) C." *Clinical Infectious Diseases* 46 (12): 1813–21. https://doi.org/10.1086/588660.

[44] Samonis, G, A Gikas, P Toloudis, S Maraki, G Vrentzos, Y Tselentis, N Tsaparas, and G Bodey. 1994. "Prospective Study of the Impact of Broad-Spectrum Antibiotics on the Yeast Flora of the Human Gut." *European Journal of Clinical Microbiology & Infectious Diseases: Official Publication of the European Society of Clinical Microbiology* 13 (8). Department of Medicine, University of Crete, Greece.: Springer: 665–67. http://survey.hshsl. umaryland.edu/?url–http://search.ebscohost.com/login.aspx?direct=true&db=cmedm&AN=7813500&site=eds-live.

[45] Smith, Julian A., Michael H. Mullerworth, George W. Westlake, and James Tatoulis. 1991. "Empyema Thoracis: 14-Year Experience in a Teaching Center." *The Annals of Thoracic Surgery* 51 (1). Elsevier: 39–42. https://doi.org/10.1016/0003-4975(91)90443-T.

In: Pleural Effusions: Causes, Types and Treatment
Editor: Rahul Khosla
ISBN: 978-1-53614-683-7

Chapter 8

PLEURAL EFFUSIONS IN RHEUMATOLOGICAL DISEASES

Georges Al-Helou[1], MD and Rahul Khosla[1,2*], MD
[1]Pulmonary, Critical Care, and Sleep Medicine,
The George Washington University, Washington DC, US
[2]Pulmonary and CCM Section, Veterans Affairs Medical Center,
Washington DC, US

ABSTRACT

Rheumatologic diseases are a broad group of immune mediated systemic diseases that often involve the lung and pleura. Pleural involvement is usually a sign of diffuse systemic involvement and can change with disease activity. Rheumatological diseases as a cause for pleural effusions are rare accounting for around 1% of all effusions. The rheumatological diseases most commonly associated with pleuropulmonary involvement are: 1) Rheumatoid Arthritis, 2) Systemic Lupus Erythematosus 3) Granulomatosis with Polyangiitis (formerly called Wegner's Syndrome) 4) Churg-Strauss Syndrome. Pleural effusions due to other rheumatological diseases (such as Systemic Sclerosis, Sjogren's Syndrome, Polymyositis/Dermatomyositis and Sarcoidosis) are rare but can still occur. Even though these diseases are usually grouped together, they are a heterogeneous group with varying clinical manifestations. In this chapter, we will discuss the different presentations, epidemiology, clinical and radiological signs as well as laboratory analysis in each of these diseases. We will also discuss the management strategies currently available.

Keywords: connective tissue disease, rheumatological disease, inflammatory pleural effusions

* Corresponding Author Email: Rahul.khosla@va.gov.

INTRODUCTION

Rheumatologic diseases are a broad group of immune mediated systemic diseases with varying manifestations and disease course. These include Rheumatoid Arthritis (RA), Systemic Lupus Erythematosus (SLE), Scleroderma, Polymyositis/Dermatomyositis (PM/DM), Sjogren's Syndrome (SS), and Sarcoidosis. They often involve the lung and pleura, with different diseases causing different pulmonary manifestations, and can be the major cause of morbidity and mortality.

Pleural involvement is common in rheumatological diseases, however, they only account for around 1% of all pleural effusion [1, 2]. Pleural involvement is usually a sign of diffuse systemic involvement and can change with disease activity. The course of this effusion depends on the duration and severity of the inflammatory process and can lead to resolution of the effusion or pleural fibrosis. The rheumatological diseases that are most commonly associated with pleural effusions are SLE and RA, however, effusions can still be seen in other rheumatological diseases like SS, PM/DM, scleroderma and sarcoidosis.

In rheumatological diseases, the development of inflammation in the pleura and the subpleural tissue causes increased capillary permeability and increased fluid extravasation. This fluid then moves along pressure gradients from the interstitium into the pleural space thus causing pleural effusions [3]. This increased permeability is the result of multiple overlapping mechanisms that culminate in endothelial injury. These include immune complex deposition, immune cell infiltration and the release of cytokines and proteolytic enzymes from neutrophils and macrophages [3, 4].

SYSTEMIC LUPUS ERYTHEMATOSUS

Pleural involvement is common in Systemic Lupus Erythematosus (SLE) with 30-50% of patients developing pleural inflammation during the disease. However, only 5% of patients have pleural effusions on initial presentation [5, 6]. Although SLE is more common in women than in men (9:1), thoracic manifestations are more common in men [7]. Pleuritis and pleural effusions are included in the criteria for the diagnosis of SLE [8].

The most common pleural manifestation of SLE is pleuritis, characterized by the development of chest pain, fever, cough and dyspnea. The development of effusions in SLE is due to the inflammatory process in the pleura with immune complex deposition and activation of the complimentary cascade [3]. Pleural biopsies have shown lymphocyte and plasma cell invasion, as well as pleural cells with a specific nuclear immune fluorescence staining with anti-IgM, anti IgG and anti-C3 [9]. However, it could also be due to other causes like infection, renal and heart failure or pulmonary embolism [10]. Pleural effusions in SLE are characteristically bilateral, small and usually symptomatic on presentation [11]. Pulmonary disease is not typically present at the same time.

Fluid analysis shows exudative effusions with high protein (greater than 3.5 g/dL) normal pH and glucose with high anti-nuclear antibody titers (usually greater than 1:160) [6]. The high anti-nuclear antibody titers are suggestive of lupus exudates but can be seen in other diseases like lymphoma. Lactate dehydrogenase is usually less than 500 U/L and cell counts can range between 500 and 15,000 /μL mostly neutrophils and lymphocytes [12, 13]. The presence of lupus erythematosus cells is highly specific for the presence of lupus effusions; however, the sensitivity is low, and this test is rarely conducted due to the long processing time needed [11, 14].

Treatment of SLE associated pleural effusions differs based on the severity of symptoms and the presence of systemic manifestations. Most small asymptomatic effusions do not require treatment and will usually resolve spontaneously [6]. Mildly symptomatic patients with no other manifestations usually respond well to non-steroidal anti-inflammatory, while more severe cases or patients with systemic SLE manifestations will require treatment with corticosteroids or other immune suppressive modalities [2]. In refractory cases, talc, tetracycline and mechanical pleurodesis have been described [15, 16, 17].

Rheumatoid Arthritis

Rheumatoid arthritis (RA) is a chronic inflammatory disease that mostly affects the small joints usually of hand and feet. Up to 5% of patients develop pleural effusions making it the most common intra-thoracic manifestation of RA [18, 19]. Autopsy studies on patients with RA, have shown even higher incidence of pleuritis with up to 70% involvement, however, this involvement is usually asymptomatic or masked by immune suppressive therapy [20]. Pleural effusions are seen mostly in male patients with long standing history of active joint disease and rheumatoid nodules [10, 11]. However, pleuritis and effusion can occur before joint involvement is evident in up to 30% of patients [21, 22]. Genetic predisposition plays a role in the development of pleural effusions in RA as an association was found with HLA-B8 and HLA-Dw3 [23].

Pleural effusions associated with RA are usually unilateral in more than 70% of cases [24]. Furthermore, they are small to moderate in size and asymptomatic [6], but massive effusions have been described. Patients can present with chest pain, shortness of breath or asymptomatic with radiographic evidence of an effusion. RA effusions are waxing and waning in nature and tend to resolve spontaneously [1]. Unlike effusions in patients with SLE, RA effusions can be associated with underlying lung involvement in up to 30% of patients [25]. This is especially so when symptoms are out of proportion to size of effusion or if severe cough or dyspnea develop [2].

Fluid analysis shows exudative effusions with high level of and lactate dehydrogenase. Typically, chronic effusions have very low pH (<7.2), glucose levels (<50mg/dL) and complement levels, as well as elevated immune complexes. The low glucose is mostly due to the glucose consumption by the inflammatory cells and the pleura. The high level of anaerobic metabolism in the effusion leads to accumulation of lactate and low pH. Rheumatoid factor levels are usually elevated due to the production by pleural tissues and mononuclear cells in the effusion, however, this is not diagnostic of a rheumatoid pleural effusion. On the other hand, glucose and pH might be normal in acute effusions [26]. Adenosine deaminase can be elevated similar to tuberculous pleural effusions [27]. Cytology can be helpful in diagnosing rheumatoid pleural effusions. The characteristic cytological pattern seen in chronic rheumatoid effusions are giant multinucleated macrophages, elongated tadpole-like macrophages, and a necrotic background material in the absence of mesothelial cells [28]. However, neutrophils are more common in acute effusions.

Fluid appearance can vary between serous, cloudy, milky, greenish and rarely hemorrhagic appearance. Empyema can occur in RA due to either infection or the massive inflammatory reaction and fibrinous deposition. Necrosis of rheumatoid nodules can cause bronchopleural fistulae alongside the empyema. Chylothorax and pseudochylothorax have been described in rheumatoid arthritis effusions. They can occur in both acute and chronic effusions and are due to the high lipid levels with cholesterol levels above 1000 mg/dL and triglycerides above 110 mg/dL [29, 30]. There are multiple factors that cause these high levels of lipids and cholesterol. The breakdown of the neutrophils and other inflammatory cells releases lipids and cholesterol. These are not readily absorbed due to the thick inflamed and fibrotic pleura, as well as the occasional lymphatic obstruction from secondary amyloidosis.

Small asymptomatic effusions do not require intervention unless another diagnosis is suspected. These effusions will resolve over few weeks to several months. Large effusions can be treated with therapeutic thoracentesis and intra-pleural corticosteroid infusions [6]. Sometimes, systemic immune suppression may be necessary to control these large effusions. Refractory pleural effusions may require surgical intervention particularly in cases of trapped lungs or empyema. Decortication and pleurodesis may be considered if effusions persist despite intensive medical treatment. Pneumothoraces occur in up to 6% of patient from rupture of rheumatoid nodules and formation of bronchopleural fistulae. These can be difficult to treat and require several weeks to resolve despite chest tube placement. Open thoracotomy may be indicated in such cases [31].

Sjogren's Syndrome

Sjogren's Syndrome (SS) is a chronic inflammatory condition which can be seen in association with other connective tissue diseases as secondary SS or alone as primary SS. SS is an auto-immune disease characterized by lymphocyte infiltration of the exocrine glands and epithelium. Salivary and lacrimal glands are most commonly involved. Up to 60% of patients with SS will develop pulmonary complications however, pleural disease is uncommon and ranges between 1-2% of patients [1]. Most pleural effusions are seen in secondary SS in association with RA or SLE. Effusions in primary SS are rarely seen.

Pleural effusions can be unilateral or bilateral and pleural adhesions can develop. The effusions are exudative with a high number of B-lymphocytes. These lymphocytes are positive for CD-3 and CD-20. Glucose and pH are usually normal. Since SS patients are at risk of developing non-Hodgkin's lymphomas, pleural biopsies should be done in SS patients who develop effusions.

Pleural effusions in SS, like those of RA and SLE can resolve spontaneously or with corticosteroid treatment [2]. Complete resolution with immune suppressive treatment is the norm.

SYSTEMIC SCLEROSIS

Systemic sclerosis is a rare auto-immune disease that involves diffuse fibrous deposition in connective tissue and small blood vessels with eventual organ failure. There are various sub-types of systemic sclerosis each with its own diagnostic criteria. Although systemic sclerosis can affect the pleura, it causes more fibrosis than effusions. The latter only occur in up to 5% of patients and are more commonly seen in the diffuse cutaneous subtype and the scleroderma overlap syndromes [32]. It is frequently associated with pericardial effusion.

Systemic sclerosis associated effusions are usually exudative. However, transudative effusions can be seen especially in the presence of renal or cardiac failure. It is important to rule out infection as a cause especially that esophageal involvement can increase the risk of reflux and aspiration. Treatment of systemic sclerosis is often difficult with multiple medications used. The most commonly used drugs are corticosteroids and cyclophosphamide.

POLYMYOSITIS/DERMATOMYOSITIS

Polymyositis and dermatomyositis (PM/DM) are a group of rare auto-immune diseases that cause an inflammatory reaction in the skeletal muscles. They are associated with underlying malignancy and involve the proximal muscles preferentially. DM has more skin manifestations and less severe myopathy. Pulmonary manifestations occur in up to 50% of patients [1] most commonly interstitial lung disease and pulmonary hypertension. Pleural involvement is rare but can be seen in the setting of interstitial lung disease or infections (either because of immune suppression or aspiration). Given the association with malignancy, all patients with pleural effusions must undergo thoracentesis. Treatment for PM/DM associated effusions is usually with corticosteroids with or without other cytotoxic agents.

Granulomatosis with Polyangiitis (Formerly Called Wegner's Syndrome)

Granulomatosis with polyangiitis (GPA) is a chronic necrotizing small vessel vasculitis that involves the respiratory tract and kidneys preferentially. It is characterized by chronic granulomatous inflammation involving the small blood vessels that damages these vessels and causes ischemia and necrosis. Patients with GPA usually test positive for cytoplasmic anti-neutrophil cytoplasmic antibodies (c-ANCA) with most common protein target being proteinase-3. Respiratory system is frequently involved and ranges between 12 and 55% [33, 34]. Pathogenesis of effusions in GPA is not well understood and includes pleuritic inflammation with subpleural vasculitis causing pulmonary infarction, renal failure, heart failure and infections. Effusions in GPA are usually small and unilateral but bilateral effusions can occur. They are frequently exudative and non-hemorrhagic with a dominantly neutrophilic cell presence [35]. Pleural biopsies show acute or chronic fibrinous pleuritis with granulomas [33]. These effusions usually are small, asymptomatic and resolve spontaneously or with immunosuppression. The most commonly used medications are corticosteroids.

Churg-Strauss Syndrome

Churg-Strauss Syndrome (CSS) is a chronic auto-immune multi-system disease characterized by the triad of asthma, eosinophilia and vasculitis. Pathogenesis of the disease involves an eosinophilic and granulomatous inflammation in the small to medium blood vessels causing a necrotizing vasculitis mostly in the respiratory tract and kidneys. Patients with CSS usually test positive for Perinuclear Anti-Neutrophil Cytoplasmic Antibodies (p-ANCA). It is estimated that 30% of patients develop pleural effusions [36] mainly due to the increased vascular permeability and pulmonary infarction. Pleural fluids are usually bloody with a high eosinophil count. Pleural biopsies show eosinophilic infiltration with subpleural necrotizing vasculitis, pleural thickening, and adhesive pleuritis [36]. Pleural effusions usually respond well to corticosteroid treatment.

SARCOIDOSIS

Sarcoidosis is a chronic inflammatory disease that is characterized by non-caseating granulomas that involve multiple organ systems. Thoracic involvement is common, however, pleural effusions due to sarcoid are very rare [36]. The underlying pathogenesis of effusions in sarcoidosis is increased vascular permeability from active inflammation. These effusions are usually small and unilateral, but bilateral effusions can occur. These effusions are usually exudative with mostly lymphocytic infiltrates. The CD4/CD8 ratio is elevated like what is seen on broncho-alveolar lavage [37, 38]. Definitive diagnosis requires pleural biopsy showing non-caseating granulomas. These effusions can resolve spontaneously, but symptomatic effusions can be treated with corticosteroids with good response.

ADULT-ONSET STILL'S DISEASE

Adult-onset Still's disease (ASD) is a rare, multi-system auto-immune disease that was first described in 1971 [39]. The disease is characterized by high spiking fevers, arthritis and high ferritin. Pleuritis occurrence is very common and has been included in the diagnostic criteria for the disease [40]. Pleural effusions from ASD are usually bilateral and exudative. The most predominant cells present are neutrophils. Pericarditis is sometimes present simultaneously. These effusions improve with immune suppressive therapy.

CONCLUSION

Pleural effusions due to auto-immune rheumatological diseases are rare causing less than 1% of effusions. The most common pathological mechanism is through increased vascular permeability causing fluid extravasation into the interstitium. In turn, this fluid tracks along pressure gradients into the pleural space. These effusions are usually exudative, and they can resolve spontaneously or with immune suppressive treatment.

REFERENCES

[1] Frankel, Stephen K., and Kevin K. Brown. "Collagen vascular diseases of the lung." *Clinical Pulmonary Medicine* 13, no. 1 (2006): 25-36. doi:10.1097/01.cpm.0000197403.64631.de.

[2] Ferreiro, Lucía, José Manuel Álvarez-Dobaño, and Luis Valdés. "Systemic diseases and the pleura." *Archivos de Bronconeumología* (English Edition) 47, no. 7 (2011): 361-370. DOI: 10.1016/j.arbr.2011.02.009.

[3] Antony, V. B. "Immunological mechanisms in pleural disease." *European Respiratory Journal* 21, no. 3 (2003): 539-544. DOI: 10.1183/09031936.03.00403902.

[4] Halla, James T., Ralph E. Schrohenloher, and John E. Volanakis. "Immune complexes and other laboratory features of pleural effusions: a comparison of rheumatoid arthritis, systemic lupus erythematosus, and other diseases." *Annals of internal medicine* 92, no. 6 (1980): 748-752.

[5] Kamen, Diane L., and Charlie Strange. "Pulmonary manifestations of systemic lupus erythematosus." *Clinics in chest medicine* 31, no. 3 (2010): 479-488. doi:10.1016/j.ccm.2010.05.001.

[6] Porcel, José M., and Richard W. Light. "Pleural effusions." *Disease-a-Month* 59, no. 2 (2013): 29-57. DOI: 10.1016/j.disamonth.2012.11.002.

[7] Alarcon, G. S., A. W. Friedman, K. V. Straaton, J. M. Moulds, J. Lisse, H. M. Bastian, G. McGwin Jr, A. A. Bartolucci, J. M. Roseman, and J. D. Reveille. "Systemic lupus erythematosus in three ethnic groups: III A comparison of characteristics early in the natural history of the LUMINA cohort." *Lupus* 8, no. 3 (1999): 197-209. DOI: 10.1191/096120399678847704.

[8] Hochberg, M. C. for the Diagnostic and Therapeutic Criteria Committee of the American College of Rheumatology. "Updating the American College of Rheumatology revised criteria for the classification of systemic lupus erythematosus." *Arthritis Rheum* 40, no. 9 (1997): 1725. DOI: https://doi.org/10.1002/art.1780400928.

[9] Chandrasekhar, A. J., John Robinson, and Lewis Barr. "Antibody deposition in the pleura: a finding in drug-induced lupus." *Journal of Allergy and Clinical Immunology* 61, no. 6 (1978): 399-402. DOI: https://doi.org/10.1016/0091-6749(78)90120-3.

[10] Balbir-Gurman, Alexandra, Mordechai Yigla, Abraham Menahem Nahir, and Yolanda Braun-Moscovici. "Rheumatoid pleural effusion." In *Seminars in arthritis and rheumatism*, vol. 35, no. 6, pp. 368-378. Elsevier, 2006. DOI: https://doi.org/10.1016/j.semarthrit.2006.03.002.

[11] Bouros, Demosthenes, Ioannis Pneumatikos, and Argyris Tzouvelekis. "Pleural involvement in systemic autoimmune disorders." *Respiration* 75, no. 4 (2008): 361-371. DOI: 10.1159/000119051.

[12] Good, James T., Talmadge E. King, Veena B. Antony, and Steven A. Sahn. "Lupus pleuritis: clinical features and pleural fluid characteristics with special reference to pleural fluid antinuclear antibodies." *Chest* 84, no. 6 (1983): 714-718. DOI: https://doi.org/10.1378/chest.84.6.714.

[13] Keane, Michael P., and Joseph P. Lynch. "Pleuropulmonary manifestations of systemic lupus erythematosus." *Thorax* 55, no. 2 (2000): 159-166. DOI: 10.1136/thorax.55.2.159.

[14] Maskell, N., and R. Butland. "BTS guidelines for the investigation of a unilateral pleural effusion in adults." *Thorax* 58, no. Suppl 2 (2003): ii8. DOI: 10.1136/thorax.58.suppl_2.ii8.

[15] Kaine, JEFFREY L. "Refractory massive pleural effusion in systemic lupus erythematosus treated with talc poudrage." *Annals of the rheumatic diseases* 44, no. 1 (1985): 61.

[16] Loddenkemper, R., P. N. Mathur, P. Lee, and M. Noppen. "History and clinical use of thoracoscopy/pleuroscopy in respiratory medicine." *Breathe* 8, no. 2 (2011): 144-155. DOI: 10.1183/20734735.011711.

[17] Elborn, J. S., P. Conn, and S. D. Roberts. "Refractory massive pleural effusion in systemic lupus erythematosus treated by pleurectomy." *Annals of the rheumatic diseases* 46, no. 1 (1987): 77.

[18] Avnon, L. Sølling, M. Abu-Shakra, D. Flusser, D. Heimer, and N. Sion-Vardy. "Pleural effusion associated with rheumatoid arthritis: what cell predominance to anticipate?" *Rheumatology international* 27, no. 10 (2007): 919-925. DOI: 10.1007/s00296-007-0322-9.

[19] Cohen, Mark, and Steven A. Sahn. "Resolution of pleural effusions." *Chest* 119, no. 5 (2001): 1547.

[20] Baggenstoss, A. H. "Visceral lesions associated with chronic infectious (rheumatoid) arthritis." *Arch Pathol* 35 (1943): 503-516.

[21] Horler, A. R., and Malcolm Thompson. "The pleural and pulmonary complications of rheumatoid arthritis." *Annals of internal medicine* 51, no. 6 (1959): 1179-1203.

[22] Faurschou, P., D. Francis, and P. Faarup. "Thoracoscopic, histological, and clinical findings in nine cases of rheumatoid pleural effusion." *Thorax* 40, no. 5 (1985): 371-375. DOI: 10.1136/thx.40.5.371.

[23] Hakala, Markku, Anja Tiilikainen, Risto Hämeenkorpi, Jorma Ilonen, Seppo Jalava, Pekka Ruuska, and Reino Mäkitalo. "Rheumatoid arthritis with pleural effusion includes a subgroup with autoimmune features and HLA-B8, Dw3 association." *Scandinavian journal of rheumatology* 15, no. 3 (1986): 290-296. DOI: 10.3109/03009748609092595.

[24] Lillington, Glen A., David T. Carr, and John G. Mayne. "Rheumatoid pleurisy with effusion." *Archives of internal medicine* 128, no. 5 (1971): 764-768. Stanford, Ray E. "Rheumatoid and other collagen lung diseases." In *Seminars in Respiratory Medicine*, vol. 4, no. 02, pp. 107-112. DOI: 10.1001/archinte.1971.00310230094008.

[25] Stanford, Ray E. "Rheumatoid and other collagen lung diseases." In *Seminars in Respiratory Medicine*, vol. 4, no. 02, pp. 107-112.1982.

[26] Sahn, Steven A., Robin L. Kaplan, Robert M. Maulitz, and James T. Good. "Rheumatoid pleurisy: observations on the development of low pleural fluid pH and glucose level." *Archives of internal medicine* 140, no. 9 (1980): 1237-1238. DOI:10.1001/archinte.1980.00330200113031.

[27] Pettersson, Tom, Kaarina Ojala, and Theodor H. Weber. "Adenosine deaminase in the diagnosis of pleural effusions." *Journal of Internal Medicine* 215, no. 4 (1984): 299-304. DOI: https://doi.org/10.1111/j.0954-6820.1984.tb05011.x.

[28] Naylor, B. "The pathognomonic cytologic picture of rheumatoid pleuritis. The 1989 Maurice Goldblatt Cytology award lecture." *Acta cytologica* 34, no. 4 (1990): 465-473.

[29] Wrightson, John M., Andrew E. Stanton, Nicholas A. Maskell, Robert JO Davies, and YC Gary Lee. "Pseudochylothorax without pleural thickening: time to reconsider pathogenesis?" *Chest* 136, no. 4 (2009): 1144-1147. DOI: https://doi.org/10.1378/chest.09-0445.

[30] Calatayud, J., G. Candelas, A. Gómez, C. Morado, and F. Hernando Trancho. "Nodular pulmonary amyloidosis in a patient with rheumatoid arthritis." *Clinical rheumatology* 26, no. 10 (2007): 1797-1798. DOI: https://doi.org/10.1007/s10067-007-0552-y.

[31] Rueth, Natasha, Rafael Andrade, Shawn Groth, Jonathan D'cunha, and Michael Maddaus. "Pleuropulmonary complications of rheumatoid arthritis: a thoracic surgeon's challenge." *The Annals of thoracic surgery* 88, no. 3 (2009): e20-e21. DOI:10.1016/j.athoracsur.2009.06.093.

[32] Taormina, V. J., W. T. Miller, W. B. Gefter, and D. M. Epstein. "Progressive systemic sclerosis subgroups: variable pulmonary features." *American Journal of Roentgenology* 137, no. 2 (1981): 277-285. DOI: 10.2214/ajr.137.2.277.

[33] Bambery, P., V. Sakhuja, D. Behera, and S. D. Deodhar. "Pleural effusions in Wegener's granulomatosis: report of five patients and a brief review of the literature." *Scandinavian journal of rheumatology* 20, no. 6 (1991): 445-447. DOI: 10.3109/03009749109096825.

[34] Manganelli, P., P. Fietta, M. Carotti, A. Pesci, and F. Salaffi. "Respiratory system involvement in systemic vasculitides." *Clinical and experimental rheumatology* 24, no. 2 (2006): S48.

[35] Cordier, Jean-François, Dominique Valeyre, Loïc Guillevin, Robert Loire, and Jeanne-Marie Brechot. "Pulmonary Wegener's granulomatosis: a clinical and imaging study of 77 cases." *Chest* 97, no. 4 (1990): 906-912. DOI: https://doi.org/10.1378/chest.97.4.906.

[36] Joseph, Jose, and Steven A. Sahn. "Connective tissue diseases and the pleura." *CHEST-CHICAGO-* 104 (1993): 262-262.

[37] Huggins, John T., Peter Doelken, Steven A. Sahn, Lydia King, and Marc A. Judson. "Pleural effusions in a series of 181 outpatients with sarcoidosis." *Chest* 129, no. 6 (2006): 1599-1604. DOI: https://doi.org/10.1378/chest.129.6.1599.

[38] Groman, George S., Robert J. Castele, Murray D. Altose, James Scillian, Mary E. Kleinhenz, and Rolf Ehlers. "Lymphocyte subpopulations in sarcoid pleural effusion." *Annals of internal medicine* 100, no. 1 (1984): 75-76.

[39] Gerfaud-Valentin, Mathieu, Yvan Jamilloux, Jean Iwaz, and Pascal Sève. "Adult-onset Still's disease." *Autoimmunity Reviews* 13, no. 7 (2014): 708-722. DOI: http://dx.doi.org/10.1016/j.autrev.2014.01.058.

[40] Cush, John J., Thomas A. Medsger, Wallace C. Christy, David C. Herbert, and Lawrence A. Cooperstein. "Adult-onset still's disease." *Arthritis & Rheumatology* 30, no. 2 (1987): 186-194. DOI: https://doi.org/10.1002/art.1780300209.

In: Pleural Effusions: Causes, Types and Treatment ISBN: 978-1-53614-683-7
Editor: Rahul Khosla

Chapter 9

MISCELLANEOUS CAUSES OF PLEURAL EFFUSIONS

Kewakebt Lemma[1,*], MD, Ivana Milojevic[1], MD, Akshay Bhatnagar[1], MD and Rahul Khosla[2], MD

[1]Pulmonary, Critical Care, and Sleep Medicine,
The George Washington University, Washington DC, US
[2]Pulmonary and CCM Section, Veterans Affairs Medical Center,
Washington DC, US

ABSTRACT

Apart from the conventionally appreciated and commonly encountered etiologies of a pleural effusion, as discussed in other chapters of this book, there are numerous other less frequent, or miscellaneous scenarios which can result in the development of a pleural effusion that should be considered, depending on the appropriate clinical context. In some of these cases, a pleural effusion develops as a consequence of post-surgical injury and/or inflammatory response, while in other cases an effusion is just one clue towards diagnosis of an underlying syndrome.

Keywords: viral pneumonia, parasitic infections, pulmonary embolus, urinothorax, uremia, abscess, drug reaction

INTRODUCTION

Most transudative pleural effusions result from congestive heart failure, hepatic cirrhosis and hypoalbuminemia, whereas exudative pleural effusions are often linked to bacterial, fungal or tuberculous infection, connective tissue disease or malignancy. Pleural

[*] Corresponding Author Email: Lemmak@gmail.com.

effusions due to these causes, hemothorax and chylothorax are discussed in the preceding chapters. Section on pleural manometry reviews pathophysiology of trapped and entrapped lung, along with management of resulting pleural effusions. In this chapter, we focus on additional clinical scenarios in which pleural effusion(s) can present as an isolated finding, or part of a systemic process.

VIRAL PNEUMONIA

10-15% of small, exudative effusions that spontaneously resolve without a formal etiologic diagnosis could be due to a viral infection [1]. Convalescent antibody titers and viral cultures are not routinely performed in clinical practice because they seldom inform real-time clinical decision-making. Nucleic acid amplification tests for rapid simultaneous detection of multiple viral pathogens are changing the etiologic landscape of pneumonia and have potential to influence patient management [2–4]. Clinical context remains of utmost importance, because detection of viral genetic material in respiratory secretions does not prove causality. In fact, asymptomatic viral carriage, viral co-infection and bacterial superinfection should all be considered [5], making viral parapneumonic effusion still a diagnosis of exclusion. Moreover, currently commercially available multiplex nucleic acid amplification tests are not approved for use on pleural fluid specimens. Most effusions secondary to viral infection are small [6] exudative with mononuclear cell predominance [7]. Viral etiology of a given exudative pleural effusion typically portends an excellent prognosis and does not warrant aggressive drainage, if there is evidence of clinical improvement. Adenovirus is a prototypical agent for viral pneumonia complicated by simple pleural effusion. Hantavirus and dengue are endemic infections with systemic presentation including pleural effusions.

Adenovirus

Pleural effusion develops in around 10-40% of all adenoviral pneumonias, most commonly with serotypes 3 and 7 [8]. These are typically pediatric infections, although adults can be affected, especially the immunocompromised and hosts living in crowded conditions, such as, students and military recruits [9]. Adenovirus is known to cause focal or lobar consolidation (the typical manifestation of bacterial pneumonia) as its main imaging abnormality [10]. Life-threatening infections can be treated with ribavirin [11] or cidofovir [12].

Influenza Virus

Finding of a new pleural effusion during the course of influenza A infection classically points toward staphylococcal superinfection. It seems that pleural effusions in H1N5 influenza A (avian influenza) and H1N1 influenza A (swine flu) develop without bacterial co-infection and have a more benign clinical course [13, 14].

Hepatitis Viruses

Sympathetic pleural effusions develop in 14% of children with hepatitis A infection and should be managed conservatively [15]. Exudative pleural fluid accumulation has been reported in correlation with acute exacerbations of chronic hepatitis B [16]. Hepatitis B surface and e antigens, and intact viral particles can be detected in pleural fluid [17], rendering it infective with documented cases of needle stick injury transmission [18]. Chronic hepatitis C infection has been associated with primary effusion lymphoma in HIV negative, HHV-8 negative patients [19].

Latent Herpes Viruses

Cytomegalovirus (CMV), Epstein-Barr virus (EBV) and Herpes simplex virus (HSV) are usually directly implicated in pleural effusion development only after exhaustive workup has eliminated alternative causes. Clinical spectrum of primary infection can range from asymptomatic to severe systemic disease. Reactivation is typically seen in immunocompromised hosts and it is often challenging to differentiate among latent infection, low-level active infection, and true active disease.

CMV, the "troll of transplantation medicine" [20] and frequent opportunistic pathogen in AIDS exhibits significant pulmonary tropism. CMV pneumonitis can be accompanied by pleural effusions in 20-60% of cases in different series [21, 22]. CMV pneumonitis, a form of tissue invasive disease, is not a straightforward diagnosis, since virus is commonly shed in respiratory secretions of asymptomatic patients, making isolated positive culture or viral load difficult to interpret. On the other hand, histopathological pattern of CMV cytotoxicity may not be entirely specific. Gold standard diagnosis of CMV pneumonitis therefore requires 2 elements: positive viral load and/or viral culture and CMV inclusions and/or positive CMV specific immunohistochemistry staining on histopathology [23]. Isolation of virus from pleural fluid [24, 25] is reported more frequently than identification of CMV infected cells on pleural fluid cytology [26, 27].

After primary infection, EBV persists in the organism in latently infected memory B-cells with intermittent local oropharyngeal reactivation and shedding into saliva [28]. Systemic reactivation with lytic replication occurs in immunocompromised hosts. Interstitial pneumonitis has been associated with primary infection and chronic active EBV infection, both in children and in adults [29, 30]. Pleural effusions have been described during primary EBV infection [29]. EBV-DNA was detected in 40% of unselected pleural effusions and 59% of effusions of unclear etiology using real-time PCR [31]. 66% of patients had a positive effusion EBV-PCR with a negative serum EBV-PCR, suggestive of local reactivation of the virus in the pleural space [31]. EBV- DNA was also found in pleural fluid of 15% of patients with a clear alternative diagnosis behind the pleural effusion [31]. Two patients with the highest EBV viral loads died from unexplained interstitial pneumonia, likely EBV-related. It can be more difficult to discern whether low positive EBV-PCR results are caused by the mere presence of latently infected B-cells in the pleural fluid or actual viral lytic replication [31, 32]. The precise triggers of EBV reactivation in vivo are not known. Presumption is that reactivation occurs when latently infected B cells respond to another infection, given that B-cell receptor stimulation triggers reactivation in B-cell lines [33]. It is not known whether pleural mesothelial cells are susceptible to EBV infection [34]. Cytologically, polymorphous lymphocytosis is the most common feature, although mixed inflammatory or neutrophilic pattern can be seen as well as occasional mesothelial and/or lymphocytic atypia [34]. Despite the fact that no known effective treatment exists, one should consider EBV-DNA testing in all apparently idiopathic pleural effusions in order to possibly avoid additional invasive diagnostic procedures [34]. Due to its oncogenic potential, EBV infection has been associated with specific B-cell lymphomas such as primary effusion lymphoma, pyothorax-associated lymphoma [35] and primary pleural effusion post transplant lymphoproliferative disorder [36]. HSV pneumonitis can be associated with small pleural effusions [37].

Pleural Effusions in Patients with AIDS

Most effusions in hospitalized AIDS patients are a result of bacterial pneumonia or tuberculosis [38]. Pneumocystis pneumonia does not often present with pleural effusions [39]. Malignant effusions can be seen in human herpesvirus 8 (HHV-8)-associated malignancies affecting AIDS population: pleuropulmonary Kaposi Sarcoma (KS) [40], Primary Effusion Lymphoma (PEL) [41] and Multicentric Castleman's Disease (MCD) [42]. Finding of serosanguinous exudative mononuclear effusion in an AIDS patient with cutaneous KS is suggestive of pleural KS, while cytology and closed pleural biopsy are helpful in excluding alternative causes. Cytology is not confirmatory because KS diagnosis is based on tissue architecture, not a specific neoplastic cell type. KS does not affect parietal pleura, thus favoring thoracoscopy as means of examining the visceral pleura for characteristic violaceous lesions [40]. Chylothorax can result from thoracic duct involvement by KS [43]. PEL is a rare subtype of diffuse large B-cell lymphoma originnating on serosal surfaces that presents as lymphomatous effusion without an identifiable tumor mass. Hallmark of PEL is underlying HHV-8 infection, and, in most cases, EBV coinfection, implying viral cooperation in lymphoma genesis [44]. The key diagnostic criterion is the presence of HHV-8 in the nuclei of the malignant cells.

Parasitic Infections

Parasites like *Entamoeba histolytica, Echinococcus granulosus,* and *Paragonimus westermani* can sometimes involve the pleural space and should be considered when evaluating effusion, especially in areas where parasites are prevalent.

Amebiasis

Amebiasis is a common pathogen that can involve extra-intestinal organs. Liver abscesses are common and can cause the development of pleural effusion in one of two ways. The liver abscess can cause irritation of the diaphragm which can result in the development of reactive or sympathetic effusion. The abscess can also directly rupture across the diaphragm. Symptoms can be severe and can manifest as sepsis, shock, and respiratory failure [45]. The abscess is classically described as "anchovy paste" and has a dark brown appearance with low pH, low glucose, and high LDH. Amebic trophozoites are not always isolated from the fluid and culture is often negative unless superinfection occurs. Treatment is typically directed to treatment of the parasite.

Echinococcosis

Echinococcosis or Hydatidosis is a parasite infection secondary to the larvae of Echinococcus species. Humans are infected by consumption of particles that contain fecal material of an infected dog [46]. The most common organ involved is the liver, followed by the lung. Once infected, cysts form in the organ involved. The cysts formed in the lungs can rupture within the pleural cavity forming an eosinophil rich effusion. Treatment generally includes thoracotomy and percutaneous drainage if respiratory status is limiting. Targeted therapy of the parasite should also be included in conjunction with the above interventions [47].

Paragonimiasis

Paragonimiasis is a parasite infection caused by the lung fluke acquired via consumption of undercooked or raw crustaceans. It is commonly encountered in areas of Southeast Asia and can involve the lung in a variety of ways. It can present as hydro-pneumothorax or a simple pleural effusion in endemic regions. The effusion is typically exudative with eosinophil predominance, a low pH, low glucose and high LDH. Treatment includes fluid drainage and praziquantel [48, 49].

Subphrenic Abscess

Intraabdominal surgical procedures serve as the inciting event for approximately 80% of subphrenic abscesses, with splenectomy and gastrectomy usually leading to left-sided abscesses [50]. The remainder of the abscesses are a result of complications such as gastrointestinal perforation, cholecystitis, diverticulitis, pancreatitis, and trauma [51]. The pathophysiology of pleural effusion associated with sub-phrenic abscess is likely related to diaphragmatic inflammation. Pleural effusions are seen in 60-80% of patients with sub-phrenic abscess [52]. Analysis of the pleural fluid reveals an exudative process with predominantly polymorphonuclear leukocytes. Notably, it is very uncommon for the pleural fluid itself to become infected [53].

Esophageal Perforation

Esophageal perforation is most commonly iatrogenic in nature, encountered as a result of esophageal instrumentation. In terms of non-iatrogenic etiologies, spontaneous rupture (Boerhaave's syndrome), foreign body ingestion, trauma and malignancy are most frequent [54]. Injury to the intrathoracic esophagus will be the focus here, as it leads to contamination of the mediastinal cavity. In regard to spontaneous rupture, the injury typically affects the left posterolateral aspect of the distal intrathoracic esophagus, resulting in mediastinal emphysema and inflammation, with subsequent penetration of the overlying pleura. As the distal esophagus lies next to the left pleura, a pleural effusion develops on the left. On the other hand, injury to the midesophagus generally leads to a right-sided pleural effusion given that this part of the esophagus abuts the right pleura [55, 56]. Laboratory analysis of the pleural effusion may demonstrate the presence of undigested food, a low pH, and an increased salivary amylase level [57].

Pancreatic Disease

Pancreatitis is the most common gastrointestinal disease associated with pleural effusions. Other pancreatic diseases associated with pleural effusions include pancreatic abscess and chronic pancreatitis with pseudocyst. Lymphatic drainage is responsible for connecting pancreatic inflammatory fluid with the pleural space through the diaphragm, and thus a pleural effusion accompanying pancreatitis is exudative in nature [58]. Pancreatic inflammatory exudate is rich in pancreatic enzymes, and thus when the fluid reaches the pleural lymphatics, the permeability of the vessels is increased, and fluid leaks into the pleural space [59]. If thoracentesis is performed, then laboratory analysis reveals an elevated pleural amylase level that is higher than serum amylase level [59, 60], serosanguinous and sometimes bloody fluid, with a white blood cell differential predominantly polymorphonuclear leukocyte in nature. As the episode of pancreatic inflammation subsides, the pleural effusion usually resolves as well [61]. Pancreatic abscess usually results two to three weeks after an episode of acute pancreatitis, with the patient developing fever, leukocytosis, and abdominal pain. Pleural effusion occurs commonly in these patients [62]. On the contrary, pleural effusions are relatively uncommon (approximately 5 percent) in patients with chronic pancreatic pseudocyst [63]. In this case, as the pancreatic ducts are disrupted from inflammation and exudate is released, a direct sinus tract (pancreaticopleural fistula) develops between the pancreas and pleural space [64]. As in other pancreatic disease-related pleural effusions, the effusion is usually unilateral and left-sided with an elevated amylase of the pancreatic subtype [63].

Ovarian Hyperstimulation Syndrome

Pleural effusions can develop, albeit not very frequently, with ovarian hyperstimulation syndrome. The syndrome is a severe complication of the use of assisted reproduction technologies [65]. Fertility treatments result in overstimulation leading to cystic enlargement of the ovaries [66]. Enhanced vascular permeability ensues secondary to a variety of vasoactive factors, causing intravascular fluid to third space. Ovarian enlargement produces abdominal pain and third spacing of fluid causes ascites formation. Dyspnea may be present as a consequence of diaphragmatic restriction from ascites, or pulmonary edema or pleural effusion formation [65].

Meigs Syndrome

The diagnosis of Meigs' syndrome is clinical in nature and requires the presence of ascites, benign ovarian fibroma, and pleural effusion(s) [67]. Meigs' original description of the syndrome also included the stipulation that the patient should be cured with removal of the tumor; thus the importance of identifying the syndrome lies in the fact that the presence of pleural effusion and ascites henceforth did not necessitate that the accompanying pelvic mass had to be malignant [68]. Meigs' syndrome accounts for approximately 1% of ovarian tumors, the majority of the pleural effusions associated with the syndrome are right-sided, and patients most commonly present between the third and seventh decades of life. The exact pathogenesis of ascites and pleural effusion formation has yet to be determined, however, multiple hypotheses exist. Interstitial fluid may filter through the tumor capsule into the peritoneum and then into the pleural cavity via diaphragmatic defects versus lymphatic drainage [67]. Other theories center around increased capillary permeability with resulting third-spacing secondary to involvement by inflammatory cytokines [69] versus vascular endothelial growth factor [70].

URINOTHORAX

Urinothorax marks the presence of urine in the pleural space. It typically occurs secondary to obstructive uropathy or injury to the genitourinary (GU) tract [71]. Fluid is typically transudative, in most cases with a pH < 7.4 [72]. Elevated pH can be found if infection with an urea splitting pathogen occurs. Diagnosis is typically established by pleural fluid to serum creatinine ratio > 1 [73]. Additional diagnostic studies include CT and abdominal ultrasound to identify GU tract pathology. A technetium-99m renal scan confirms the diagnosis by demonstrating translocation of 99-Tc labeled albumin from the GU tract into the pleural space [74]. Management is typically by treating the underlying pathology i.e., addressing obstruction or repairing GU tract defects. Pleurodesis is generally not recommended [72].

POSTCARDIAC INJURY SYNDROME (PCIS)

Pleural effusions are common in pericardial diseases [75], either from contiguous spread of inflammation from pericardium to pleura or simultaneous pleuropericardial involvement by the same disease process [76]. PCIS accounts for immune-mediated pericarditis in the following clinical contexts: post pericardiotomy (coronary artery bypass grafting, valve surgery), post invasive cardiac interventions (percutaneous coronary intervention, ablation of arrhythmias, pacemaker implantation), after myocardial infarction (Dressler's syndrome) and after blunt or penetrating chest trauma [77]. In the era of aggressive cardiac revascularization, Dressler's syndrome is a rare occurrence and most PCIS cases are pericardiotomy related [76]. Initial injury of pericardium, pleura, or both, exposes pleuropericardial antigens and activates immune response, followed by the inflame-matory cascade. Prospective cohort substudy of the Colchicine for the Prevention of the Post Pericardiotomy Syndrome (COPPS) trial concluded that intentional or accidental pleural incision and manipulation during cardiac surgery may stimulate the immune response even more than pericardial incision itself [78]. Pleural effusions were noted in 62% of patients in Dressler's series [79] and 93% of patients in postpericardiotomy syndrome (PPS) series [78]. PCIS is associated with small, left-sided, lymphocyte predominant, exudative pleural effusions [80]. Treatment of PPS is empirical with aspirin and non-steroidal anti-inflammatory drugs, while corticosteroids are reserved for refractory cases [81]. Colchicine can also be used for PPS treatment [82] and prevention [81].

SUPERIOR VENA CAVA SYNDROME

Superior Vena Cava (SVC) syndrome is characterized by obstruction of SVC blood flow, either from extrinsic or intrinsic causes. Thoracic malignancies are most commonly implicated, followed by intravascular devices [83, 84]. Other benign causes include fibrosing mediastinitis, primary SVC thrombosis, aortic aneurysm and hematoma [83, 84]. During the past three decades benign etiologies have been on the rise, accounting for up to 40% of cases [83, 84]. Various intravascular devices are responsible for 70% of benign etiologies [83, 84]. Animal studies show that elevated hydrostatic pressure in the SVC results in pleural fluid accumulation [85, 86]. Similar concept was illustrated by case series of infants who developed pleural effusions after central venous catheter insertion [87]. In patients undergoing hemodialysis, ipsilateral recurrent effusions are described in context of subclavian vein stenosis [88]. Effusions in non-malignant SVC syndrome are traditionally considered transudative, resulting from increased venous hydrostatic pressure [89]. In patients with malignant SVC syndrome and exudative pleural effusion(s) it may be challenging to discern the exact etiology of the effusion, given relatively low sensitivity of pleural fluid cytology. In other words, effusion may be malignant in nature and unrelated to increase in hydrostatic pressure. In a large case series of 78 adults with SVC syndrome 44 patients (56%) developed pleural effusions, half of which were sampled. Most effusions were small and neither side was preferentially involved, with bilateral effusions in 39% of cases [83, 84]. Surprisingly, no transudates were documented regardless of etiology and all samples were exudative with or without a chylous component [83, 84]. Concealed malignancy, diuretic use and pulmonary emboli showers have been proposed to explain those findings, although the exact pathophysiology of exudative effusions in SVC syndrome remains unknown [90].

Chylous effusions are relatively common in SVC syndrome [83, 84], and are caused by the occlusion of lymphatic flow from hydrostatic pressure [85]. Non-traumatic rupture of the thoracic duct seems a less likely mechanism, as suggested by rapid resolution of chylothorax after SVC stenting [90].

PULMONARY EMBOLISM

Pulmonary embolism (PE) is a common cause of pleural effusion and can occur in up to 32-47% of patients who present with a PE [91]. The effusion occurs following a PE due to increase in permeability of the pulmonary vasculature and increased cytokine release [92]. If thoracentesis is performed, fluid studies almost always reveal an exudative effusion [93]. Cell count shows neutrophil or mononuclear cell predominance and typically also includes eosinophils and mesothelial cells. Pleural effusion associated with pulmonary embolism tends to be small in size and typically resolves with treatment of the PE. A bloody effusion is not a contraindication for anticoagulation unless fluids studies are consistent with hemothorax.

YELLOW NAIL SYNDROME

First described in 1964, yellow nail syndrome (YNS) is a very rare entity characterized by a triad of yellow thickened nails, lymphedema and pleural effusions.

The disorder can also be associated with upper and lower respiratory infections. The exact etiology remains unclear, however, it is believed that lymphatic drainage impairment might play a role in the pathogenesis. The estimated prevalence of YNS is <1/1,000,000. It typically presents as bilateral effusions in about 68.4% of the cases. Fluid appears to be serous but can also be milky or purulent in rare cases. Analysis of fluid shows a lymphocytic predominance [94]. Pleurodesis and decortication have been shown to be effective in majority of the cases. Pleural-peritoneal shuts have also been utilized but are less effective. In addition to this, the somatostatin analogue octreotide has been used for treatment of pleural effusions with some response. The mechanism is unclear but thought to be due to reduction of intestinal lipid absorption and ultimately triglyceride concentration in the thoracic duct. However, this does not explain the non-chylous nature of effusions present in most YNS patients [95].

GORHAM-STOUT SYNDROME

Gorham Stout syndrome is a rare disease which is also commonly referred to as "vanishing bone disease," "phantom bone disease" and "spontaneous bone absorption." Exact mechanism is unclear but thought to be due to proliferation of vascular and lymphatic capillaries resulting in destruction and resorption of surrounding tissue [96]. Involvement of the chest wall can lead to injury to the lymphatic system leading to chylothorax. Diagnosis is based on fluid analysis demonstrating elevated triglyceride levels. Management is typically with drainage and low fat diet. In addition, pegylated interferon alpha 2b has been used [97]. Use of propranolol has also been attempted in some patients who have been unable to tolerate other therapies with some promising result [98].

UREMIA

Pleural effusion is common among patients with End-Stage Renal Disease (ESRD). Hypervolemia is the most common cause and presents as a transudative effusion. Less commonly, uremia can cause accumulation of serosanguinous effusion. Uremic effusion is typically a diagnosis of exclusion since other common causes of effusion can also be seen with ESRD. The effusion is characteristically exudative and serosanguinous in appearance with lymphocyte predominance on cell count [99]. Pleural biopsy shows chronic fibrinous pleuritis [100]. Effusion typically resolves with drainage of effusion, however, surgical decortication might be required if the patient has persistent effusion or constrictive pleural thickening develops [101].

PERITONEAL DIALYSIS (PD)

Pleural effusion has been identified in up to 2% of patients who undergo peritoneal dialysis. Owing to the high concentration of glucose, it is also often referred to as "sweet effusion." It typically presents as a right sided unilateral transudative effusion and can occur at anytime after peritoneal dialysis has been initiated. The pathogenesis is not clear but could be due to a pleuroperitoneal defect. Thoracentesis reveals transudative effusion with low protein and high glucose. A glucose gradient of > 50 is diagnostic. In addition, peritoneal scintigraphy, CT peritoneography and MR peritoneography can be used to establish a diagnosis of pleuro-peritoneal leak. Management can include interruption of PD for a few weeks and also pleurodesis for definitive management if recurrent effusion is seen [102].

SARCOIDOSIS

The overall prevalence of pleural involvement in sarcoidosis (pleural thickening, pleural nodules, pleural effusions, and pneumothorax) is not low [103] but is hard to determine due to incomplete reporting, despite our ability to detect discrete lesions on high-resolution CT scans. Notably, pleural involvement usually does not translate into pleural disease, as most pleural lesions are clinically insignificant [103]. In clinical practice most diagnoses of pleural sarcoidosis are made in context of non-caseating granulomas present elsewhere, without pursuing pleural biopsy as ultimate proof [103, 104]. On the other hand, most patients with pleural effusions and noncaseating granulomas found on pleural biopsy in fact have tuberculosis (or fungal infection) rather than sarcoidosis, which should not be surprising if one considers prevalence of these diseases.

Prevalence of pleural effusions in patients with sarcoidosis is variably cited [103–106]. They are often unilateral, small-to-moderate in size, and rarely loculate [103]. Pleural fluid analysis typically shows an exudate, with CD4 T-lymphocytic predominance, and CD4/CD8 ratio ranging from 2.35 to 8.6 [103, 107, 108]. Pleural fluid CD4/CD8 ratios seem to correlate with bronchoalveolar lavage CD4/CD8 ratios [103, 107, 108]. Eosinophilic effusions [109] and chylothorax [110, 111] have also been reported.

Chylothorax can be associated with significant mediastinal and hilar adenopathy causing obstruction of the thoracic duct [111]. Presumed mechanism of effusion development in pleural sarcoidosis is obstruction of the lymphatic and venous drainage from pleural surface due to granulomatous inflammation. However, in rare clinical scenarios on the sarcoidosis spectrum such as SVC syndrome [112] or middle lobe atelectasis caused by an endobronchial lesion [113], effusions can develop without direct pleural involvement. In such cases, as well as in cardiac sarcoidosis with heart failure, pleural fluid may more often be transudative. From practical standpoint, even though effusions are no longer considered rare in sarcoidosis, any sizeable pleural effusion should not be automatically attributed to sarcoidosis, without diagnostic thoracentesis. Due diligence in exploring alternative causes, such as, heart failure, pneumonia and especially tuberculosis or fungal infection is strongly recommended [103, 104]. Clinical course of sarcoidosis-related effusions varies from spontaneous or steroid-induced resolution to progressive pleural thickening.

Radiation-Induced Pleural Effusions (RIPE)

Isolated pleural effusion or effusion associated with pleural thickening [114] represents a potential side effect of chest radiation therapy (CRT), a common treatment modality for lung, breast, esophageal cancer and Hodgkin's lymphoma. Radiation induced pleural effusion (RIPE) can be defined as a new effusion or increase in size of the existing effusion post CRT, in absence of underlying tumor progression [115]. Although RIPE definition varies across literature, it is typically assumed that such effusion is non-infectious and is not caused by the primary malignancy. Pathogenesis of RIPE is quite heterogeneous and not fully understood. Acute effusions typically appear simultaneously with radiation pneumonitis, commonly during breast cancer treatment [116]. Late developing effusions result from fibrosis of the pleural lymphatics, months after CRT completion. Cardiac toxicity often develops during esophageal cancer treatment [117]. Radiation effects on the heart seem to be dose-dependent and can be attenuated by concurrent ACE-inhibition [118]. Radiation induced pleural angiosarcoma with recurrent effusions has also been described [119]. Thoracentesis is not commonly performed due to small size of RIPE effusions. In a series of 34 patients who underwent CRT for lung cancer and subsequently developed RIPE, 26% underwent thoracentesis with fluid studies showing both exudative and transudative characteristics [120]. 12% of patients from the same series had a loculated pleural effusion [120].

Benign Asbestos Pleural Effusion (BAPE)

Benign Asbestosis Pleural Effusion is one of the pulmonary manifestations related to asbestos exposure. It can occur independently or in combination with other asbestos related pulmonary diseases [121]. Unlike other asbestosis related diseases, BAPE can occur early after exposure to asbestosis [122]. Presentation is non-specific and other etiologies have to be excluded before the diagnosis can be established. The effusion can remit spontaneously but drainage and pleurodesis might be considered for symptomatic treatment.

DRUG-INDUCED PLEURAL EFFUSIONS

Drug-induced pleural disease is relatively uncommon compared to drug-induced parenchymal lung disease [123]. The most common manifestation of drug-induced pleural disease is a pleural effusion which may be isolated, in combination with parenchymal lung involvement or part of a systemic process such as drug-induced lupus erythematosus (DILE), drug reaction with eosinophilia and systemic symptoms (DRESS), retinoic acid differentiation syndrome, capillary leak syndrome with IL-2 [124] or G-CSF [125], ovarian hyperstimulation syndrome (OHS). Patients on therapeutic anticoagulation for pulmonary embolism with infarction and those receiving adequate thrombolytic doses rarely develop spontaneous hemothorax [126–128]. Drug-related pleural fibrosis occurs less frequently with or without associated effusion. Pleural fibrosis is a prominent feature of amiodarone and ergot derivatives toxicity [129, 130]. Proposed mechanisms of drug-induced pleural toxicity include: chemical inflammation, hypersensitivity, fluid retention, oxidative stress [131]. Acute hypersensitivity reactions tend to occur within hours to days, whereas late toxicity presentations (months to years) are common with dose-related effects. To prove causal relationship between the drug and the effusion is often challenging. Detailed history including temporal association between drug exposure and symptom development is essential. The invariable first step is to exclude other reasonable causes, followed by drug discontinuation, and rechallenge. Resolution of pleural effusion with drug withdrawal and its recurrence after rechallenge is highly supportive of a drug-induced effusion, although no specific biologic markers are available to clinch the diagnosis. Except for overwhelming prevalence of exudates, pleural fluid characteristics are highly variable and non-specific, and rarely support the diagnosis beyond exclusion of alternative causes. Although pleural fluid eosinophilia is often regarded as a clue pointing towards drug-induced pleural disease, its presence or absence is non-specific [132]. If the cause of an exudative pleural effusion is not clinically obvious after initial workup including pleural fluid analysis, discontinuation of any suspicious drug should be considered, if clinically appropriate, to potentially avoid further invasive procedures [132, 133]. Clinical scenarios in which implicated drugs (cardiovascular agents, antibiotics, chemotherapeutics) are used to treat disease states frequently associated with pleural effusions are particularly difficult to decipher. There is scarcity of evidence in support of steroid rescue for refractory cases after drug withdrawal or if one is unable to discontinue the implicated drug due to lack of therapeutic alternatives [134–136]. Colchicine has anecdotally been used with success in a case of ergotamine-induced pleural and pericardial effusions [137].

Drug-Induced Eosinophilic Pleural Effusions

Eosinophil count of at least 10% of total nucleated cells constitutes an eosinophilic pleural effusion. Drugs aside, there are many different causes of eosinophilic effusions: pneumothorax, hemothorax, Hodgkin's lymphoma, pulmonary embolism with infarction, benign asbestos pleural effusion, parasitic and fungal infections [138]. Pleural fluid eosinophilia at initial thoracentesis should not be used as predictor of benign disease, since in some series malignancy was among leading causes [139, 140]. List of currently prescribed drugs that are implicated in development of eosinophilic pleural effusions in case reports/series is long: nitrofurantoin, penicillin, mesalamine, acyclovir, valproic acid, dantrolene, warfarin, diltiazem, propylthiouracil, isotretinoin [141–147] and ever growing. Nitrofurantoin, valproic acid, dantrolene and warfarin may also be associated with systemic eosinophilia [147, 148]. More than 60% of patients with daptomycin-induced eosinophilic pneumonia may present with pleural effusions [149]. Nitrofurantoin has been implicated in more than 2000 cases of pulmonary adverse effects [141]. Bilateral pleural effusions are never isolated and occur in about one third of patients with parenchymal involvement. Acute hypersensitivity reaction to nitrofurantoin is not dose-dependent whereas chronic pneumonitis and pleural fibrosis are time and dose-dependent. Whenever a pleural effusion increases in size during warfarin use, one should consider a warfarin-induced side effect in the differential [150].

Amiodarone

Pulmonary parenchymal and pleural toxicity are dose dependent [129]. Exudative effusions with lymphocytic predominance are not a prominent finding but may accompany interstitial infiltrates and pleural thickening [129]. Foamy macrophages similar to those seen in bronchoalveolar lavage samples may be present in pleural fluid [129].

Dasatinib

Tyrosine Kinase Inhibitors (TKI) imatinib, dasatinib and nilotinib are used for treatment of chronic myeloid leukemia (CML) and Philadelphia chromosome positive acute lymphoblastic leukemia (ALL), targeting BCR-ABL gene product. Dasatinib is the "dirtiest" TKI considering its off-target inhibition profile, while imatinib and nilotinib have a more limited range of protein kinase targets [151]. It does not seem surprising that clinical consequences of serosal inflammation, including pleural and pericardial effusions, have emerged as a frequent adverse event associated with dasatinib while occurring much less frequently (<1%) during imatinib [151, 152] and nilotinib [151, 153] therapy. Dasatinib is

[10] Tan D, Zhu H, Fu Y, et al. Severe Community-Acquired Pneumonia Caused by Human Adenovirus in Immunocompetent Adults: A Multicenter Case Series. *PloS One* 2016; **11**:e0151199.

[11] Yoon BW, Song YG, Lee SH. Severe community-acquired adenovirus pneumonia treated with oral ribavirin: a case report. *BMC Res Notes* 2017; **10**:47.

[12] Kim SJ, Kim K, Park SB, Hong DJ, Jhun BW. Outcomes of early administration of cidofovir in non-immunocompromised patients with severe adenovirus pneumonia. *PloS One* 2015; **10**:e0122642.

[13] Soepandi PZ, Burhan E, Mangunnegoro H, et al. Clinical course of avian influenza A(H5N1) in patients at the Persahabatan Hospital, Jakarta, Indonesia, 2005-2008. *Chest* 2010; **138**:665–673.

[14] McEwen RE, Scriven JE, Green CA, Bailey MS, Banerjee AK. Chest radiography findings in adults with pandemic H1N1 2009 influenza. *Br J Radiol* 2010; **83**:499–504.

[15] Kumar KJ, Kumar HCK, Manjunath VG, Anitha C, Mamatha S. Hepatitis A in children- clinical course, complications and laboratory profile. *Indian J Pediatr* 2014; **81**:15–19.

[16] Lee HS, Yang PM, Liu BF, et al. Pleural effusion coinciding with acute exacerbations in a patient with chronic hepatitis B. *Gastroenterology* 1989; **96**:1604–1606.

[17] Tabor E, Russell RP, Gerety RJ, Barker LF, Hillis WD, Jackson DR. Hepatitis B surface antigen and e antigen in pleural effusion: a case report. *Gastroenterology* 1977; **73**:1157–1159.

[18] Hess G, Dienes HP, Hess A, Arnold W, Meyer zum Bäuschenfelde KH. Transmission of hepatitis-B-virus by pleural effusion containing Dane particles. *Hepatogastroenterology* 1981; **28**:151–154.

[19] Dai H, Cherian R, Mathur S. Primary body cavity-based large B-cell lymphoma in an HIV and HHV-8 negative, HCV positive patient: a case report and literature review. *Lab Med* 2014; **45**:136–140.

[20] Balfour HH. Cytomegalovirus: the troll of transplantation. *Arch Intern Med* 1979; **139**:279–280.

[21] Abe K, Suzuki K, Kamata N, et al. [High-resolution CT findings in cytomegalovirus pneumonitis after bone marrow transplantation]. *Nihon Igaku Hoshasen Gakkai Zasshi Nippon Acta Radiol* 1998; **58**:7–11.

[22] Moon JH, Kim EA, Lee KS, Kim TS, Jung KJ, Song JH. Cytomegalovirus pneumonia: high-resolution CT findings in ten non-AIDS immunocompromised patients. *Korean J Radiol* 2000; **1**:73–78.

[23] Kotton CN, Kumar D, Caliendo AM, et al. The Third International Consensus Guidelines on the Management of Cytomegalovirus in Solid-organ Transplantation. *Transplantation* 2018; **102**:900–931.

[24] Rees AP, Meadors M, Ventura HO, Pankey GA. Diagnosis of disseminated cytomegalovirus infection and pneumonitis in a heart transplant recipient by skin biopsy: case report. *J Heart Lung Transplant Off Publ Int Soc Heart Transplant* 1991; **10**:329–332.

[25] Friedman HM, Grossman RA, Plotkin SA, Perloff LJ, Barker CF. Relapse of pneumonia caused by cytomegalovirus in two recipients of renal transplants. *J Infect Dis* 1979; **139**:465–473.

[26] Delfs-Jegge S, Dalquen P, Hurwitz N. Cytomegalovirus-infected cells in a pleural effusion from an acquired immunodeficiency syndrome patient. A case report. *Acta Cytol* 1994; **38**:70–72.

[27] Goodman ZD, Gupta PK, Frost JK, Erozan YS. Cytodiagnosis of viral infections in body cavity fluids. *Acta Cytol* 1979; **23**:204–208.

[28] Babcock GJ, Decker LL, Volk M, Thorley-Lawson DA. EBV persistence in memory B cells in vivo. *Immunity* 1998; **9**:395–404.

[29] Alpert G, Fleisher GR. Complications of infection with Epstein-Barr virus during childhood: a study of children admitted to the hospital. *Pediatr Infect Dis* 1984; **3**:304–307.

[30] Kimura H, Hoshino Y, Kanegane H, et al. Clinical and virologic characteristics of chronic active Epstein-Barr virus infection. *Blood* 2001; **98**:280–286.

[31] Thijsen SFT, Luderer R, van Gorp JMH, Oudejans SJG, Bossink AWJ. A possible role for Epstein-Barr virus in the pathogenesis of pleural effusion. *Eur Respir J* 2005; **26**:662–666.

[32] Martró E, Ausina V. The role of Epstein-Barr virus in pleural effusions of unknown aetiology: an interesting clinical perspective. *Eur Respir J* 2005; **26**:566–568.

[33] Odumade OA, Hogquist KA, Balfour HH. Progress and problems in understanding and managing primary Epstein-Barr virus infections. *Clin Microbiol Rev* 2011; **24**:193–209.

[34] Takei H, Mody D. Epstein-Barr virus-positive pleural effusion: Clinical features, cytomorphologic characteristics, and flow cytometric immunophenotyping. *Am J Clin Pathol* 2014; **142**:788–794.

[35] Nakatsuka S-I, Yao M, Hoshida Y, Yamamoto S, Iuchi K, Aozasa K. Pyothorax-associated lymphoma: a review of 106 cases. *J Clin Oncol Off J Am Soc Clin Oncol* 2002; **20**:4255–4260.

[36] Ohori NP, Whisnant RE, Nalesnik MA, Swerdlow SH. Primary pleural effusion posttransplant lymphoproliferative disorder: Distinction from secondary involvement and effusion lymphoma. *Diagn Cytopathol* 2001; **25**:50–53.

[37] Umans U, Golding RP, Duraku S, Manoliu RA. Herpes simplex virus 1 pneumonia: conventional chest radiograph pattern. *Eur Radiol* 2001; **11**:990–994.

[38] Joseph J, Strange C, Sahn SA. Pleural effusions in hospitalized patients with AIDS. *Ann Intern Med* 1993; **118**:856–859.

[39] Horowitz ML, Schiff M, Samuels J, Russo R, Schnader J. Pneumocystis carinii pleural effusion. Pathogenesis and pleural fluid analysis. *Am Rev Respir Dis* 1993; **148**:232–234.

[40] O'Brien RF, Cohn DL. Serosanguineous pleural effusions in AIDS-associated Kaposi's sarcoma. *Chest* 1989; **96**:460–466.

[41] Nador RG, Cesarman E, Chadburn A, et al. Primary effusion lymphoma: a distinct clinicopathologic entity associated with the Kaposi's sarcoma-associated herpes virus. *Blood* 1996; **88**:645–656.

[42] Guihot A, Couderc L-J, Agbalika F, et al. Pulmonary manifestations of multicentric Castleman's disease in HIV infection: a clinical, biological and radiological study. *Eur Respir J* 2005; **26**:118–125.

[43] Judson MA, Postic B. Chylothorax in a patient with AIDS and Kaposi's sarcoma. *South Med J* 1990; **83**:322–324.

[44] Gloghini A, Volpi CC, Gualeni AV, et al. Multiple viral infections in primary effusion lymphoma: a model of viral cooperation in lymphomagenesis. *Expert Rev Hematol* 2017; **10**:505–514.

[45] Aggarwal R, Aggarwal M, Dwivedi S. Giant liver abscess with bilateral pleural effusion: An unfamiliar association. *Trop Parasitol* 2012; **2**:129–130.

[46] Morar R, Feldman C. Pulmonary echinococcosis. *Eur Respir J* 2003; **21**:1069–1077.

[47] Arıbaş BK, Dingil G, Köroğlu M, Ungül U, Zaralı AC. Liver hydatid cyst with transdiaphragmatic rupture and lung hydatid cyst ruptured into bronchi and pleural space. *Cardiovasc Intervent Radiol* 2011; **34** Suppl 2:S260-265.

[48] Vidamaly S, Choumlivong K, Keolouangkhot V, Vannavong N, Kanpittaya J, Strobel M. Paragonimiasis: a common cause of persistent pleural effusion in Lao PDR. *Trans R Soc Trop Med Hyg* 2009; **103**:1019–1023.

[49] DTM&H WPMDsDHCRDPF, FRCPE GPMMCDpF, Pasvol G. *Tropical Medicine and Parasitology*. 5 edition. London: Mosby; 2002.

[50] Connell TR, Stephens DH, Carlson HC, Brown ML. Upper abdominal abscess: a continuing and deadly problem. *AJR Am J Roentgenol* 1980; **134**:759–765.

[51] Sherman NJ, Davis JR, Jesseph JE. Subphrenic abscess. A continuing hazard. *Am J Surg* 1969; **117**:117–123.

[52] van der Sluis RF. Subphrenic abscess. *Surg Gynecol Obstet* 1984; **158**:427–430.

[53] Carter R, Brewer LA. Subphrenic abscess: a thoracoabdominal clinical complex: the changing picture with antibiotics. *Am J Surg* 1964; **108**:165–174.

[54] Brinster CJ, Singhal S, Lee L, Marshall MB, Kaiser LR, Kucharczuk JC. Evolving options in the management of esophageal perforation. *Ann Thorac Surg* 2004; **77**:1475–1483.

[55] Razi E, Davoodabadi A, Razi A. Spontaneous esophageal perforation presenting as a right-sided pleural effusion: a case report. *Tanaffos* 2013; **12**:53–57.

[56] Katsetos MC, Tagbo AC, Lindberg MP, Rosson RS. Esophageal perforation and mediastinitis from fish bone ingestion. *South Med J* 2003; **96**:516–520.

[57] Porcel JM, Light RW. Diagnostic approach to pleural effusion in adults. *Am Fam Physician* 2006; **73**:1211–1220.

[58] Gumaste V, Singh V, Dave P. Significance of pleural effusion in patients with acute pancreatitis. *Am J Gastroenterol* 1992; **87**:871–874.

[59] Kaye MD. Pleuropulmonary complications of pancreatitis. *Thorax* 1968; **23**:297–306.

[60] Roseman DM, Kowlessar OD, Sleisenger MH. Pulmonary manifestations of pancreatitis. *N Engl J Med* 1960; **263**:294–296.

[61] Light RW, Ball WC. Glucose and amylase in pleural effusions. *JAMA* 1973; **225**:257–260.

[62] Miller TA, Lindenauer SM, Frey CF, Stanley JC. Proceedings: Pancreatic abscess. *Arch Surg Chic Ill 1960* 1974; **108**:545–551.

[63] Rockey DC, Cello JP. Pancreaticopleural fistula. Report of 7 patients and review of the literature. *Medicine* (Baltimore) 1990; **69**:332–344.

[64] Anderson WJ, Skinner DB, Zuidema GD, Cameron JL. Chronic pancreatic pleural effusions. *Surg Gynecol Obstet* 1973; **137**:827–830.

[65] Kumar P, Sait SF, Sharma A, Kumar M. Ovarian hyperstimulation syndrome. *J Hum Reprod Sci* 2011; **4**:70–75.

[66] Whelan JG, Vlahos NF. The ovarian hyperstimulation syndrome. *Fertil Steril* 2000; **73**:883–896.

[67] Saha S, Robertson M. Meigs' and Pseudo-Meigs' syndrome. *Australas J Ultrasound Med* 2012; **15**:29–31.

[68] Meigs JV, Cass JW. Fibroma of the Ovary with Ascites and Hydrothorax: With a Report of Seven Cases. *Am J Obstet Gynecol* 1937; **33**:249–267.

[69] Abramov Y, Anteby SO, Fasouliotis SJ, Barak V. The role of inflammatory cytokines in Meigs' syndrome. *Obstet Gynecol* 2002; **99**:917–919.

[70] Ishiko O, Yoshida H, Sumi T, Hirai K, Ogita S. Vascular endothelial growth factor levels in pleural and peritoneal fluid in Meigs' syndrome. *Eur J Obstet Gynecol Reprod Biol* 2001; **98**:129–130.

[71] Garcia-Pachon E, Romero S. Urinothorax: a new approach. *Curr Opin Pulm Med* 2006; **12**:259–263.

[72] Austin A, Jogani SN, Brasher PB, Argula RG, Huggins JT, Chopra A. The Urinothorax: A Comprehensive Review With Case Series. *Am J Med Sci* 2017; **354**:44–53.

[73] Stark DD, Shanes JG, Baron RL, Koch DD. Biochemical features of urinothorax. *Arch Intern Med* 1982; **142**:1509–1511.

[74] Bhattacharya A, Venkataramarao SH, Kumar S, Mittal BR. Urinothorax demonstrated on 99mTc ethylene dicysteine renal scintigraphy. *Nephrol Dial Transplant Off Publ Eur Dial Transpl Assoc - Eur Ren Assoc* 2007; **22**:1782–1783.

[75] Porcel JM, Esquerda A, Vives M, Bielsa S. Etiology of pleural effusions: analysis of more than 3,000 consecutive thoracenteses. *Arch Bronconeumol* 2014; **50**:161–165.

[76] Porcel JM. Pleural effusions in acute idiopathic pericarditis and postcardiac injury syndrome. *Curr Opin Pulm Med* 2017; **23**:346–350.

[77] Khan AH. The postcardiac injury syndromes. *Clin Cardiol* 1992; **15**:67–72.

[78] Imazio M, Brucato A, Rovere ME, et al. Contemporary features, risk factors, and prognosis of the post-pericardiotomy syndrome. *Am J Cardiol* 2011; **108**:1183–1187.

[79] Dressler W. The post-myocardial-infarction syndrome: a report on forty-four cases. *AMA Arch Intern Med* 1959; **103**:28–42.

[80] Bielsa S, Corral E, Bagüeste P, Porcel JM. Characteristics of Pleural Effusions in Acute Idiopathic Pericarditis and Post–Cardiac Injury Syndrome. *Ann Am Thorac Soc* 2016; **13**:298–300.

[81] Imazio M, Trinchero R, Brucato A, et al. COlchicine for the Prevention of the Post-pericardiotomy Syndrome (COPPS): a multicentre, randomized, double-blind, placebo-controlled trial. *Eur Heart J* 2010; **31**:2749–2754.

[82] Molad Y. Update on colchicine and its mechanism of action. *Curr Rheumatol Rep* 2002; **4**:252–256.

[83] Rice TW, Rodriguez RM, Light RW. The superior vena cava syndrome: clinical characteristics and evolving etiology. *Medicine* (Baltimore) 2006; **85**:37–42.

[84] Rice TW, Rodriguez RM, Barnette R, Light RW. Prevalence and characteristics of pleural effusions in superior vena cava syndrome. *Respirol Carlton Vic* 2006; **11**:299–305.

[85] Blalock A, Cunningham RS, Robinson CS. Experimental production of chylothorax by occlusion of the superior vena cava. *Ann Surg* 1936; **104**:359–364.

[86] Allen SJ, Laine GA, Drake RE, Gabel JC. Superior vena caval pressure elevation causes pleural effusion formation in sheep. *Am J Physiol* 1988; **255**:H492-495.

[87] Dhande V, Kattwinkel J, Alford B. Recurrent bilateral pleural effusions secondary to superior vena cava obstruction as a complication of central venous catheterization. *Pediatrics* 1983; **72**:109–113.

[88] Muthuswamy P, Alausa M, Reilly B. Clinical problem-solving. The effusion that would not go away. *N Engl J Med* 2001; **345**:756–759.

[89] Good JT, Moore JB, Fowler AA, Sahn SA. Superior vena cava syndrome as a cause of pleural effusion. *Am Rev Respir Dis* 1982; **125**:246–247.

[90] Rice TW. Pleural effusions in superior vena cava syndrome: prevalence, characteristics, and proposed pathophysiology. *Curr Opin Pulm Med* 2007; **13**:324–327.

[91] Porcel JM, Madroñero AB, Pardina M, Vives M, Esquerda A, Light RW. Analysis of pleural effusions in acute pulmonary embolism: radiological and pleural fluid data from 230 patients. *Respirol Carlton Vic* 2007; **12**:234–239.

[92] Light RW. Pleural effusion due to pulmonary emboli. *Curr Opin Pulm Med* 2001; **7**:198–201.

[93] Romero Candeira S, Hernández Blasco L, Soler MJ, Muñoz A, Aranda I. Biochemical and cytologic characteristics of pleural effusions secondary to pulmonary embolism. *Chest* 2002; **121**:465–469.

[94] Valdés L, Huggins JT, Gude F, et al. Characteristics of patients with yellow nail syndrome and pleural effusion. *Respirol Carlton Vic* 2014; **19**:985–992.

[95] Brooks KG, Echevarria C, Cooper D, Bourke SC. Case-based discussion from North Tyneside General Hospital: somatostatin analogues in yellow nail syndrome associated with recurrent pleural effusions. *Thorax* 2014; **69**:967–968.

[96] Nikolaou VS, Chytas D, Korres D, Efstathopoulos N. Vanishing bone disease (Gorham-Stout syndrome): A review of a rare entity. *World J Orthop* 2014; **5**:694–698.

[97] Hagberg H, Lamberg K, Aström G. Alpha-2b interferon and oral clodronate for Gorham's disease. *Lancet Lond Engl* 1997; **350**:1822–1823.

[98] Nir V, Guralnik L, Livnat G, et al. Propranolol as a treatment option in Gorham-Stout syndrome: a case report. *Pediatr Pulmonol* 2014; **49**:417–419.

[99] Berger HW, Rammohan G, Neff MS, Buhain WJ. Uremic pleural effusion. A study in 14 patients on chronic dialysis. *Ann Intern Med* 1975; **82**:362–364.

[100] Agustí C, Campistol JM, Xaubet A, et al. [Characteristics and evolution of uremic pleural effusion]. *Med Clin (Barc)* 1988; **90**:693–695.

[101] Maher JF. Uremic pleuritis. *Am J Kidney Dis Off J Natl Kidney Found* 1987; **10**:19–22.

[102] Chow KM, Szeto CC, Li PK-T. Management options for hydrothorax complicating peritoneal dialysis. *Semin Dial* 2003; **16**:389–394.

[103] Soskel NT, Sharma OP. Pleural involvement in sarcoidosis. *Curr Opin Pulm Med* 2000; **6**:455–468.

[104] Soskel NT, Sharma OP. Pleural Involvement in Sarcoidosis: Case Presentation and Detailed Review of the Literature. *Semin Respir Med* 1992; **13**:492–514.

[105] Iyer S, Afshar K, Sharma OP. Peritoneal and pleural sarcoidosis: an unusual association - review and clinical report. *Curr Opin Pulm Med* 2008; **14**:481–487.

[106] Chusid EL, Siltzbach LE. Sarcoidosis of the pleura. *Ann Intern Med* 1974; **81**:190–194.

[107] Flammang d'Ortho MP, Cadranel J, Milleron BJ, Akoun GM. Pleural, alveolar and blood T-lymphocyte subsets in pleuropulmonary sarcoidosis. *Chest* 1990; **98**:782–783.

[108] Mizushima Y, Sassa K, Fujishita T, Iwai H, Yasumura S, Kobayashi M. Sarcoidosis accompanied by pleural effusion and multiple bronchial stenoses. *Intern Med Tokyo Jpn* 1997; **36**:637–639.

[109] Tudela P, Haro M, Martí S, Roig J. [Eosinophilic pleuritis as the presenting form of sarcoidosis]. *Med Clin (Barc)* 1992; **99**:558.

[110] Jarman PR, Whyte MK, Sabroe I, Hughes JM. Sarcoidosis presenting with chylothorax. *Thorax* 1995; **50**:1324–1325.

[111] Lengyel RJ, Shanley DJ. Recurrent chylothorax associated with sarcoidosis. *Hawaii Med J* 1995; **54**:817–818.

[112] Gordonson J, Trachtenberg S, Sargent EN. Superior vena cava obstruction due to sarcoidosis. *Chest* 1973; **63**:292–293.

[113] Poe RH. Middle-lobe atelectasis due to sarcoidosis with pleural effusion. *N Y State J Med* 1978; **78**:2095–2097.

[114] Veiga C, Landau D, McClelland JR, et al. Long term radiological features of radiation-induced lung damage. *Radiother Oncol J Eur Soc Ther Radiol Oncol* 2018; **126**:300–306.

[115] Zhao J, Day RM, Jin J-Y, et al. Thoracic radiation-induced pleural effusion and risk factors in patients with lung cancer. *Oncotarget* 2017; **8**:97623–97632.

[116] Hietala SO, Hahn P. Pulmonary radiation reaction in the treatment of carcinoma of the breast. *Radiography* 1976; **42**:225–230.

[117] Shirai K, Tamaki Y, Kitamoto Y, et al. Dose-volume histogram parameters and clinical factors associated with pleural effusion after chemoradiotherapy in esophageal cancer patients. *Int J Radiat Oncol Biol Phys* 2011; **80**:1002–1007.

[118] van der Veen SJ, Ghobadi G, de Boer RA, et al. ACE inhibition attenuates radiation-induced cardiopulmonary damage. *Radiother Oncol J Eur Soc Ther Radiol Oncol* 2015; **114**:96–103.

[119] Miller R, Mudambi L, Vial MR, Kalhor N, Grosu HB. Radiation-induced Angiosarcoma as a Cause of Pleural Effusion. *Am J Respir Crit Care Med* 2017; **196**:e10–e11.

[120] Deek MP, Nagarajan S, Kim S, et al. Clinical characteristics and dose-volume histogram parameters associated with the development of pleural effusions in non-small cell lung cancer patients treated with chemoradiation therapy. *Acta Oncol Stockh Swed* 2016; **55**:1029–1035.

[121] Fujimoto N, Gemba K, Aoe K, et al. Clinical Investigation of Benign Asbestos Pleural Effusion. *Pulm Med* 2015; **2015**:416179.

[122] American Thoracic Society. Diagnosis and initial management of nonmalignant diseases related to asbestos. *Am J Respir Crit Care Med* 2004; **170**:691–715.

[123] Cooper JA, White DA, Matthay RA. Drug-induced pulmonary disease. Part 2: Noncytotoxic drugs. *Am Rev Respir Dis* 1986; **133**:488–505.

[124] Vogelzang PJ, Bloom SM, Mier JW, Atkins MB. Chest roentgenographic abnormalities in IL-2 recipients. Incidence and correlation with clinical parameters. *Chest* 1992; **101**:746–752.

[125] Vial T, Descotes J. Clinical toxicity of cytokines used as haemopoietic growth factors. *Drug Saf* 1995; **13**:371–406.

[126] Ganguli A, Walker L, FitzGerald RJ, Pirmohamed M. Spontaneous hemothorax following anticoagulation with low-molecular-weight heparin. *Ann Pharmacother* 2009; **43**:1528–1531.

[127] Varnholt V, Ringe H, Nietsch L, Gaedicke G. Hemothorax under thrombolytic therapy with recombinant tissue: plasminogen activator (rt-PA) in a 16-year-old girl. *Eur J Pediatr* 1999; **158 Suppl 3**:S140-142.

[128] Simon HB, Daggett WM, DeSanctis RW. Hemothorax as a complication of anticoagulant therapy in the presence of pulmonary infarction. *JAMA* 1969; **208**:1830–1834.

[129] Stein B, Zaatari GS, Pine JR. Amiodarone pulmonary toxicity. Clinical, cytologic and ultrastructural findings. *Acta Cytol* 1987; **31**:357–361.

[130] McElvaney NG, Wilcox PG, Churg A, Fleetham JA. Pleuropulmonary disease during bromocriptine treatment of Parkinson's disease. *Arch Intern Med* 1988; **148**:2231–2236.

[131] Antony VB. Drug-induced pleural disease. *Clin Chest Med* 1998; **19**:331–340.

[132] Huggins JT, Sahn SA. Drug-induced pleural disease. *Clin Chest Med* 2004; **25**:141–153.

[133] Morelock SY, Sahn SA. Drugs and the pleura. *Chest* 1999; **116**:212–221.

[134] Cudzilo C, Aragaki A, Guitron J, Benzaquen S. Methotrexate-induced pleuropericarditis and eosinophilic pleural effusion. *J Bronchol Interv Pulmonol* 2014; **21**:90–92.

[135] Chakraborty K, Bossaer JB, Patel R, Krishnan K. Successful treatment of nilotinib-induced pleural effusion with prednisone. *J Oncol Pharm Pract Off Publ Int Soc Oncol Pharm Pract* 2013; **19**:175–177.

[136] Felz MW, Haviland-Foley DJ. Eosinophilic pleural effusion due to dantrolene: resolution with steroid therapy. *South Med J* 2001; **94**:502–504.

[137] Helsen V, Decoutere L, Spriet I, Fagard K, Boonen S, Tournoy J. Ergotamine-induced pleural and pericardial effusion successfully treated with colchicine. *Acta Clin Belg* 2013; **68**:113–115.

[138] Kalomenidis I, Light RW. Eosinophilic pleural effusions. *Curr Opin Pulm Med* 2003; **9**:254–260.

[139] Martínez-García MA, Cases-Viedma E, Cordero-Rodríguez PJ, et al. Diagnostic utility of eosinophils in the pleural fluid. *Eur Respir J* 2000; **15**:166–169.

[140] Oba Y, Abu-Salah T. The prevalence and diagnostic significance of eosinophilic pleural effusions: a meta-analysis and systematic review. *Respir Int Rev Thorac Dis* 2012; **83**:198–208.

[141] Rosenow EC. Drug-induced bronchopulmonary pleural disease. *J Allergy Clin Immunol* 1987; **80**:780–787.

[142] Anshelevich IV, Svistunova AA. [Eosinophilic exudative pleurisy as a manifestation of drug allergy]. *Ter Arkh* 1986; **58**:142–143.

[143] Trisolini R, Dore R, Biagi F, et al. Eosinophilic pleural effusion due to mesalamine. Report of a rare occurrence. *Sarcoidosis Vasc Diffuse Lung Dis Off J WASOG* 2000; **17**:288–291.

[144] Kamenetsky Z, Da'as N, Esayag Y, Kleinman Y, Samuels N. Valproic acid-induced eosinophilic pleural effusion: a case report and review of the literature. *The Neurologist* 2012; **18**:39–40.

[145] Raptis L, Pappas G, Katsanou A, Koutsouka F, Petrakis D, Akritidis N. Diltiazem-induced eosinophilic pleural effusion. *Pharmacotherapy* 2007; **27**:600–602.

[146] Foucher P, Biour M, Blayac JP, et al. Drugs that may injure the respiratory system. *Eur Respir J* 1997; **10**:265–279.

[147] Kuwahara T, Hamada M, Inoue Y, Aono S, Hiwada K. Warfarin-induced eosinophilic pleurisy. *Intern Med Tokyo Jpn* 1995; **34**:794–796.

[148] Kaufman J, O'Shaughnessy IM. Eosinophilic pleural effusion associated with valproic acid administration. *South Med J* 1995; **88**:881–882.

[149] Hirai J, Hagihara M, Haranaga S, et al. Eosinophilic pneumonia caused by daptomycin: Six cases from two institutions and a review of the literature. *J Infect Chemother Off J Jpn Soc Chemother* 2017; **23**:245–249.

[150] Jo YM, Park TH, Jeong IH, et al. Warfarin-induced eosinophilic pleural effusion. *Korean Circ J* 2011; **41**:109–112.

[151] Kelly K, Swords R, Mahalingam D, Padmanabhan S, Giles FJ. Serosal inflammation (pleural and pericardial effusions) related to tyrosine kinase inhibitors. *Target Oncol* 2009; **4**:99–105.

[152] Druker BJ, Guilhot F, O'Brien SG, et al. Five-year follow-up of patients receiving imatinib for chronic myeloid leukemia. *N Engl J Med* 2006; **355**:2408–2417.

[153] Kantarjian HM, Giles F, Gattermann N, et al. Nilotinib (formerly AMN107), a highly selective BCR-ABL tyrosine kinase inhibitor, is effective in patients with Philadelphia chromosome-positive chronic myelogenous leukemia in chronic phase following imatinib resistance and intolerance. *Blood* 2007; **110**:3540–3546.

[154] Brixey AG, Light RW. Pleural effusions due to dasatinib. *Curr Opin Pulm Med* 2010; **16**:351–356.

[155] Goldblatt M, Huggins JT, Doelken P, Gurung P, Sahn SA. Dasatinib-induced pleural effusions: a lymphatic network disorder? *Am J Med Sci* 2009; **338**:414–417.

[156] Bergeron A, Réa D, Levy V, et al. Lung abnormalities after dasatinib treatment for chronic myeloid leukemia: a case series. *Am J Respir Crit Care Med* 2007; **176**:814–818.

[157] Novartis Pharmaceuticals. *Sprycel, prescribing information*. 2007.

[158] de Lavallade H, Punnialingam S, Milojkovic D, et al. Pleural effusions in patients with chronic myeloid leukaemia treated with dasatinib may have an immune-mediated pathogenesis. *Br J Haematol* 2008; **141**:745–747.

[159] Nagata Y, Ohashi K, Fukuda S, Kamata N, Akiyama H, Sakamaki H. Clinical features of dasatinib-induced large granular lymphocytosis and pleural effusion. *Int J Hematol* 2010; **91**:799–807.

[160] Porkka K, Khoury HJ, Paquette RL, Matloub Y, Sinha R, Cortes JE. Dasatinib 100 mg once daily minimizes the occurrence of pleural effusion in patients with chronic myeloid leukemia in chronic phase and efficacy is unaffected in patients who develop pleural effusion. *Cancer* 2010; **116**:377–386.

[161] Shah NP, Kantarjian HM, Kim D-W, et al. Intermittent target inhibition with dasatinib 100 mg once daily preserves efficacy and improves tolerability in imatinib-resistant and -intolerant chronic-phase chronic myeloid leukemia. *J Clin Oncol Off J Am Soc Clin Oncol* 2008; **26**:3204–3212.

[162] Kim D, Goh H-G, Kim S-H, Cho B-S, Kim D-W. Long-term pattern of pleural effusion from chronic myeloid leukemia patients in second-line dasatinib therapy. *Int J Hematol* 2011; **94**:361–371.

[163] Cortes JE, Jimenez CA, Mauro MJ, Geyer A, Pinilla-Ibarz J, Smith BD. Pleural Effusion in Dasatinib-Treated Patients With Chronic Myeloid Leukemia in Chronic Phase: Identification and Management. *Clin Lymphoma Myeloma Leuk* 2017; **17**:78–82.

[164] Light RW, Lee YCG eds. *Textbook of Pleural Diseases,* Third Edition. 3 edition. Boca Raton: CRC Press; 2016.

[165] Good JT, King TE, Antony VB, Sahn SA. Lupus pleuritis. Clinical features and pleural fluid characteristics with special reference to pleural fluid antinuclear antibodies. *Chest* 1983; **84**:714–718.

[166] He Y, Sawalha AH. Drug-induced lupus erythematosus: an update on drugs and mechanisms. *Curr Opin Rheumatol* 2018.

[167] Vasoo S. Drug-induced lupus: an update. *Lupus* 2006; **15**:757–761.

[168] Borchers AT, Keen CL, Gershwin ME. Drug-induced lupus. *Ann N Y Acad Sci* 2007; **1108**:166–182.

[169] Magno Pereira V, Andrade C, Figueira R, Faria G, Jasmins L. Infliximab-Induced Lupus: A Case Report. *GE Port J Gastroenterol* 2017; **24**:84–88.

[170] Porfyridis I, Kalomenidis I, Psallidas I, et al. Etanercept-induced pleuropericardial lupus-like syndrome. *Eur Respir J* 2009; **33**:939–941.

[171] Ozkan H, Cetinkaya AS, Yildiz T, Bozat T. A Rare Side Effect due to TNF-Alpha Blocking Agent: Acute Pleuropericarditis with Adalimumab. *Case Rep Rheumatol* 2013; **2013**:985914.

[172] Bukhari M. Drug-induced rheumatic diseases: a review of published case reports from the last two years. *Curr Opin Rheumatol* 2012; **24**:182–186.

[173] Hiraoka K, Nagata N, Kawajiri T, et al. Paradoxical pleural response to antituberculous chemotherapy and isoniazid-induced lupus. Review and report of two cases. *Respir Int Rev Thorac Dis* 1998; **65**:152–155.

[174] Varenika V, Blanc PD. A patient on RIPE therapy presenting with recurrent isoniazid-associated pleural effusions: a case report. *J Med Case Reports* 2011; **5**:558.

In: Pleural Effusions: Causes, Types and Treatment ISBN: 978-1-53614-683-7
Editor: Rahul Khosla

Chapter 10

CLOSED PLEURAL BIOPSY AND PLEUROSCOPY

Justin Segraves, MD, Venkata Bandi, MD and Donald R. Lazarus*, MD
Pulmonary, Critical Care, and Sleep Section
Baylor College of Medicine and the Michael E. DeBakey
VA Medical Center, Houston, TX, US

ABSTRACT

Undiagnosed exudative pleural effusions are a commonly encountered clinical problem. The differential diagnosis is broad, and in the absence of positive pleural fluid cytology or cultures additional testing is indicated to evaluate for malignancy or infection. Closed pleural biopsy using an Abrams needle or a Cope needle is most useful in evaluating patients who are at high risk of pleural tuberculosis with good diagnostic yield. Closed pleural biopsy is much less sensitive for diagnosing malignant pleural effusion. Pleuroscopy (also known as medical thoracoscopy) is a procedure in which the pleural space is visualized with a camera. It is most often performed with local analgesia and light sedation in the outpatient setting. Pleuroscopy is used primarily for the diagnosis of exudative pleural effusions when thoracentesis with fluid analysis has been unrevealing, but therapeutic pleuroscopy with talc poudrage for pleurodesis is also a common indication for this procedure. Pleuroscopy allows visually guided biopsies of abnormal areas of the pleura, increasing the diagnostic yield beyond what can be obtained with closed pleural biopsy. Both rigid and flexible instruments are available. In contrast with closed pleural biopsy, pleuroscopy has a high sensitivity for diagnosing malignant pleural effusion as well as tuberculous effusions.

Keywords: pleural biopsy, pleuroscopy, medical thoracoscopy, exudate, malignant pleural effusion, pleurodesis, pleural tuberculosis

* Corresponding Author Email: Donald.Lazarus@va.gov.

INTRODUCTION

As many as 20-25% of pleural effusions remain undiagnosed after an initial evaluation to include thoracentesis with pleural fluid analysis [1, 2]. In those cases of persistent exudative effusion in which pleural analysis is not diagnostic and malignancy or tuberculosis (TB) are suspected additional testing to determine the presence of malignancy or infection is indicated [1]. Closed needle biopsy of the pleura or pleuroscopy (also known as medical thoracoscopy) with direct visualization of the pleura with biopsy of abnormal appearing areas are very useful procedures for this indication. In this chapter we will discuss the equipment and technique of both closed pleural biopsy and pleuroscopy as well as indications, contraindications, and relative advantages for both procedures.

CLOSED PLEURAL BIOPSY

Closed pleural biopsy, first introduced in the 1950s, is a percutaneous biopsy of the parietal pleura using a specialized cutting needle [3]. The procedure is usually performed blindly, although guidance with CT or ultrasound may be used. Imaging guidance may increase the yield over blind biopsy if pleural abnormalities are able to be seen [4-7].

Equipment

Closed pleural biopsy is performed using a specialized cutting needle. Several types of needle are available including Vim-Silverman and Tru-Cut needles, but the Abrams and Cope needles are probably the most commonly used for closed pleural biopsy [3, 8-13]. The Abrams needle [Figure 1] is composed of two concentric metal tubes. The outer trocar, which is 4 mm in diameter, has a hooked notch just proximal to its tip and is used to enter the pleural space and grip the tissue. The inner cannula is used to cut the tissue in the grip of the outer trocar as well as for aspirating fluid since it can be connected to a syringe [8]. The Cope needle [Figure 2] is also made of concentric metal tubes with a maximum diameter of 2.4 mm. They are a short outer cannula used to maintain location in the pleural space, a beveled needle which fits inside the cannula and is used to introduce it into the pleural space, and a blunt-tipped needle with a hooked curet in a side slot which is used to scrape the tissue specimen from the pleural lining [10]. The other equipment needed includes disinfectant for sterilizing the skin, local anesthetic medication such as lidocaine with needles for administration, syringes for aspiration, and a scalpel. Ultrasound is also recommended to optimally localize a site for biopsy with adequate pleural fluid for safe biopsy.

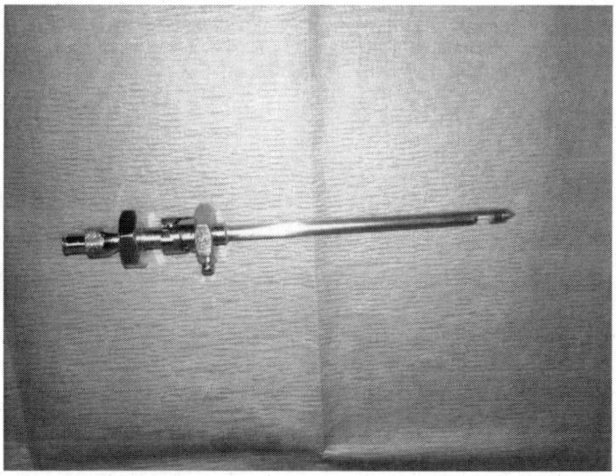

Figure 1. Abrams needle used for closed pleural biopsy.

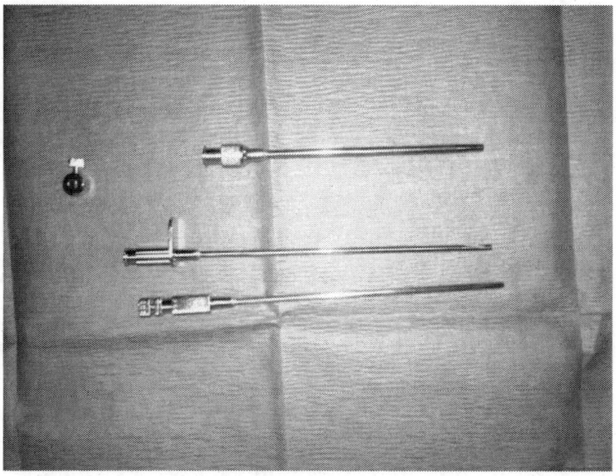

Figure 2. Cope needle used for closed pleural biopsy.

Technique

The technique for closed pleural biopsy is similar for both the Abrams and Cope needles. After informed consent the patient is positioned as for a thoracentesis. Ultrasound should ideally be used to localize the pleural effusion and select an appropriate site for pleural entry. In order to safely perform closed pleural biopsy some pleural fluid should be present. After the site is marked and the area is sterilized and draped appropriately local analgesia with lidocaine should be obtained. The biopsy site should be numbed until the pleural space is reached [11]. In addition to allowing optimal analgesia this also allows the operator to estimate the depth of tissue that must be traversed to reach the pleura. Once the patient is adequately numbed a small skin incision is made and the biopsy needle is introduced until the tip is just within the pleural space.

For the Abrams needle the inner cannula can then be rotated counterclockwise to allow aspiration of fluid if desired and also to open the hooked notch which will be used to obtain the pleural tissue. The needle is then angled so that the notch is in contact with the pleura and withdrawn with mild pressure until it "bites" the inner wall of the chest. Then the outer tube is held firmly in place while the inner cannula is rotated clockwise, shearing off the tissue captured by the hooked notch. The entire needle is then withdrawn, the outer cannula is removed, and the tissue sample taken from inside the hooked notch [8]. For the Cope needle the beveled needle is placed within the outer cannula and used to access the pleural space with some aspiration of fluid. Then the beveled needle is removed and the outer cannula withdrawn until its tip is just inside the pleura. The blunt-tipped curet needle is then introduced through the outer cannula with a syringe attached. Once its tip is within the pleural space the needle is then angled with the hooked curet toward the chest wall and withdrawn slowly until it is felt to engage the parietal pleura. The hooked curet is held steady with one hand while the outer cannula is advanced with the other, cutting a small plug of tissue which can be removed by withdrawing the blunt-tipped curet needle without removing the outer cannula [10, 11]. At least four to six biopsies are recommended to optimize yield [14].

Indications, Contraindications, and Complications of Closed Pleural Biopsy

The primary indication for closed pleural biopsy is for the diagnosis of exudative pleural effusions [1]. Prior to undertaking pleural biopsy a diagnostic thoracentesis should be performed with appropriate pleural fluid analysis including cytology and microbiologic studies. If the thoracentesis is non-diagnostic and there is suspicion for malignancy or tuberculosis then pleural biopsy—whether closed or thoracoscopic—should be pursued. Closed pleural biopsy has few contraindications—namely the absence of a pleural effusion, an uncooperative patient, and severe coagulopathy [1].

Complications of closed pleural biopsy are similar to the complications seen in thoracentesis, and are listed in Table 1. Pain at the biopsy site is probably the most common, followed by pneumothorax and vasovagal reaction [4].

Table 1. Complications of closed pleural biopsy

Pain
Pneumothorax
Vasovagal reaction
Bleeding/hemothorax
Local hematoma
Fever
Death from severe bleeding

Diagnostic Yield of Closed Pleural Biopsy

The yield of closed pleural biopsy varies with the underlying condition [14]. Because the parietal pleura is typically diffusely involved in pleural tuberculosis, closed pleural biopsy has a fairly high sensitivity for diagnosing this condition. When histology, acid fast staining, and culture are all used on the acquired biopsy specimens, the sensitivity for pleural TB is between 50% and 90% [2, 3, 15, 16]. When biopsy was combined with pleural fluid analysis with cytology, cell count, and adenosine deaminase measurement the sensitivity for pleural TB exceeded 90% [15].

The diagnostic yield of closed pleural biopsy for malignant effusion is lower than for tuberculosis, with sensitivity ranging from 44-74% in various studies [2, 4, 17]. When added to pleural fluid cytology the yield is only increased over cytology alone by 7-27% [2, 4, 18, 19]. The use of imaging guidance increases the sensitivity of closed pleural biopsy to 97% when a pleural abnormality is visible [5, 7]. This is still lower than the sensitivity of thoracoscopy for malignant pleural involvement.

PLEUROSCOPY

Pleuroscopy, also called medical thoracoscopy, is a procedure in which a camera is inserted into the pleural cavity to allow direct visualization of the pleural space in a patient who is breathing spontaneously [20]. It was introduced by Jacobeus, a Swedish internist, in 1910 for the purpose of diagnosing tuberculous pleurisy [2]. This allows biopsies to be taken under direct visualization to facilitate the diagnosis of pleural diseases. While primarily a diagnostic procedure, limited therapeutic interventions such as talc poudrage pleurodesis, lysis of pleural adhesions in loculated effusions, and chest tube placement under visual guidance can also be completed using this technique [20, 21]. It is typically performed in the bronchoscopy suite under moderate sedation or monitored anesthesia care (MAC) by pulmonologists [20, 21]. This is in contrast to video assisted thoracoscopic surgery (VATS), which is performed in the operating room under general anesthesia with a double-lumen endotracheal tube [21]. While pleuroscopy is generally limited in scope to diagnostic pleural procedures and simple therapeutic interventions, VATS encompasses the gamut of more extensive thoracic surgical procedures performed in a minimally invasive way [20, 21].

Equipment

Pleuroscopy can be performed with either rigid or semirigid instruments. The rigid instruments are generally similar to those used in VATS. Since the pleural space is entered in the same manner as is used when placing a chest tube antiseptic scrub for sterilizing the skin, lidocaine for local analgesia, a scalpel, and hemostats or scissors for blunt dissection into the pleural space are required. The other necessary items include an endoscopic telescope, a light source, a camera, a sterile suction catheter, and a trocar. Telescopes of differing viewing angles can be used to optimize inspection of the pleural space. The standard 0-degree telescope is used for biopsies, but the 30-degree, 60-degree, and 90-degree telescopes may aid in the visual inspection of the pleural cavity. The diameter of the trocar varies from 3 to 13 mm, with 7 mm trocars most commonly used [20, 21]. Optical forceps or standard thoracoscopy forceps are used for biopsy. The use of optical forceps allows the procedure to be done using a single port in most cases [20, 21].

The semirigid pleuroscope (LTF-160, Olympus, Japan) is an alternative pleuroscope designed to look and feel much like a flexible bronchoscope. It can also utilize the same processor and light source as the Olympus flexible bronchoscope. The instrument is 27 cm in length with an outer diameter of 7 mm [21, 22]. The distal 5 cm of the shaft is able to be flexed and retroflexed using a lever on the handle [20]. The working channel diameter is 2.8 mm and accommodates the same instruments as the standard therapeutic bronchoscope, and integrated suction is used in a fashion identical to the flexible bronchoscope. It is introduced through a disposable 8-10 mm plastic trocar [20]. Pleuroscopy using the semirigid pleuroscope also typically uses a single port of entry.

Technique

The technique of pleuroscopy using rigid and semirigid instrument is quite similar, with the major difference being in the way the biopsies are taken. The first consideration must be to ensure that the patient is fit for the procedure. Since pleuroscopy is performed with the ipsilateral lung deflated to allow visualization of the pleural cavity, the patient must be able to tolerate single lung ventilation. This is not often limiting as evacuation of the pleural effusion typically present in the hemithorax of interest will frequently improve the patient's dyspnea rather than worsening it. Most patients undergoing pleuroscopy should have a pleural effusion present in the ipsilateral side, although in some cases experienced proceduralists may induce pneumothorax to perform pleuroscopy in the absence of effusion [23]. The patient must also be able to lie in the decubitus position for the duration of the procedure and not have severe hypoxemia unrelated to the pleural effusion [21, 23]. Pleuroscopy is typically performed using local analgesia and moderate sedation administered by the pulmonologist performing the procedure or monitored anesthesia care (MAC) administered by an anesthesia practitioner [20].

The patient is positioned in the lateral decubitus position with the affected side up. The arm is extended above the head and the standard monitoring equipment used for moderate sedation procedures is applied, taking care to keep electrocardiogram leads out of the sterile field [20]. Then the site for pleural entry is selected, usually with the help of ultrasound [20]. While ultrasound is not strictly required for pleuroscopy, it does decrease the risk of an inaccurate entry site and should be used routinely when available [23-25]. Pleural entry is typically made in the mid-axillary line. For the evaluation of exudative effusions insertion in the 6th or 7th intercostal space is usual to allow optimal visualization of the lower pleural cavity. For recurrent pneumothorax a higher entry point, nearer to the 4th intercostal space, is often selected [20, 21]. Once the site is selected the area is prepped and draped in the usual sterile fashion. Sterile technique is required and the operator is gowned and gloved just as in a procedure in the operating room. Then local analgesia with lidocaine is obtained. A small skin incision is made and then the pleural space is entered using blunt dissection just as in chest tube placement. The trocar is then inserted into the pleural space at an angle perpendicular to the chest wall and the lung is allowed to collapse [20, 21]. A suction catheter is then used to evacuate the pleural fluid allowing for adequate inspection of the pleural cavity. At this point the pleuroscope—either the rigid telescope or the semirigid pleuroscope—is introduced via the trocar. The pleural space should be carefully and completely examined, and note made of any abnormalities along with photographic documentation if possible [20]. When present, adhesions can be lysed using the pleuroscope, forceps, or cautery taking care not to damage any vessels or the visceral pleura in the process [Figure 3] [20, 23].

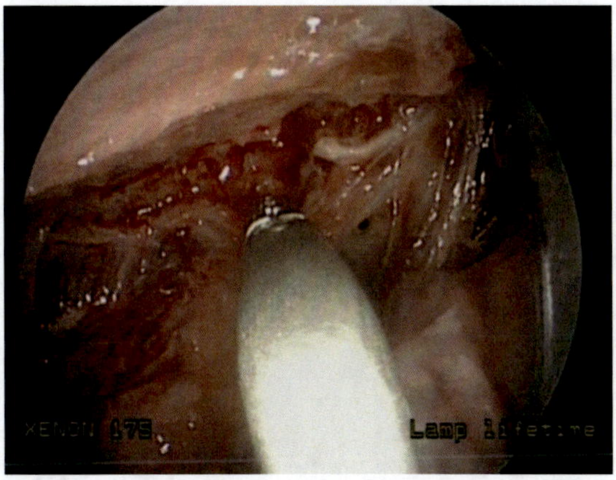

Figure 3. Optical forceps with thick pleural adhesions.

Once adequate visualization and inspection of the pleural space has been achieved, biopsy is then undertaken. If focally abnormal areas of pleura or tumor implants are seen then these are obvious targets for biopsy [Figure 4]. If the pleura is diffusely thickened or no focal abnormalities are seen then biopsy is usually started over the ribs to avoid inadvertent damage to the intercostal vessels [20]. When using the rigid instruments with optical forceps the pleura over the rib is located by gently pressing the forceps against the pleura until the hard rib can be felt. Then the jaws of the forceps are opened and the pleura is grasped. The forceps are then used to peel the pleura in a plane parallel to the inner chest wall. This allows for long strips of tissue to be removed with the biopsy so that larger samples are obtained and fewer biopsies must be taken. The use of the flexible forceps makes this technique more difficult to do with the semirigid pleuroscope, but the same general principle holds. The pleura over the rib is grasped with the forceps and then the instruments are used to peel off samples for analysis. After biopsies are completed talc may be insufflated if chemical pleurodesis is indicated. A typical dose is 3 to 5 grams of asbestos-free talc, and it should be spread evenly throughout the pleural cavity [20]. At the conclusion of the procedure a chest tube is placed to allow for re-expansion of the lung [20]. Either large or small bore chest tubes can be used. Additionally, tunneled indwelling pleural catheters can also be used post-pleuroscopy to re-expand the lung and are especially appropriate in those patients with malignant pleural effusion who have unexpandable lung or decline talc pleurodesis. If pleurodesis is undertaken the chest tube should stay in place for at least 24 hours and preferably for 72 hours and until the chest tube fluid output is less than 150 mL/day [20]. If pleurodesis is not done with pleuroscopy then the tube can be removed as soon as the lung is shown to be fully inflated post-procedure as long as no persistent air leak is present. Patients who undergo pleuroscopy with pleurodesis are usually admitted until the chest tube is removed. However, those patients who do not have pleurodesis and have a tunneled pleural catheter or whose chest tubes are removed post-procedure are often able to have pleuroscopy done as an outpatient day procedure.

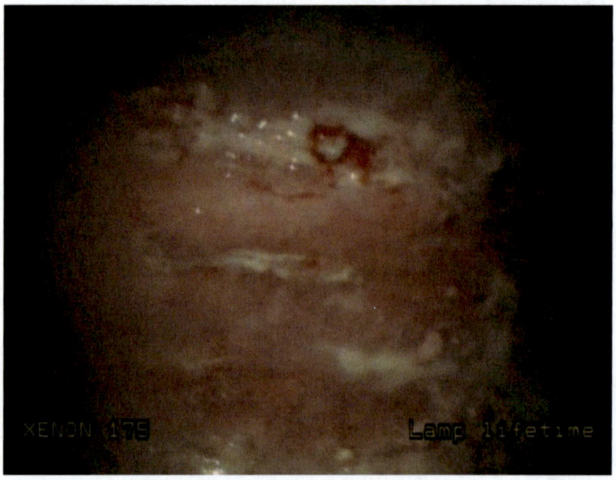

Figure 4. Parietal pleura with tumor implant.

Indications, Contraindications, and Complications of Pleuroscopy

The primary indication for pleuroscopy is for the diagnosis of exudative pleural effusions of unknown etiology, particularly when malignancy or tuberculosis is suspected

[20, 21, 23]. Because it is an invasive procedure thoracentesis with pleural fluid analysis should be performed first, and only if that initial testing is not diagnostic is pleuroscopy indicated [2]. While pleuroscopy is primarily a diagnostic tool, it also has therapeutic indications. The most important is probably palliation of malignant pleural effusion. Pleurodesis with talc poudrage is a particularly attractive option for patients with suspected malignant effusion in whom the diagnosis is not yet known. Pleurodesis with talc poudrage is more effective than with talc slurry for malignant pleural effusion [26]. In a single procedure pleuroscopy can offer both biopsy for diagnosis and pleurodesis for palliation via talc poudrage [21, 26]. Pleuroscopy can also be used to help treat pleural infections. It is most effective if used early in the clinical course when adhesions are not as thick and organized to facilitate drainage, place chest tubes optimally under visual guidance, and thereby aid in lung expansion. If a very complex multiloculated pleural space with a thick pleural rind is seen, however, pleuroscopy is better deferred in favor of surgical management with decortication [21, 27, 28]. Pleuroscopy may also be used to treat recurrent spontaneous pneumothorax. Although it is inferior to VATS or thoracotomy for intervening upon parenchymal lesions which are a source of air leaks, it may remain useful for pleural abrasion and talc poudrage for recurrence prevention in those patients who are poor candidates for general anesthesia or lung resection [21, 23, 29].

Table 2. Complications of pleuroscopy

Major complications	Minor complications
Empyema	Subcutaneous emphysema
Hemorrhage	Skin site infection
Bronchopleural fistula	Intra-procedure hypotension
Tumor seeding of port site	Fever
Post-procedure pneumothorax	Atrial fibrillation
Pneumonia	
Shock	
Death	

Contraindications for pleuroscopy include the absence of a pleural space secondary to thick adhesions, cardiovascular instability, uncorrected coagulopathy, and inadequate oxygenation and ventilation not attributable to the ipsilateral effusion being intervened upon [21]. Relative contraindications include severe obesity, the known presence of an obstructing airway tumor, lack of pleural effusion in the hemithorax of interest, inability of the patient to lie flat, and severe loculations [21, 23, 30].

Major complications of pleuroscopy are uncommon and occur in less than 3% of cases [23]. Mortality is extremely rare, with only 16 deaths reported in pooled analysis of over 4700 cases, with an estimated mortality rate of pleuroscopy of 0.34% [23]. All 16 deaths occurred in the 2315 patients who had received talc poudrage, for a rate in that subgroup of 0.69% [23]. Minor complications are more common and may occur in up to 8% of patients. These include subcutaneous emphysema, minor bleeding, skin infections, intraprocedural hypotension, and atrial fibrillation [23]. Table 2 summarizes the complications of pleuroscopy.

Diagnostic Yield of Pleuroscopy

The diagnostic yield of pleuroscopy is superior to that of closed pleural biopsy for pleural conditions because it allows biopsy to be targeted to the abnormal areas of the pleura. Pleuroscopy has a diagnostic yield for pleural tuberculosis of 70% when tissue culture alone is used [4]. When culture is combined with histologic examination, sensitivity is even higher and typically is between 90-100% [4, 15, 31].

The diagnostic yield of pleuroscopy for malignant pleural effusion is excellent, with sensitivity of 85% to 95% for this indication [21, 23, 32, 33]. This high yield persists even when previous closed pleural biopsy was not diagnostic. Pooled results of 8 studies including 337 patients with negative closed pleural biopsy who underwent pleuroscopy for the diagnosis of malignant effusions still demonstrated a sensitivity of 90% [23, 34-40].

Conclusion

Undiagnosed exudative pleural effusions are a common problem encountered in pulmonary medicine. Closed pleural biopsy and pleuroscopy are very useful techniques for diagnosing the cause of exudative pleural effusions when thoracentesis is not diagnostic, especially when malignancy or tuberculosis is suspected. Closed pleural biopsy has a higher sensitivity for TB than malignancy, and is probably best used when the prevalence or clinical suspicion for tuberculosis is much higher than for malignancy. Alternatively in settings where pleuroscopy is not available or if the patient is unable to tolerate single lung ventilation closed pleural biopsy is an acceptable alternative for suspected malignant pleural disease as well.

Pleuroscopy has a very high sensitivity for both pleural infection and malignancy, and may be used when either diagnosis is highly suspected. It can also be used to facilitate pleurodesis and the lysis of intrapleural adhesions. Because of its superior diagnostic yield and therapeutic versatility as well pleuroscopy when available is therefore recommended as the next step after non-diagnostic thoracentesis for exudative effusions in patients who are acceptable candidates [23].

REFERENCES

[1] Sokolowski, JW; Jr. Burgher, LW; Jones, FL; Jr. Patterson, JR; Selecky, PA. "Guidelines for Thoracentesis and Needle Biopsy of the Pleura. This Position Paper of the American Thoracic Society Was Adopted by the Ats Board of Directors, June 1988." *Am Rev Respir Dis*, 140, no. 1, (Jul 1989), 257-8.

[2] Loddenkemper, R. "Thoracoscopy--State of the Art." *Eur Respir J*, 11, no. 1, (Jan 1998), 213-21.

[3] Koegelenberg, CF; Bolliger, CT; Theron, J; Walzl, G; Wright, CA; Louw, M; Diacon, AH. "Direct Comparison of the Diagnostic Yield of Ultrasound-Assisted Abrams and Tru Cut Needle Biopsies for Pleural Tuberculosis." *Thorax*, 65, no. 10, (Oct 2010), 857-62.

[4] Hooper, C; Lee, YC; Maskell, N; B. T. S. Pleural Guideline Group. "Investigation of a Unilateral Pleural Effusion in Adults: British Thoracic Society Pleural Disease Guideline 2010." *Thorax*, 65 Suppl 2, (Aug 2010), ii4-17.

[5] Maskell, NA; Gleeson, FV; Davies, RJ. "Standard Pleural Biopsy Versus Ct-Guided Cutting-Needle Biopsy for Diagnosis of Malignant Disease in Pleural Effusions: A Randomised Controlled Trial." *Lancet*, 361, no. 9366, (Apr 19 2003), 1326-30.

[6] Adams, RF; Gray, W; Davies, RJ; Gleeson, FV. "Percutaneous Image-Guided Cutting Needle Biopsy of the Pleura in the Diagnosis of Malignant Mesothelioma." *Chest*, 120, no. 6, (Dec 2001), 1798-802.

[7] Adams, RF; Gleeson, FV. "Percutaneous Image-Guided Cutting-Needle Biopsy of the Pleura in the Presence of a Suspected Malignant Effusion." *Radiology*, 219, no. 2, (May 2001), 510-4.

[8] Abrams, LD. "A Pleural-Biopsy Punch." *Lancet*, 1, no. 7010, (Jan 4 1958), 30-1.

[9] Defrancis, N; Klosk, E; Albano, E. "Needle Biopsy of the Parietal Pleura; a Preliminary Report." *N Engl J Med*, 252, no. 22, (Jun 2 1955), 948-51.

[10] Cope, C. "New Pleural Biopsy Needle; Preliminary Study." *J Am Med Assoc*, 167, no. 9, (Jun 28 1958), 1107-8.

[11] Kettel, LJ; Cugell, DW. "Pleural Biopsy." *JAMA*, 200, no. 4, (Apr 24 1967), 317-20.

[12] Schools, GS. "Needle Biopsy of Parietal Pleura: Current Status." *Tex State J Med*, 59, (Nov 1963), 1056-61.

[13] McLeod, DT; Ternouth, I; Nkanza, N. "Comparison of the Tru-Cut Biopsy Needle with the Abrams Punch for Pleural Biopsy." *Thorax*, 44, no. 10, (Oct 1989), 794-6.

[14] Chakrabarti, B; Ryland, I; Sheard, J; Warburton, CJ; Earis, JE. "The Role of Abrams Percutaneous Pleural Biopsy in the Investigation of Exudative Pleural Effusions." *Chest*, 129, no. 6, (Jun 2006), 1549-55.

[15] Diacon, AH; Van de Wal, BW; Wyser, C; Smedema, JP; J. Bezuidenhout, C. T. Bolliger, and G. Walzl. "Diagnostic Tools in Tuberculous Pleurisy: A Direct Comparative Study." *Eur Respir J*, 22, no. 4, (Oct 2003), 589-91.

[16] Levine, H; Metzger, W; Lacera, D; Kay, L. "Diagnosis of Tuberculous Pleurisy by Culture of Pleural Biopsy Specimen." *Arch Intern Med*, 126, no. 2, (Aug 1970), 269-71.

[17] Tomlinson, JR. "Invasive Procedures in the Diagnosis of Pleural Disease." *Semin Respir Med*, 9, (1987), 30-60.

[18] Nance, KV; Shermer, RW; Askin, FB. "Diagnostic Efficacy of Pleural Biopsy as Compared with That of Pleural Fluid Examination." *Mod Pathol*, 4, no. 3, (May 1991), 320-4.

[19] Prakash, UB; Reiman, HM. "Comparison of Needle Biopsy with Cytologic Analysis for the Evaluation of Pleural Effusion: Analysis of 414 Cases." *Mayo Clin Proc*, 60, no. 3, (Mar 1985), 158-64.

[20] Casal, RF; Eapen, GA; Morice, RC; Jimenez, CA. "Medical Thoracoscopy." *Curr Opin Pulm Med*, 15, no. 4, (Jul 2009), 313-20.

[21] Lee, P; Colt, HG. "State of the Art: Pleuroscopy." *J Thorac Oncol*, 2, no. 7, (Jul 2007), 663-70.

[22] Lee, P; Hsu, A; Lo, C; Colt, HG. "Prospective Evaluation of Flex-Rigid Pleuroscopy for Indeterminate Pleural Effusion: Accuracy, Safety and Outcome." *Respirology*, 12, no. 6, (Nov 2007), 881-6.

[23] Rahman, NM; Ali, NJ; Brown, G; Chapman, SJ; Davies, RJ; Downer, NJ; Gleeson, FV; et al. "Local Anaesthetic Thoracoscopy: British Thoracic Society Pleural Disease Guideline 2010." *Thorax*, 65 Suppl 2, (Aug 2010), ii54-60.

[24] Macha, HN; Reichle, G; von Zwehl, D; Kemmer, HP; Bas, R; Morgan, JA. "The Role of Ultrasound Assisted Thoracoscopy in the Diagnosis of Pleural Disease. Clinical Experience in 687 Cases." *Eur J Cardiothorac Surg*, 7, no. 1, (1993), 19-22.

[25] Hersh, CP; Feller-Kopman, D; Wahidi, M; Garland, R; Herth, F; Ernst, A. "Ultrasound Guidance for Medical Thoracoscopy: A Novel Approach." *Respiration*, 70, no. 3, (May-Jun 2003), 299-301.

[26] Shaw, P; Agarwal, R. "Pleurodesis for Malignant Pleural Effusions." *Cochrane Database Syst Rev*, no. 1, (2004), CD002916.

[27] Cameron, RJ. "Management of Complicated Parapneumonic Effusions and Thoracic Empyema." *Intern Med J*, 32, no. 8, (Aug 2002), 408-14.

[28] Colice, GL; Curtis, A; Deslauriers, J; Heffner, J; Light, R; Littenberg, B; Sahn, S; Weinstein, RA; Yusen, RD. "Medical and Surgical Treatment of Parapneumonic Effusions: An Evidence-Based Guideline." *Chest*, 118, no. 4, (Oct 2000), 1158-71.

[29] Lee, P; Yap, WS; Pek, WY; Ng, AW. "An Audit of Medical Thoracoscopy and Talc Poudrage for Pneumothorax Prevention in Advanced Copd." *Chest*, 125, no. 4, (Apr 2004), 1315-20.

[30] Michaud, G; Berkowitz, DM; Ernst, A. "Pleuroscopy for Diagnosis and Therapy for Pleural Effusions." *Chest*, 138, no. 5, (Nov 2010), 1242-6.

[31] Hansen, M; Faurschou, P; Clementsen, P. "Medical Thoracoscopy, Results and Complications in 146 Patients: A Retrospective Study." *Respir Med*, 92, no. 2, (Feb 1998), 228-32.

[32] Boutin, C; Cargnino, P; Viallat, JR. "Thoracoscopy in the Early Diagnosis of Malignant Pleural Effusions." *Endoscopy*, 12, no. 4, (Jul 1980), 155-60.

[33] Weissberg, D; Kaufman, M; Zurkowski, Z. "Pleuroscopy in Patients with Pleural Effusion and Pleural Masses." *Ann Thorac Surg*, 29, no. 3, (Mar 1980), 205-8.

[34] Blanc, FX; Atassi, K; Bignon, J; Housset, B. "Diagnostic Value of Medical Thoracoscopy in Pleural Disease: A 6-Year Retrospective Study." *Chest*, 121, no. 5, (May 2002), 1677-83.

[35] Menzies, R; Charbonneau, M. "Thoracoscopy for the Diagnosis of Pleural Disease." *Ann Intern Med*, 114, no. 4, (Feb 15 1991), 271-6.

[36] Davidson, AC; George, RJ; Sheldon, CD; Sinha, G; Corrin, B; Geddes, DM. "Thoracoscopy: Assessment of a Physician Service and Comparison of a Flexible Bronchoscope Used as a Thoracoscope with a Rigid Thoracoscope." *Thorax*, 43, no. 4, (Apr 1988), 327-32.

[37] Munavvar, M; Khan, MA; Edwards, J; Waqaruddin, Z; Mills, J. "The Autoclavable Semirigid Thoracoscope: The Way Forward in Pleural Disease?". *Eur Respir J*, 29, no. 3, (Mar 2007), 571-4.

[38] Oldenburg, FA; Jr. Newhouse, MT. "Thoracoscopy. A Safe, Accurate Diagnostic Procedure Using the Rigid Thoracoscope and Local Anesthesia." *Chest*, 75, no. 1 (Jan 1979), 45-50.

[39] Wilsher, ML; Veale, AG. "Medical Thoracoscopy in the Diagnosis of Unexplained Pleural Effusion." *Respirology*, 3, no. 2 (Jun 1998), 77-80.

[40] Tscheikuna, J. "Medical Thoracoscopy: Experiences in Siriraj Hospital." *J Med Assoc Thai*, 89, Suppl 5 (Nov 2006), S62-6.

In: Pleural Effusions: Causes, Types and Treatment
Editor: Rahul Khosla
ISBN: 978-1-53614-683-7

Chapter 11

INTERVENTIONAL MANAGEMENT OF PLEURAL EFFUSIONS

Hyeon Yu*[*]*, MD and Ari J. Isaacson, MD
Division of Vascular and Interventional Radiology,
Department of Radiology,
University of North Carolina at Chapel Hill,
Chapel Hill, NC, US

ABSTRACT

Pleural effusion can result from various etiologies including infection, organ failure, numerous systemic conditions, malignancy, trauma, and underlying lung disease. If not treated properly and promptly, pleural fluid can significantly impair respiration, resulting in life-threatening complications and/or poor quality of life. Pleural effusion can be managed medically, surgically or with minimally invasive interventional procedures. Image-guided procedures in interventional radiology have become well-established treatment tool for pleural effusion. These procedures include thoracentesis, non-tunneled pigtail catheter placement, tunneled catheter placement, intrapleural fibrinolytic therapy, and image-guided pleurodesis. This chapter aims to review the current imaging modalities for diagnosis, describe minimally invasive interventional radiology treatments for pleural effusion and summarize the literature.

Keywords: pleural effusion, empyema, image-guidance, interventional radiology, thoracentesis, nontunneled pleural catheter, tunneled pleural catheter, intrapleural fibrinolytic therapy, pleurodesis, tube thoracostomy, ultrasound, computed tomography, magnetic resonance imaging, PET CT

[*] Corresponding Author Email: hyeon_yu@med.unc.edu.

INTRODUCTION

Pleural effusion is a common and nonspecific manifestation of various pleural diseases that are frequently encountered by clinicians in daily practice [1]. Approximately 1.5 million new pleural effusions develop each year in the United States, with nonmalignant etiologies accounting for up to 86% [2]. Congestive heart failure is by far the most common cause for all nonmalignant effusions, with an incidence rate up to 87% in patients with decompensated heart failure requiring diuresis [3, 4]. Other etiology of nonmalignant pleural effusion includes hepatic failure, renal failure, pleural infections (empyema, simple and complex parapneumonic effusions, and tuberculous pleuritis), post-CABG, BAPE (benign asbestosis pleural effusion)/DPT (diffuse pleural thickening), pulmonary embolism, rheumatic disease, trauma, drug-induced, and lymphatic injuries [4]. More than 50% of patients with disseminated malignant tumors develop pleural effusion during the course of their disease [5]. Malignant etiologies include lung cancer, breast cancer, lymphoma, ovarian cancer, gastrointestinal cancer, mesothelioma, and others. Lung cancer, breast cancers and lymphoma account for 75% of malignant pleural effusions [6-8]. In about 6% of patients, the primary source is not identified [9]. Although the exact incidence rate of malignant pleural effusion is unknown, it is estimated to be more than 150,000 new cases per year in the United States [10].

The pleural space normally contains 5–10 mL of serous fluid that separates the visceral and parietal pleura, minimizing friction between the two layers. Normally, the fluid is secreted from the parietal pleura at a rate of 0.01 mL/kg/h. However, the rate of secretion is dependent on the hydrostatic and oncotic pressure gradients between the capillaries and the pleural space. The fluid is subsequently absorbed by the lymphatic capillaries in the parietal pleura [11, 12]. Pleural effusion occurs as a result of an imbalance between fluid secretion and absorption. Traditionally, pleural effusion is classified as either transudative or exudative based on the total protein and lactate dehydrogenase, as described in Light's Criteria [13]. Transudate is resulted from an imbalance between hydrostatic and oncotic pressures in the pleural space [12]. Exudate is caused by increased permeability of the damaged capillary beds in patients with pleural infections or malignancies [14].

The clinical presentation of pleural effusion is largely dependent on the underlying lung or pleural conditions. Pleural effusion itself can be asymptomatic and physical examination findings can also be subtle or non-existant if the volume of fluid is less than 300 mL [11]. Most common respiratory symptoms related to pleural effusion are dyspnea, pleuritic chest pain, and cough. Patients with malignant pleural effusion may develop constitutional symptoms such as fever, chills, and weight loss. Significant hypoxemia rarely occurs if the respiratory function and the compliance of the lung/chest walls are normal because ventilation and perfusion are diminished simultaneously in the adjacent compressed lung parenchyma. The heart, however, can be affected by the mass effect of a large pleural effusion, resulting decreased cardiac distension and filling. In this scenario, clinical signs can suggest cardiac tamponade [15].

Diagnosis of Pleural Effusion

Chest Radiography

Conventional chest radiography is widely accepted as the initial imaging modality for patients with suspected pleural effusion. In general, free pleural fluid tends to accumulate in the most dependent portions of the thorax, initially in the subpulmonic space and subsequently in the costophrenic recesses when the patient is upright. Although upright posterior-anterior chest radiograph is the most commonly used diagnostic technique for various lung and pleural diseases, its sensitivity for detecting small amounts of pleural fluid is limited; the costophrenic recess is no longer visible when 200 mL is present and the hemidiaphragm is obscured with 400 mL [16, 17]. On lateral upright chest radiograph, however, blunting of the costophrenic recess can be detected when only 50 mL of fluid have accumulated [17]. The lateral decubitus chest radiograph is even more sensitive and can reliably demonstrate as little as 10 mL of fluid in the pleural space [18]. On supine anterior-posterior chest radiograph it can be difficult to detect a small effusion, as air is dispersed anteriorly and fluid posteriorly [19, 17]. In general, chest radiography has significant limitations when evaluating pleural effusions, and they are as follows: 1) inability to differentiate free flowing from septated effusions, 2) inability to differentiate pleural fluid from pleural thickening, and 3) inability to distinguish between fluid, dense lung parenchymal consolidations, and elevated hemidiaphragm [20].

Ultrasonography

Thoracic ultrasound (US) has become an inexpensive, reliable and easy to use imaging modality for the evaluation of pleural diseases not only in radiology departments, but at the bedside in intensive care units and emergency departments [21, 22]. For the detection of small volume pleural effusion, US is more accurate when compared to chest radiography [23-27]. Detection of physiologic pleural fluid (<5 mL) is possible with US, although the sensitivity of detection is considerably improved when >20 mL are present [28, 29]. Reported diagnostic accuracy for pleural effusion is 91%–93% for US compared to 56% and 33% for physical examination and upright posterior-anterior chest radiograph, respectively [30, 27]. In a meta-analysis, sensitivity and specificity of US for detection of pleural effusions were reported as 93% and 96%, respectively [27, 30-32].

US is frequently used to differentiate pleural fluid from atelectasis, pneumonia, elevated hemidiaphragm, and lung/ pleural masses [33, 34]. US also allows for evaluation of the type of fluid. Although a definitive diagnosis of transudate vs. exudate requires a fluid analysis using Light's criteria, US allows for visualization of debris, septations or loculations [35]. Increased echogenicity and the presence of septations typically suggests exudative effusion, whereas a homogeneous, anechoic fluid is more typically transudative (Figure 1A) [36]. Empyema and hemothorax usually have homogenously increased echogenicity on US.

The incidence of thoracentesis-related complications, such as pneumothorax or bleeding increases when the pleural effusion is small [37]. US evaluation for quantifying the volume of fluid can be useful to stratify risk prior to thoracentesis. Fluid volume can be reliably estimated by using formulas based on either interpleural distance (IPD) or maximal distance between the visceral pleura and diaphragm (PDD): 1) volume (mL) = 20 x IPD (mm) and 2) volume (mL) = 16 x PDD (mm) [38, 39]. For aspiration of pleural effusion or placement of drainage catheters, US plays an important role for real-time procedural guidance.

Computed Tomography

Computed tomography (CT) can be also used to characterize pleural fluid [40]. Suggested CT features for differentiating exudates from transudates include pleural nodules, pleural thickening, loculation, extrapleural fat tissue, changes in lung or mediastinum, and CT attenuation (Hounsfield unit; HU) of the fluid [40, 41]. Among these features, CT attenuation is the most controversial. Cullu et al. reported in a retrospective study that CT attenuation values of >15 HU may be a useful indicator for exudates, although there was an overlap in most effusions [40]. Nandalur et al. demonstrated that the mean attenuation values of exudates were significantly higher than those of transudates (17.1 ± 4.4 HU vs. 12.5 ± 6.3 HU; $p = 0.001$) [42]. Abramowitz et al. also found that the mean attenuation values of transudates were lower than those of exudates (7.2 ± 9.4 HU vs. 10.1 ± 6.9 HU; $p = 0.24$), but there was no statistically significant difference [43]. In these studies, the authors concluded that the use of CT attenuation alone is not reliable and clinical correlation is important for proper management of pleural effusions [40, 42, 43]. Thickening of parietal pleura is another CT feature that has been suggested as a reliable indicator for exudates. In a retrospective study with 86 effusions evaluating the appearance of parietal pleural and extrapleural fat thickening on contrast-enhanced CT, Aquino et al. reported that the parietal pleural thickening was found in all cases of parapneumonic exudates and empyema with a specificity of 96% [44]. Arenas-Jimenez et al. also found that the presence of pleural thickening, pleural nodules and loculations were highly specific for exudates and empyema [41]. Pleural separation, or the "split pleura" sign on CT, has been considered a diagnostic sign for empyema. If both visceral and parietal pleura are thickened and separated by effusion, it is defined as the "split pleura sign." In a retrospective study with a total of 83 patients, Tsujimoto et al. found that the split pleura sign was highly indicative of complicated parapneumonic effusion and empyema vs simple parapneumonic effusion prior to diagnostic thoracentesis [45].

For patients with suspected malignant pleural effusion, contrast-enhanced CT is the standard imaging technique for the evaluation of pleural space as well as the surrounding lung parenchyma, mediastinum, thoracic soft tissues and abdomen. The CT features highly suggestive of malignant pleural disease are circumferential pleural thickening, nodular pleural thickening, pleural irregularity, parietal pleural thickness > 1 cm, and mediastinal pleural involvement [46-48]. Reported overall sensitivity and specificity of these CT findings are 36%–51% and 88%–100%, respectively [46]. In 2014, Hallifax et al. evaluated the role of CT in detecting pleural malignancy [49]. They reviewed all CT findings from 211 patients with confirmed malignant pleural disease and found that the reported sensitivity, specificity, positive predictive value, and negative predicted value for CT were 68%, 78%, 80%, and 65% respectively [49]. Porcel et al. conducted a similar study in 2015 using a CT-based scoring system, which included: 1) any pleural lesion ≥ 1 cm (5 points), 2) the presence of liver metastases, an abdominal mass, or lung mass or nodule ≥ 1 cm (3 points each), 3) the absence of either pleural loculations, pericardial effusions, or cardiomegaly (2 points each) [50]. In this study, they found the sensitivity for a score ≥ 7 was 88% and the specificity was 94%. CT is also frequently used for imaging guidance while accessing the pleural space either for thoracentesis or drainage catheter placement in situations in which ultrasonographic visualization is difficult.

Magnetic Resonance Imaging

Magnetic resonance imaging (MRI) is the preferred diagnostic modality for the detection of lung and pleural disease without ionizing radiations [51]. MRI can be used for determining if a pleural effusion has malignant features as well as for evaluating changes after treatment [52]. With greatly improved soft-tissue resolution and higher flow sensitivity, MRI provides valuable information of the pleura-chest wall interfaces, cardiovascular system, diaphragm, mediastinal structures, and chest wall [53]. Accurate evaluation of tumor invasion of the chest wall, diaphragm, heart, great vessels, airways, and other mediastinal structures are critical for determining surgical resectability of primary and secondary pleural tumors [53, 54].

Various MRI techniques are used to help identify the nature of the pleural fluid and evaluate the relationship between tissues. T1-weighted imaging (T1WI) of MRI enables identification of hemorrhage in the pleural space using different paramagnetic characteristics of hemoglobin, methemogralobin, and hemosiderin [51]. Due to its excellent anatomic resolution, T1WI is used to differentiate pleural space from extrapleural fat [53].

Intravenous administration of Gadolinium on fat-saturated T1WI can further enhance tissue contrast between lesions and adjacent normal structures. On T2-weighted imaging (T2WI), signal intensity of pleural fluid is increased compared to the pleura, lung or extrapleural fat. This allows for differentiation of pleural thickening and nodularity from effusion and helps delineate pleural tumor from adjacent muscles or extrapleural fat. Short tau inversion recovery (STIR) can reliably detect tumor or infection in a bone because the pathologic tissue will have bright signal intensity within the dark-to-intermediate signal bone [53]. Diffusion-weighted imaging (DWI), a more advanced MRI technique, based on random motion of water molecules which is restricted in a tissue environment of high cellularity. In most malignancies, diffusion is decreased and signal intensity is increased due to high cellularity on DWI [52].

18-Fluorodeoxyglucose Positron Emission Tomography-Computed Tomography

The combination of 18-Fluorodeoxyglucose Positron Emission Tomography and CT (18-FDG PET-CT) has been increasingly used to stage malignant tumors and evaluate responses after chemotherapy. The technique is based on the increased uptake of 18-FDG in metabolically active tissue, such as a malignant tumor, compared with surrounding normal tissues [55]. In the diagnosis of malignant pleural effusion, reported sensitivity, specificity, and negative predictive values of PET-CT are 93%–100%, 67%–89% and 94%–100%, respectively [46]. However, its diagnostic value is limited due to false positive results from increased uptake in infectious or inflammatory lesions. Further, increased FDG uptake in the pleura is also seen in patients with uremic or parapneumonic effusions and following pleurodesis [56]. In a meta-analysis performed by Porcel et al. PET-CT had a sensitivity of 81% and specificity of 74% [55]. With the moderate accuracy and high false positive rates, PET-CT is not recommended for differentiating malignant from benign pleural effusions [55, 57]. In cases with complex pleural lesions which are not easily separable on CT or MRI, PET-CT can be helpful for detecting a metabolically active area as a target for biopsy [58].

Interventional Management of Pleural Effusions

Thoracentesis

Thoracentesis is a safe and effective procedure that can result in the immediate relief of respiratory symptoms. The ability to perform thoracentesis at the bedside under US guidance is especially useful in intensive care units or emergency departments. Regardless of the amount of pleural effusion or experience of the operator, US guidance is strongly recommended for a needle access into the pleural space in order to avoid potential injury to the underlying lung parenchyma, diaphragm, heart, intercostal arteries, or other vital organs. It is recommended to perform a diagnostic thoracentesis when there is a clinically significant pleural effusion of >1 cm in thickness on US or lateral decubitus chest radiograph with an unknown etiology [59]. However, if there is a suspected underlying cause likely associated with a transudative pleural effusion, the underlying disease should be treated before thoracentesis. Diagnostic thoracentesis is not recommended in a patient who has bilateral symmetrical pleural effusions associated with congestive heart failure without fever or chest pain [60]. Congestive heart failure related pleural effusions are almost always transudative and in 75% of cases resolve within 48 hours of diuretic administration [60]. However, if the pleural effusion persists >72 hours despite initial treatment of the underlying disease, diagnostic thoracentesis can be performed [59]. Although most transudates resolve by managing the underlying medical condition, if significant respiratory symptoms related to the effusion persist, therapeutic thoracentesis is recommended for immediate symptomatic relief [61].

Although there is no consensus in regard to maximum volume of fluid that can be safely removed during thoracentesis, the most common recommendation is to remove no more than 2,000 mL due to the risk of reexpansion pulmonary edema (RPE) and hypotension. RPE is a life-threatening condition that occurs after rapid expansion of a chronically collapsed lung [62-64]. Etiology of chronically collapsed lung includes pneumothorax, pleural effusion, and large mediastinal mass. Reported incidence and mortality rates associated with RPE are ~33% and ~20%, respectively [65, 66]. Risk factors associated with RPE are: 1) large pneumothorax or pleural effusion, 2) younger age, and 3) a rapid rate of reexpansion [64]. To minimize the risk of RPE, thoracentesis should be stopped immediately when the patient starts developing a cough or chest pain. Other complications from thoracentesis include pain at the puncture site, pneumothorax, hemothorax, empyema and organ laceration [67]. The incidences of pneumothorax and hemothorax are 2%–6% and 1%, respectively. Only a half of pneumothoraces require chest tube insertion [68]. It is not recommended to obtain chest radiograph routinely after thoracentesis unless procedure-related complications are suspected.

Procedure

The patient is placed in a sitting position on the edge of the bed, leaning forward with the patient's arms resting on a bedside table. If the sitting position is not possible, the lateral decubitus or supine position can be used. Preprocedural US evaluation is essential for localizing proper entry site to the pleural effusion at the posterior or posterolateral intercostal space. The skin at the needle entry site is prepared and draped using all elements of maximum sterile barrier technique. The skin entry site is then anesthetized using 1%

lidocaine and a small incision is made. The needle entry site should be at the upper margin of the rib in order to avoid an injury to the intercostal artery, which runs along the inferior border of the rib. There are several types of 18-gauge over-the-needle sheath systems available for thoracentesis including; 1) One-Step Centesis catheter (Merit Medical Systems, South Jordan, UT), 2) Yueh needle (Cook, Bloomington, IN), and 3) Safe-T-Centesis drainage system (Control Alt Design, Elgin, IL). The diameters of the outer sheath range from 4 Fr to 8 Fr and there are multiple side holes at the distal portion of the sheath to facilitate fluid drainage. The One-Step Centesis catheter and the Safe-T-Centesis drainage systems both have a self-sealing valve at the hub to minimize the chance for air infiltration or fluid leakage. Through the skin incision, the over-the-needle sheath system is advanced until the tip of the needle is identified inside the pleural effusion under continuous US guidance (Figure 1).

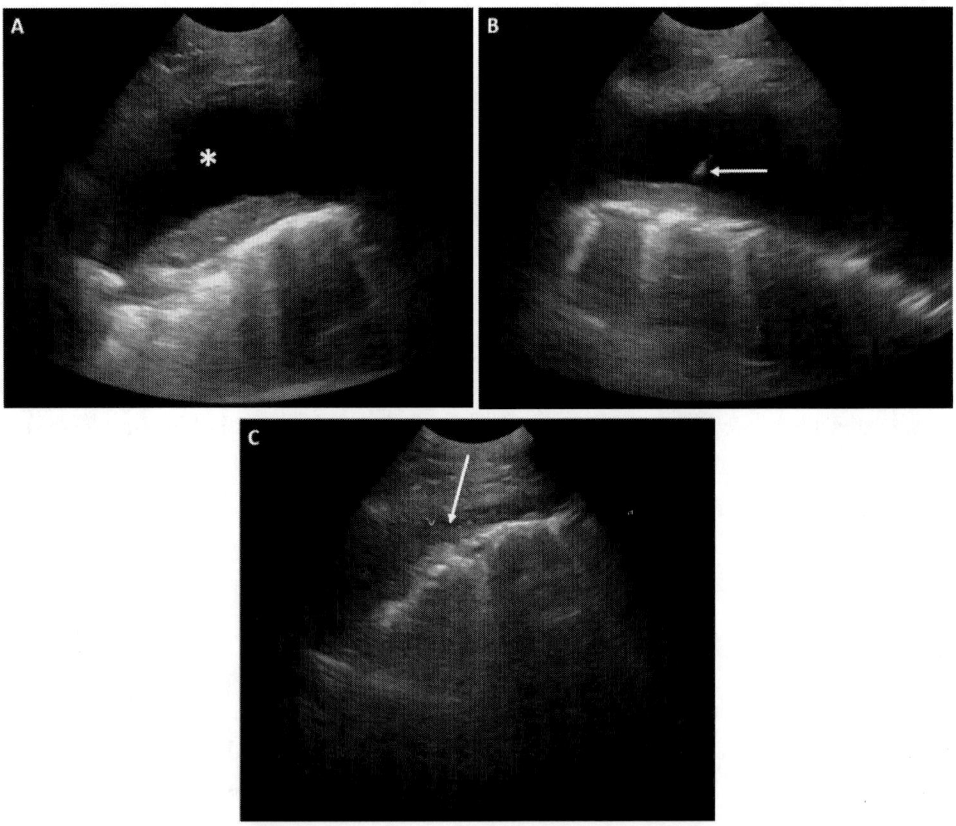

Figure 1 (a-c). US-guided thoracentesis of transudative pleural effusion. Thoracentesis in a 16-year-old female with history of anoxic brain injury from cardiac arrest caused by non-obstructive hypertrophic cardiomyopathy complicated by right pleural effusion with intermittent low grade fever. Figure 1a. Ultrasound image shows a large volume of anechoic pleural fluid (*). Figure 1b. Under US guidance, an 18-G needle is advanced into the fluid. The tip of the needle (arrow) is confirmed in the center of the fluid. Figure 1c. After removing 900 mL of fluid, US image shows no residual effusion (arrow) in the pleural space.

Once the position of the needle tip is confirmed, the outer sheath is advanced over the needle, and the needle is removed. As the needle is withdrawn, the open hub of the sheath needs to be covered with a finger if there is no valve. A stopcock is then connected to the hub and a fluid sample can be obtained without the risk of air coursing into the pleural space. In diagnostic thoracentesis, 50 mL of fluid is typically aspirated and placed immediately in the appropriate specimen container. The fluid sample is properly sealed, labeled, and sent for a laboratory analysis; the analysis should include protein and LDH levels for comparison to those in serum. If malignant pleural effusion is suspected, the fluid sample is sent for a cytologic analysis. If therapeutic thoracentesis is necessary, the sheath is attached to an extension tubing system, which is connected to a vacuum bottle or wall-suction system. Once the procedure is completed, the sheath is removed at end expiration. The skin entry site should then be covered using a sterile occlusive dressing.

Tube Thoracostomy

Placement of a large-bore chest tube is referred to as tube thoracostomy and is usually performed by surgeons. If the outer diameter of a chest tube is greater than 20 Fr, it is considered a large-bore chest tube [69]. Based on recommendations from the British Thoracic Society, indications for placement of a large-bore chest tube include pneumothorax, malignant pleural effusion, empyema, complicated parapneumonic effusion, traumatic hemothorax or hemopneumothorax, and postoperative pleural fluid collections [69, 70]. Although there are no absolute contraindications for tube thoracostomy, it is generally recommended to correct coagulopathy or thrombocytopenia before the procedure to avoid bleeding complications. Complications associated with a tube thoracostomy include malposition, malfunction, hemorrhage, infection, and underlying organ injuries [69]. A chest radiograph should be obtained after tube thoracostomy to evaluate the tube position and changes in pleural fluid volume or resolution of pneumothorax. Complications such as pneumothorax or soft tissue emphysema should also be excluded [70]. When the chest tube is removed, the patient should perform Valsalva's maneuver during expiration to prevent pneumothorax. If the initial indication was pneumothorax, the chest tube can be removed when bubbling into the water-sealed collection chamber has stopped and chest radiograph shows optimal lung expansion.

Procedure

A tube thoracostomy is usually performed by a surgeon at the bedside. The patient is placed in the supine position with the tube insertion side slightly elevated (30°~45°). The arm on the tube insertion side is positioned behind the patient's head in order to expose the axillary region [71, 72]. The patient can also be sitting-up, leaning over a table or in the lateral decubitus position [73]. The common tube insertion site is along the midaxillary line, inside the "safe tringle" to minimize the risk of an injury to underlying structures such as the internal mammary artery, muscles and breast tissue. The area between the anterior border of the latissimus dorsi, the lateral border of the pectoralis major muscle and a line superior to the horizontal level of the nipple is defined as the "safe triangle" [70]. Once the tube insertion site is prepared and draped with a full sterile technique, local anesthetic (1% Lidocaine) is injected into the skin and an incision is made above and parallel to the superior border of the rib. The size of the incision is slightly bigger than the operator's finger or the chest tube diameter. To avoid any damage to underlying structures, blunt dissection of the subcutaneous tissue and muscle should be performed using a hemostat and a finger before advancing the tube [74]. It is essential to create a complete track from the skin through the subcutaneous tissue and muscles into the pleural cavity, to ensure easy insertion of the chest tube without excessive force. Once the pleural cavity is entered, soft pleural adhesions can be removed using a finger. Dissection of thick adhesions is not recommended because the tissues may contain vessels and can result in significant hemorrhage [69]. The chest tube is then advanced through the dissected tract using a curved clamp. The tip of the tube is advanced posteriorly and superiorly towards to the apex of the lung to drain any potential pneumothorax. At the completion of the procedure, the skin incision site is closed and the tube is secured to the skin using sutures. The chest tube is connected to a single flow drainage system.

Non-Tunneled Pleural Catheter Placement

In the past, large-bore tube thoracostomy was believed to be less prone to obstruction by fibrin plugs or blood clots than smaller tubes, despite the lack of published evidence [75]. Optimal size and type of pleural drainage catheters remain controversial, but, a growing body of evidence suggests that small-bore (10~14Fr) pigtail catheters are as effective, safe, and well-tolerated as conventional large-bore stiff chest tubes [6, 76, 75, 77-80]. The 2010 British Thoracic Society guidelines recommended that small-bore pigtail catheters should be considered as the treatment of choice for drainage and pleurodesis of pleural effusions [75]. Similar to tube thoracostomy, indications for a small-bore pigtail catheter placement include pneumothorax, parapneumonic effusion, complicated pleural effusion, malignant pleural effusion, chylothorax, hemopneumothorax, and leakages into the pleural space from esophageal or gastric rupture [5, 69]. There is no absolute contraindication for non-tunneled small-bore pigtail catheter placement. Relative contra-indications may include coagulopathy and thrombocytopenia, which should be corrected before the procedure.

Potential advantages of small, soft, flexible pigtail catheters are: 1) relatively easy catheter insertion, 2) less pain during and after the procedure, 3) lower risk of complications,

4) faster recovery, and 5) decreased hospital stay [77]. In a multicenter study that included 405 patients with pleural infections, Rahman et al. found that a small-bore, guide-wire-inserted catheters resulted in substantially less pain than blunt-dissection-inserted large-bore chest tubes [81]. There was no significant difference in clinical outcome between the two groups. The authors concluded that small-bore pigtail catheters should be the initial treatment of choice for pleural infection. Kulvatunyou et al. also reported similar results from a prospective randomized trial comparing 14-Fr pigtail catheters and 28-Fr chest tubes in patients with traumatic pneumothorax [82]. They found that the patients with 14-Fr pigtail catheters had reduced pain at the insertion site without clinically significant differences in indwelling catheter time, success rate or procedure-related complications.

Complications associated with small-bore catheters include drain blockage, drain malposition, underlying tissue injury, post-procedural hemothorax/pneumothorax, empyema, and drain site infection [83, 84]. In a retrospective study evaluating complication rates related to small-bore catheter placement using a guide-wire technique, Davies et al. reported the incidence of catheter displacement and obstruction to be 21% and 9%, respectively. The rate of repeat procedure was 13%. The study, however, did not focus on comparing small-bore catheters to large-bore catheters and not all catheters were placed by interventional radiologist under imaging guidance [83]. In several other studies, complication rates associated with large-bore chest tube insertion were reported to be up to 31% and included post-removal pneumothorax, drain obstruction/displacement, lung laceration, diaphragmatic perforation, visceral organ perforation, vascular injury, wound site infection, and empyema [84-87]. In the 2010 British Thoracic Society Guidelines, Havelock et al. summarized that the highest reported complication rates are associated with large-bore chest tubes inserted in trauma patients using a trocar technique, while lowest complication rates were seen in studies where small-bore pigtail catheters were inserted by consultant radiologists [84]. The guidelines also mentioned that complications are likely reduced by using US guidance. In order to decrease the risk of complications, small-bore catheters should be secured to the skin with a suture and when draining hemothorax, complicated pleural effusions or empyema, flushed with saline regularly to avoid occlusion [5].

Procedure

The patient is either positioned sitting-up/leaning forward, lateral decubitus or in a semidecubitus position. After localization of the pleural fluid and the skin entry site using US or CT, the patient is prepared and draped using all elements of sterile barrier technique. Local anesthesia is achieved with 1% Lidocaine and a small skin incision is made. The pleural fluid is accessed using an 18-gauge entry needle under continuous US guidance similar to that of thoracentesis or intermittent CT guidance. If the location of the fluid collection is not seen using US (due to its location, surrounding anatomic structures, loculated nature, or air in the pleural space), intermittent CT imaging should be used as an alternative option (Figure 2).

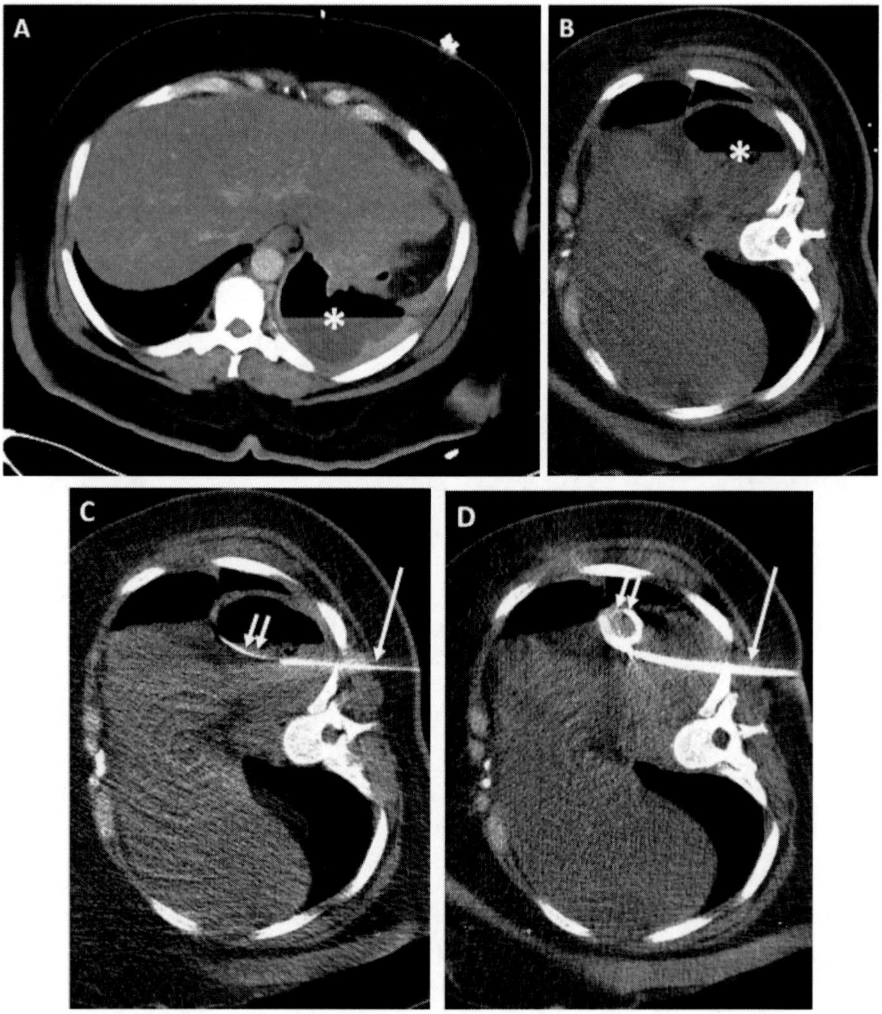

Figure 2. (a-d). CT-guided pigtail pleural catheter placement for empyema. Nontunneled pigtail pleural catheter placement in a 44-year-old female with acute pancreatitis and pancreatic pseudocyst complicated by a loculated empyema. Figure 2a. Axial contrast-enhanced CT image demonstrates a loculated empyema (*) with air-fluid in the left pleural space. Figure 2b. For CT-guided drainage catheter placement, the patient is placed in a right lateral decubitus position to identify an optimal access site. Loculated empyema with air-fluid level is seen in the left pleural space (*). Figure 2c. An 18-G needle (long arrow) is inserted into the pleural cavity under CT guidance. A 0.038-inch Newton J guidewire (double short arrows) is then advanced through the needle into the pleural cavity. Figure 2d. Over the guidewire, the track is serially dilated to 12-Fr. A dilator is then exchanged for a 12-Fr pigtail pleural drainage catheter (long arrow) and the pigtail portion (double short arrows) is positioned inside the pleural empyema.

Once the needle tip is safely positioned inside the pleural space, a 0.038-inch Newton-J or 0.035-inch Bentson (AngioDynamics, Queensbury, NY) guidewire is advanced through the needle into the pleural fluid collection. The needle is then exchanged over a guidewire for a dilator (8 Fr ~ 14 Fr), which is utilized for serial dilation of the skin and the soft tissue track. The dilator is subsequently exchanged for a locking pigtail nontunneled drainage catheter (8 Fr ~ 14 Fr), which is advanced over the guidewire and coiled in the pleural space. The catheter is secured to the skin using a suture at the exit site and covered with a sterile dressing. The external tip of the catheter is connected to a sterile pleural drainage system, such as a Pleur-evac1 (Teleflex Medical, Research Triangle Park, NC) plastic compartmentalized drainage system.

Tunneled Pleural Catheter Placement

The main indication for tunneled pleural catheter placement is malignant pleural effusion. The quality of life in most patients with malignant pleural effusion is significantly impaired due to decreased functional capacity and respiratory symptoms, such as dyspnea, cough and chest discomfort [88]. In patients with malignant pleural effusion refractory to medical management, thoracentesis is the first option for immediate symptomatic relief. However, when the effusion rapidly re-accumulates regular repeat thoracenteses can be logistically difficult and expose the patient to unnecessary risk. Therefore, additional options for malignant pleural effusions are chemical pleurodesis or placement of tunneled pleural catheters. Currently the British Thoracic Society guidelines recommend the use of tunneled catheter placement when talc pleurodesis is unsuccessful or with trapped lung [75]. Sometimes, pleurodesis and tunneled pleural catheter placement are performed concurrently to shorten the length of hospital stay [89]. In a randomized controlled study, Putnam et al. evaluated the utility of tunneled pleural catheters compared with chemical pleurodesis through traditional tube thoracostomy [90]. The length of hospital stay for the tunneled pleural catheter group was significantly shorter (1 day) than that of the pleurodesis group (6 days). Spontaneous pleurodesis was achieved in 46% of the patients in the tunneled catheter group. The rates of pleural fluid reaccumulation in the tunneled catheter and pleurodesis groups were 13% and 21%, respectively. There was a modest improvement in the quality of life and dyspnea scores in both groups. The complication rate was higher (14%) in the catheter group and included local cellulitis (most common) and, rarely, tumor seeding through the catheter tract. In a meta-analysis of 3 trials involving 307 patients with malignant pleural effusion, Kheir et al. found no significant difference in the success and complication rates between groups with tunneled pleural catheter and chemical pleurodesis [91]. The overall cost associated with pleurodesis and tunneled pleural catheters are reported to be comparable. However, initial cost for tunneled pleural catheter placement is lower as it is done as a same day outpatient procedure [91]. Complications associated with tunneled pleural catheters include loculation of pleural fluid, tunnel site infection, empyema, and tumor seeding through the catheter tract [75].

Pleural effusion associated with congestive heart failure is often unilateral and transudative. The primary management for this type of pleural effusion is treating the underlying cause. However, a significant percentage of patients with advanced congestive heart failure have dyspnea and shortness of breath from an effusion refractory to medical management [92]. Traditional treatment options include intermittent thoracenteses, "bedside" chemical pleurodesis, thoracoscopic pleurodesis and tunneled pleural catheters. In patients with rapidly accumulating pleural effusion, thoracentesis would not be an optimal treatment choice. Pleurodesis is an effective treatment for patients with this type of pleural effusion, but, causes an extended length of hospital stay [93]. As an alternative option, tunneled pleural catheters have been increasingly utilized for pleural effusions related to congestive heart failure. In 2014, Freeman el al. published a study comparing thoracoscopic pleurodesis to tunneled pleural catheter for heart failure patients with recurrent pleural effusion. In this investigation, the authors found that tunneled pleural catheters provided equal palliation effect for pleural effusions without reintervention and with a shorter hospital stay, compared to thoracoscopic pleurodesis [92].

Hepatic hydrothorax is a complication of end-stage liver disease in which portal hypertension results in recurrent fluid accumulation within the pleural space. When medical therapy fails to relieve respiratory symptoms, repeated thoracenteses, transjugular intrahepatic portosystemic shunt (TIPS) and liver transplantation are treatment options. However, for patients who are not candidates for TIPS or liver transplantation and cannot tolerate repeated thoracenteses, tunneled pleural catheters have been successfully used to palliate respiratory symptoms [94-96]. In a small prospective feasibility study, Chen et al. demonstrated that tunneled pleural catheters are an effective and safe management option in 25 patients with hepatic hydrothorax [94]. The mean number of catheter placement was 1.9 and spontaneous pleurodesis was achieved in 33% of patients. Although initial data are promising, a randomized controlled trial is required to validate the utility of tunneled pleural catheters in patients with hepatic hydrothorax.

There are two types of tunneled pleural catheters currently available: 1) PleurX Catheter (Becton, Dickinson and Company, Franklin Lakes, NJ) and 2) Aspira Pleural Drainage Catheter (Merit Medical Systems, Inc., South Jordan UT). The diameter of each catheter is 15.5 Fr and they have 30 side holes along the distal 1/3 of their entire length (66 cm). They are made of silicone with a Dacron cuff around the catheter 36 cm from the tip. The cuff is positioned inside the tunnel to prevent catheter dislodgement, infection, pericatheter fluid leakage. The external end of the catheter is connected to one-way valve system which prevents transcatheter fluid leakage and pneumothorax.

Procedure

For tunneled pleural catheter placement, intravenous moderate sedation consisting of midazolam (Roche, Nutley, NJ) and fentanyl (Elkins-Sinn, Cherry Hill, NJ) may be given in selected patients but local anesthesia along the tract suffices. Patient positioning is similar to nontunneled catheter placement depending on the location of the pleural fluid. After preparation and draping using full sterile technique, 1% lidocaine is used for local anesthesia. Through a small skin incision, an 18-gauge needle is inserted into the pleural space along the superior border of the rib just above the diaphragm with US guidance. From a lateral approach the needle is directed posteriorly in order to position the catheter tip in the posterior costophrenic angle for free-flowing fluid. The second incision is made approximately 5 cm anterior or medial and inferior to the needle entry site. Between the two incisions, the catheter is subcutaneously tunneled. The direction of the tunnel can be either antegrade or retrograde depending on operator's preference. A 0.035-inch Newton-J or 0.035-inch Bentson (AngioDynamics, Queensbury, NY) guidewire is advanced through the access needle into the pleural space either under fluoroscopic or US guidance. The needle is then exchanged for a dilator and the track is dilated to 16 Fr. The dilator is exchanged for a 16-Fr peel-away introducer sheath through which the tunneled catheter is advanced into the pleural space. While the introducer sheath is removed, it should be covered at the hub with a finger to prevent fluid spillage or air entering the pleural space. The external end of the catheter is connected to the Luer adapter. The initial pleural puncture site and tunnel exit site are closed using a suture and covered with sterile dressing. A final fluoroscopic spot image or routine chest radiograph should be obtained to evaluate the catheter position, for residual fluid, for pneumothorax, and for injury to the underlying lung parenchyma. After the procedure, up to 2,000 mL of fluid can be evacuated for immediate symptomatic relief.

Intrapleural Fibrinolytic Therapy

Reduced drainage from tunneled pleural catheters due to pleural fluid loculations occurs in up to 14% of patients [97]. Loculations also occur in parapneumonic effusion and empyema. Formation of a parapneumonic effusion is divided into three stages: 1) sterile exudative stage, 2) fibro-purulent stage, and 3) organization stage [98]. If sterile exudate is infected, the fluid starts progresses into the fibro-purulent stage. During the fibro-purulent stage, fibrin is deposited over the visceral and parietal pleural which subsequently leads to loculations and adhesions. In the organization stage, fibroblasts start to grow into the fluid to create a fibrous peel. If the fluid becomes purulent, it is called empyema. Most empyemas arise from parapneumonic effusions, but approximately 25% of empyemas can be caused by trauma or surgical injury [98]. Once, pleural fluid is loculated, drainage through pleural catheters decreases significantly.

For the treatment of complicated parapneumonic effusion with loculations, antibiotics alone may not be effective unless the loculation in the pleural space is cleared [99]. Although optimal treatment of complicated parapneumonic effusion is still controversial, it has been suggested that early disruption of loculations with fibrinolytics may avoid complications associated with them [100]. Since the first use of a streptokinase-streptodornase mixture in the pleural cavity in 1951, many studies have described the efficacy and safety of fibrinolytics for the treatment of multiloculated parapneumonic effusion, empyema, and hemothorax [97, 100-102]. Recently streptokinase, urokinase, tissue plasminogen activator (tPA), and combination of tPA and DNase have been successfully used in treating loculated pleural fluid collections. Cameron and Davies conducted a systematic review of the benefit of adding intrapleural fibrinolytics to pleural drainage catheters for the treatment of parapneumonic effusions and empyema [100]. They reviewed 6 trials and found that intrapleural fibrinolytic therapy had a significant benefit in reducing overall treatment failure (death) and the requirement for surgical intervention for patients with either empyema or loculated parapneumonic effusions. In a retrospective study, Vial et al. tested tPA in 97 patients with malignant pleural effusions and a nondraining pleural catheter [97]. They reported flow restoration rates after first and second dose of tPA as 85% and 72%, respectively. The complication rate was 5% which included hemothorax and infection. In 2009, Zuckerman et al. reported similar results from intrapleural tPA in 25 patients with loculated parapneumonic effusion [103]. Complete clinical and radiographic resolution of loculated effusions was achieved in 72% of the patients. There were no bleeding complications. Retained and coagulated hemothorax was also successfully drained using urokinase in a study that included 46 post lung surgery patients [102]. The use of intrapleural urokinase was successful in 91% of patients with complete and partial response rates of 76% and 15%, respectively.

Intrapleural fibrinolytics are instilled through nontunneled pigtail pleural catheters with sizes ranging from 8 Fr to 16 Fr. In the United States, tPA is the most commonly used agent and typical doses range from 4 mg to 10 mg [104]. The doses should be reduced to 1~4 mg in pediatric patients [105]. tPA is diluted in 50 mL of saline to make a total volume of mixture that is approximately 30%–50% of the initial pleural fluid volume. Following administration of the fibrinolytics, the catheter is clamped for 30 minutes ~ 2 hours [105, 103]. The catheter is then aspirated. This can be repeated twice daily for 3 days [105, 106] or for up to a total of 6 doses [103]. Imaging studies, such as CT or chest radiograph, are obtained within 24 hours of completion of the fibrinolytic treatment. The pleural catheter is subsequently removed if daily output is below 15 mL, a physiologic volume of the pleural fluid.

Chemical Pleurodesis

Pleurodesis is the obliteration of the pleural space by inducing adhesion between the parietal and visceral pleura. Despite repeated thoracentesis or catheter placement, pleural fluid recurs in approximately 2/3 of patients with malignant pleural effusions. To date, pleurodesis is considered the best treatment option available to prevent recurrent malignant effusion. Although there is no change in the patient's survival, the patient's quality of life can be significantly improved by pleurodesis [107]. Pleurodesis is performed either via tube thoracostomy, tunneled pleural catheter, or video-assisted thoracoscopy. Of those, tunneled pleural catheter is reported to be the best route for pleurodesis [108]. Early pleurodesis, immediately after initial diagnosis of malignant pleural effusion, may be performed to reduce the risk of trapped lung.

The International Survey of Pleurodesis Practice (ISPP) polled 859 physicians in 5 English-speaking countries to identify variations in pleurodesis practice [109]. In this survey, the reported overall success rate of pleurodesis was 66%. Sclerosing agents frequently used for pleurodesis were talc, tetracycline, and bleomycin with talc as the most effective and commonly used agent. The most common complications from pleurodesis were fever and pain. Other complications included nausea, respiratory failure and death. In the ISPP report, talc caused significantly more pain, fever, and nausea than other agents. Respiratory failure was also observed more frequently with talc. In a meta-analysis of 36 randomized controlled studies, Shaw et al. confirmed that talc was the most effective agent compared with other agents. However, talc was found to be associated with pain, nausea, and fever. Respiratory failure was also observed more frequently in patients with talc pleurodesis than other sclerosing agents [110]. Bleomycin and tetracycline derivatives also can be problematic for pleurodesis. Bleomycin is relatively ineffective and expensive compared to other sclerosing agents. Tetracycline derivatives are not always available in many countries [107]. Therefore, several alternative agents have been reported including: 1) silver nitrate, 2) quinacrine, 3) iodopovidone, 4) oral forms of doxycycline, and 5) other talc preparations [107].

For pleurodesis, the pleural cavity should be dried for a better apposition of the pleural layers. Daily output of a drainage catheter less than 150 mL is recommended for initiation of pleurodesis. Expansion of the lung on chest radiograph can also be used as an indicator regardless of the daily output of the pleural catheter. Once the pleural fluid is removed, a sclerosing agent is instilled in the pleural cavity through the pleural catheter, which is then clamped for 1– 4 hours. Rotation of the patient following instillation of a sclerosing agent was believed to encourage even dispersion of the agent in the pleural space. However, in a prospective randomized study by Mager et al. rotation of the patients did not affect the overall dispersion of talc suspension with unequal dispersion observed in 75% of the patients. In addition, there was no difference in success rates of pleurodesis between patients with and without rotation [111]. Dryzer et al. also found that rotational maneuvers did not offer a benefit to the success of pleurodesis after intrapleural instillation of tetracycline [112].

CONCLUSION

Pleural effusion is a commonly encountered medical problem that can cause serious respiratory symptoms and decreased quality of life. Knowledge of the underlying pathophysiology and etiology is essential for the diagnosis and management of pleural effusions. Chest radiography is the most widely used initial screening method for patients with suspected pleural effusion, although the sensitivity is not as high as other imaging modalities such as US and CT. US is a sensitive imaging tool not only for the detection of small pleural effusion but for guidance for percutaneous procedures. CT, MRI, and PET-CT are useful modalities especially for the differentiation and staging of more complex or malignant pleural effusions. Minimally invasive interventional procedures for pleural effusions include thoracentesis, nontunneled pigtail catheter placement and tunneled pleural catheter placement. In the past, large-bore chest tube was believed to be less prone to obstruction by fibrin plugs or blood clots, despite the lack of published evidence. However, small-bore, flexible pleural catheters have demonstrated advantages in the management of pleural effusions compared to traditional tube thoracostomy in a number of published studies. Additionally, intrapleural fibrinolytic therapy and pleurodesis may also be performed safely and effectively through small-bore pleural catheters.

REFERENCES

[1] Gasparini, S., and M. Bonifazi. (2017). Pleural diseases. *Curr Opin Pulm Med* 23 (3):269-274. doi: 10.1097/MCP.0000000000000374.

[2] Azzopardi, M., J. M. Porcel, C. F. Koegelenberg, Y. C. Lee, and E. T. Fysh. (2014). Current controversies in the management of malignant pleural effusions. *Semin Respir Crit Care Med* 35 (6):723-731. doi: 10.1055/s-0034-1395795.

[3] Kataoka, H. (2000). Pericardial and pleural effusions in decompensated chronic heart failure. *Am Heart J* 139 (5):918-923.

[4] Walker, S. P., A. J. Morley, L. Stadon, D. De Fonseka, D. T. Arnold, A. R. L. Medford, and N. A. Maskell. (2017). Nonmalignant Pleural Effusions: A Prospective Study of 356 Consecutive Unselected Patients. *Chest* 151 (5):1099-1105. doi: 10.1016/j.chest.2016.12.014.

[5] Yu, H. (2011). Management of pleural effusion, empyema, and lung abscess. *Semin Intervent Radiol* 28 (1):75-86. doi: 10.1055/s-0031-1273942.

[6] Heffner, J. E., and J. S. Klein. (2008). Recent advances in the diagnosis and management of malignant pleural effusions. *Mayo Clin Proc* 83 (2):235-250. doi: 10.4065/83.2.235.

[7] Rodriguez-Panadero, F., and B. Romero-Romero. (2011). Management of malignant pleural effusions. *Curr Opin Pulm Med* 17 (4):269-273. doi: 10.1097/MCP.0b013e3283474015.

[8] Grossi, F., M. C. Pennucci, L. Tixi, M. A. Cafferata, and A. Ardizzoni. (1998). Management of malignant pleural effusions. *Drugs* 55 (1):47-58.

[9] Anderson, C. B., G. W. Philpott, and T. B. Ferguson. (1974). The treatment of malignant pleural effusions. *Cancer* 33 (4):916-922.

[10] American Thoracic, Society. (2000). Management of malignant pleural effusions. *Am J Respir Crit Care Med* 162 (5):1987-2001. doi: 10.1164/ajrccm.162.5.ats8-00.

[11] Chung, J., and M. D. Perrot. 2010. Pleural effusion and empyema thoracis. In *Conn's Current Therapy*, edited by E. T. Bope, R. E. Rakel and R. D. Kellerman, 263-265. Philadelphia: Saunders/ Elsevier.

[12] Ferreiro, L., J. M. Porcel, and L. Valdes. (2017). Diagnosis and Management of Pleural Transudates. *Arch Bronconeumol* 53 (11):629-636. doi: 10.1016/j.arbres.2017.04.018.

[13] Broaddus, V. C., and R. W. Light. (1992). What is the origin of pleural transudates and exudates? *Chest* 102 (3):658-659.

[14] Miller, E. J., and S. Idell. (1993). Interleukin-8: an important neutrophil chemotaxin in some cases of exudative pleural effusions. *Exp Lung Res* 19 (5):589-601.

[15] Broaddus, V. C., and R. W. Light. 2010. Pleural Effusion. In *Textbook of Respiratory Medicine. 5th ed.*, edited by R. J. Mason, V. C. Broaddus and T. R. Martin, 1719-1763. Philadelphia: Saunders/ Elsevier.

[16] Colins, J. D., D. Burwell, S. Furmanski, P. Lorber, and R. J. Steckel. (1972). Minimal detectable pleural effusions. A roentgen pathology model. *Radiology* 105 (1):51-53. doi: 10.1148/105.1.51.

[17] Blackmore, C. C., W. C. Black, R. V. Dallas, and H. C. Crow. (1996). Pleural fluid volume estimation: a chest radiograph prediction rule. *Acad Radiol* 3 (2):103-109.

[18] Moskowitz, H., R. T. Platt, R. Schachar, and H. Mellins. (1973). Roentgen visualization of minute pleural effusion. An experimental study to determine the minimum amount of pleural fluid visible on a radiograph. *Radiology* 109 (1):33-35. doi: 10.1148/109.1.33.

[19] Hallifax, R. J., A. Talwar, J. M. Wrightson, A. Edey, and F. V. Gleeson. (2017). State-of-the-art: Radiological investigation of pleural disease. *Respir Med* 124:88-99. doi: 10.1016/j.rmed.2017.02. 013.

[20] Mercer, R. M., I. Psallidas, and N. M. Rahman. (2017). Ultrasound in the management of pleural disease. *Expert Rev Respir Med* 11 (4):323-331. doi: 10.1080/17476348.2017.1300531.

[21] Turner, J. P., and J. Dankoff. (2012). Thoracic ultrasound. *Emerg Med Clin North Am* 30 (2):451-473, ix. doi: 10.1016/j.emc.2011. 12.003.

[22] Inglis, A. J., M. Nalos, K. H. Sue, J. Hruby, D. M. Campbell, R. M. Braham, and S. R. Orde. (2016). Bedside lung ultrasound, mobile radiography and physical examination: a comparative analysis of diagnostic tools in the critically ill. *Crit Care Resusc* 18 (2):124.

[23] Kocijancic, I., K. Vidmar, and Z. Ivanovi-Herceg. (2003). Chest sonography versus lateral decubitus radiography in the diagnosis of small pleural effusions. *J Clin Ultrasound* 31 (2):69-74. doi: 10.1002/jcu.10141.

[24] Zanobetti, M., C. Poggioni, and R. Pini. (2011). Can chest ultrasonography replace standard chest radiography for evaluation of acute dyspnea in the ED? *Chest* 139 (5):1140-1147. doi: 10.1378/ chest.10-0435.

[25] Peris, A., L. Tutino, G. Zagli, S. Batacchi, G. Cianchi, R. Spina, M. Bonizzoli, L. Migliaccio, L. Perretta, M. Bartolini, K. Ban, and M. Balik. (2010). The use of point-of-care bedside lung ultrasound significantly reduces the number of radiographs and computed tomography scans in critically ill patients. *Anesth Analg* 111 (3):687-692. doi: 10.1213/ANE.0b013e3181e7cc42.

[26] Clec'h, C., P. Simon, A. Hamdi, L. Hamza, P. Karoubi, J. P. Fosse, F. Gonzalez, F. Vincent, and Y. Cohen. (2008). Are daily routine chest radiographs useful in critically ill, mechanically ventilated patients? A randomized study. *Intensive Care Med* 34 (2):264-270. doi: 10.1007/s00134-007-0919-1.

[27] Lichtenstein, D., I. Goldstein, E. Mourgeon, P. Cluzel, P. Grenier, and J. J. Rouby. (2004). Comparative diagnostic performances of auscultation, chest radiography, and lung ultrasonography in acute respiratory distress syndrome. *Anesthesiology* 100 (1):9-15.

[28] Gryminski, J., P. Krakowka, and G. Lypacewicz. (1976). The diagnosis of pleural effusion by ultrasonic and radiologic techniques. *Chest* 70 (1):33-37.

[29] Kalokairinou-Motogna, M., K. Maratou, I. Paianid, T. Soldatos, E. Antipa, A. Tsikkini, and C. S. Baltas. (2010). Application of color Doppler ultrasound in the study of small pleural effusion. *Med Ultrason* 12 (1):12-16.

[30] Kataoka, H., and S. Takada. (2000). The role of thoracic ultrasonography for evaluation of patients with decompensated chronic heart failure. *J Am Coll Cardiol* 35 (6):1638-1646.

[31] Grimberg, A., D. C. Shigueoka, A. N. Atallah, S. Ajzen, and W. Iared. (2010). Diagnostic accuracy of sonography for pleural effusion: systematic review. *Sao Paulo Med J* 128 (2):90-95.

[32] Xirouchaki, N., E. Magkanas, K. Vaporidi, E. Kondili, M. Plataki, A. Patrianakos, E. Akoumianaki, and D. Georgopoulos. (2011). Lung ultrasound in critically ill patients: comparison with bedside chest radiography. *Intensive Care Med* 37 (9):1488-1493. doi: 10.1007/ s00134-011-2317-y.

[33] Sajadieh, H., F. Afzali, V. Sajadieh, and A. Sajadieh. (2004). Ultrasound as an alternative to aspiration for determining the nature of pleural effusion, especially in older people. *Ann N Y Acad Sci* 1019:585-592. doi: 10.1196/annals.1297.110.

[34] Qureshi, N. R., N. M. Rahman, and F. V. Gleeson. (2009). Thoracic ultrasound in the diagnosis of malignant pleural effusion. *Thorax* 64 (2):139-143. doi: 10.1136/thx.2008.100545.

[35] Prina, E., A. Torres, and C. R. Carvalho. (2014). Lung ultrasound in the evaluation of pleural effusion. *J Bras Pneumol* 40 (1):1-5. doi: 10.1590/S1806-37132014000100001.

[36] Chen, H. J., C. Y. Tu, S. J. Ling, W. Chen, K. L. Chiu, T. C. Hsia, C. M. Shih, and W. H. Hsu. (2008). Sonographic appearances in transudative pleural effusions: not always an anechoic pattern. *Ultrasound Med Biol* 34 (3):362-369. doi: 10.1016/j.ultrasmedbio. 2007.09.009.

[37] Menger, R., G. Telford, P. Kim, M. R. Bergey, J. Foreman, B. Sarani, J. Pascual, P. Reilly, C. W. Schwab, and C. A. Sims. (2012). Complications following thoracic trauma managed with tube thoracostomy. *Injury* 43 (1):46-50. doi: 10.1016/j.injury.2011.06.420.

[38] Usta, E., M. Mustafi, and G. Ziemer. (2010). Ultrasound estimation of volume of postoperative pleural effusion in cardiac surgery patients. *Interact Cardiovasc Thorac Surg* 10 (2):204-207. doi: 10.1510/icvts.2009.222273.

[39] Balik, M., P. Plasil, P. Waldauf, J. Pazout, M. Fric, M. Otahal, and J. Pachl. (2006). Ultrasound estimation of volume of pleural fluid in mechanically ventilated patients. *Intensive Care Med* 32 (2):318. doi: 10.1007/s00134-005-0024-2.

[40] Cullu, N., S. Kalemci, O. Karakas, I. Eser, F. Yalcin, F. N. Boyaci, and E. Karakas. (2014). Efficacy of CT in diagnosis of transudates and exudates in patients with pleural effusion. *Diagn Interv Radiol* 20 (2):116-120. doi: 10.5152/dir.2013.13066.

[41] Arenas-Jimenez, J., S. Alonso-Charterina, J. Sanchez-Paya, F. Fernandez-Latorre, S. Gil-Sanchez, and M. Lloret-Llorens. (2000). Evaluation of CT findings for diagnosis of pleural effusions. *Eur Radiol* 10 (4):681-690. doi: 10.1007/s003300050984.

[42] Nandalur, K. R., A. H. Hardie, S. R. Bollampally, J. P. Parmar, and K. D. Hagspiel. (2005). Accuracy of computed tomography attenuation values in the characterization of pleural fluid: an ROC study. *Acad Radiol* 12 (8):987-991. doi: 10.1016/j.acra.2005.05.002.

[43] Abramowitz, Y., N. Simanovsky, M. S. Goldstein, and N. Hiller. (2009). Pleural effusion: characterization with CT attenuation values and CT appearance. *AJR Am J Roentgenol* 192 (3):618-623. doi: 10.2214/AJR.08.1286.

[44] Aquino, S. L., W. R. Webb, and B. J. Gushiken. (1994). Pleural exudates and transudates: diagnosis with contrast-enhanced CT. *Radiology* 192 (3):803-808. doi: 10.1148/radiology.192.3.8058951.

[45] Tsujimoto, N., T. Saraya, R. W. Light, Y. Tsukahara, T. Koide, D. Kurai, H. Ishii, H. Kimura, H. Goto, and H. Takizawa. (2015). A Simple Method for Differentiating Complicated Parapneumonic Effusion/Empyema from Parapneumonic Effusion Using the Split Pleura Sign and the Amount of Pleural Effusion on Thoracic CT. *PLoS One* 10 (6):e0130141. doi: 10.1371/journal.pone.0130141.

[46] Dixit, R., K. C. Agarwal, A. Gokhroo, C. B. Patil, M. Meena, N. S. Shah, and P. Arora. (2017). Diagnosis and management options in malignant pleural effusions. *Lung India* 34 (2):160-166. doi: 10. 4103/0970-2113.201305.

[47] Traill, Z. C., R. J. Davies, and F. V. Gleeson. (2001). Thoracic computed tomography in patients with suspected malignant pleural effusions. *Clin Radiol* 56 (3):193-196. doi: 10.1053/crad.2000.0573.

[48] Scott, E. M., T. J. Marshall, C. D. Flower, and S. Stewart. (1995). Diffuse pleural thickening: percutaneous CT-guided cutting needle biopsy. *Radiology* 194 (3):867-870. doi: 10.1148/radiology.194.3. 7862993.

[49] Hallifax, R. J., M. Haris, J. P. Corcoran, S. Leyakathalikhan, E. Brown, D. Srikantharaja, A. Manuel, F. V. Gleeson, M. Munavvar, and N. M. Rahman. (2015). Role of CT in assessing pleural malignancy prior to thoracoscopy. *Thorax* 70 (2):192-193. doi: 10.1136/thoraxjnl-2014-206054.

[50] Porcel, J. M., M. Pardina, S. Bielsa, A. Gonzalez, and R. W. Light. (2015). Derivation and validation of a CT scan scoring system for discriminating malignant from benign pleural effusions. *Chest* 147 (2):513-519. doi: 10.1378/chest.14-0013.

[51] Pessoa, F. M., A. S. de Melo, A. S. Souza, Jr., L. S. de Souza, B. Hochhegger, G. Zanetti, and E. Marchiori. (2016). Applications of Magnetic Resonance Imaging of the Thorax in Pleural Diseases: A State-of-the-Art Review. *Lung* 194 (4):501-509. doi: 10.1007/s00408 -016-9909-9.

[52] Coolen, J., J. Verschakelen, and W. De Wever. (2015). MRI of pleural diseases. *Curr Opin Pulm Med* 21 (4):399-406. doi: 10.1097/ MCP.0000000000000177.

[53] Gill, R. R., S. Patz, I. Muradyan, and R. T. Seethamraju. (2015). Novel MR Imaging Applications for Pleural evaluation. *Magn Reson Imaging Clin N Am* 23 (2):179-195. doi: 10.1016/j.mric.2015.01.006.

[54] Gill, R. R. (2011). Imaging of mesothelioma. *Recent Results Cancer Res* 189:27-43. doi: 10.1007/978-3-642-10862-4_3.

[55] Porcel, J. M., P. Hernandez, M. Martinez-Alonso, S. Bielsa, and A. Salud. (2015). Accuracy of fluorodeoxyglucose-PET imaging for differentiating benign from malignant pleural effusions: a meta-analysis. *Chest* 147 (2):502-512. doi: 10.1378/chest.14-0820.

[56] Duysinx, B., D. Nguyen, R. Louis, D. Cataldo, T. Belhocine, P. Bartsch, and T. Bury. (2004). Evaluation of pleural disease with 18-fluorodeoxyglucose positron emission tomography imaging. *Chest* 125 (2):489-493.

[57] Hooper, C., Y. C. Lee, N. Maskell, and B. T. S. Pleural Guideline Group. (2010). Investigation of a unilateral pleural effusion in adults: British Thoracic Society Pleural Disease Guideline 2010. *Thorax* 65 Suppl 2:ii4-17. doi: 10.1136/thx.2010.136978.

[58] Wang, Z. J., G. P. Reddy, M. B. Gotway, C. B. Higgins, D. M. Jablons, M. Ramaswamy, R. A. Hawkins, and W. R. Webb. (2004). Malignant pleural mesothelioma: evaluation with CT, MR imaging, and PET. *Radiographics* 24 (1):105-119. doi: 10.1148/rg.241035058.

[59] Light, R. W. (2002). Clinical practice. Pleural effusion. *N Engl J Med* 346 (25):1971-1977. doi: 10.1056/NEJMcp010731.

[60] Shinto, R. A., and R. W. Light. (1990). Effects of diuresis on the characteristics of pleural fluid in patients with congestive heart failure. *Am J Med* 88 (3):230-234.

[61] Hsu, S. L., and C. W. Tseng. (2018). Comparison of treatment of hepatic hydrothorax with catheter drainage versus serial thoracentesis. *Curr Opin Pulm Med.* doi: 10.1097/MCP.00000 00000000484.

[62] Sohara, Y. (2008). Reexpansion pulmonary edema. *Ann Thorac Cardiovasc Surg* 14 (4):205-209.

[63] Kim, Y. K., H. Kim, C. C. Lee, H. J. Choi, K. H. Lee, S. O. Hwang, J. H. Oh, Y. H. Lee, and A. J. Singer. (2009). New classification and clinical characteristics of reexpansion pulmonary edema after treatment of spontaneous pneumothorax. *Am J Emerg Med* 27 (8):961-967. doi: 10.1016/j.ajem.2008.07.036.

[64] Taira, N., T. Kawabata, T. Ichi, T. Yohena, H. Kawasaki, and K. Ishikawa. (2014). An analysis of and new risk factors for reexpansion pulmonary edema following spontaneous pneumothorax. *J Thorac Dis* 6 (9):1187-1192. doi: 10.3978/j.issn.2072-1439.2014.07.35.

[65] Mahfood, S., W. R. Hix, B. L. Aaron, P. Blaes, and D. C. Watson. (1988). Reexpansion pulmonary edema. *Ann Thorac Surg* 45 (3):340-345.

[66] Trachiotis, G. D., L. A. Vricella, B. L. Aaron, and W. R. Hix. (1997). As originally published in 1988: Reexpansion pulmonary edema. Updated in 1997. *Ann Thorac Surg* 63 (4):1206-1207.

[67] Thomsen, T. W., J. DeLaPena, and G. S. Setnik. (2006). Videos in clinical medicine. Thoracentesis. *N Engl J Med* 355 (15):e16. doi: 10.1056/NEJMvcm053812.

[68] Petersen, W. G., and R. Zimmerman. (2000). Limited utility of chest radiograph after thoracentesis. *Chest* 117 (4):1038-1042.

[69] Cooke, D. T., and E. A. David. (2013). Large-bore and small-bore chest tubes: types, function, and placement. *Thorac Surg Clin* 23 (1):17-24, v. doi: 10.1016/j.thorsurg.2012.10.006.

[70] Laws, D., E. Neville, J. Duffy, and Standards of Care Committee British Thoracic Society Pleural Diseases Group. (2003). BTS guidelines for the insertion of a chest drain. *Thorax* 58 Suppl 2:ii53-59.

[71] Iberti, T. J., and P. M. Stern. (1992). Chest tube thoracostomy. *Crit Care Clin* 8 (4):879-895.

[72] Tomlinson, M. A., and T. Treasure. (1997). Insertion of a chest drain: how to do it. *Br J Hosp Med* 58 (6):248-252.

[73] Boland, G. W., M. J. Lee, S. Silverman, and P. R. Mueller. (1995). Interventional radiology of the pleural space. *Clin Radiol* 50 (4):205-214.

[74] Millikan, J. S., E. E. Moore, E. Steiner, G. E. Aragon, and C. W. Van Way, 3rd. (1980). Complications of tube thoracostomy for acute trauma. *Am J Surg* 140 (6):738-741.

[75] Roberts, M. E., E. Neville, R. G. Berrisford, G. Antunes, N. J. Ali, and B. T. S. Pleural Disease Guideline Group. (2010). Management of a malignant pleural effusion: British Thoracic Society Pleural Disease Guideline 2010. *Thorax* 65 Suppl 2:ii32-40. doi: 10.1136/ thx.2010.136994.

[76] Mendes, M. A., N. China Pereira, C. Ribeiro, M. Vanzeller, T. Shiang, R. Gaio, and S. Campainha. (2018). Conventional versus pigtail chest tube-are they similar for treatment of malignant pleural effusions? *Support Care Cancer*. doi: 10.1007/s00520-018-4171-8.

[77] Light, R. W. (2011). Pleural controversy: optimal chest tube size for drainage. *Respirology* 16 (2):244-248. doi: 10.1111/j.1440-1843. 2010.01913.x.

[78] Parulekar, W., G. Di Primio, F. Matzinger, C. Dennie, and G. Bociek. (2001). Use of small-bore vs large-bore chest tubes for treatment of malignant pleural effusions. *Chest* 120 (1):19-25.

[79] Clementsen, P., T. Evald, G. Grode, M. Hansen, G. Krag Jacobsen, and P. Faurschou. (1998). Treatment of malignant pleural effusion: pleurodesis using a small percutaneous catheter. A prospective randomized study. *Respir Med* 92 (3):593-596.

[80] Parker, L. A., G. C. Charnock, and D. J. Delany. (1989). Small bore catheter drainage and sclerotherapy for malignant pleural effusions. *Cancer* 64 (6):1218-1221.

[81] Rahman, N. M., N. A. Maskell, C. W. Davies, E. L. Hedley, A. J. Nunn, F. V. Gleeson, and R. J. Davies. (2010). The relationship between chest tube size and clinical outcome in pleural infection. *Chest* 137 (3):536-543. doi: 10.1378/chest.09-1044.

[82] Kulvatunyou, N., L. Erickson, A. Vijayasekaran, L. Gries, B. Joseph, R. F. Friese, T. O'Keeffe, A. L. Tang, J. L. Wynne, and P. Rhee. (2014). Randomized clinical trial of pigtail catheter versus chest tube in injured patients with uncomplicated traumatic pneumothorax. *Br J Surg* 101 (2):17-22. doi: 10.1002/bjs.9377.

[83] Davies, H. E., S. Merchant, and A. McGown. (2008). A study of the complications of small bore 'Seldinger' intercostal chest drains. *Respirology* 13 (4):603-607. doi: 10.1111/j.1440-1843.2008.01296.x.

[84] Havelock, T., R. Teoh, D. Laws, F. Gleeson, and B. T. S. Pleural Disease Guideline Group. (2010). Pleural procedures and thoracic ultrasound: British Thoracic Society Pleural Disease Guideline 2010. *Thorax* 65 Suppl 2:ii61-76. doi: 10.1136/thx. 2010.137026.

[85] Bailey, R. C. (2000). Complications of tube thoracostomy in trauma. *J Accid Emerg Med* 17 (2):111-114.

[86] Deneuville, M. (2002). Morbidity of percutaneous tube thoracostomy in trauma patients. *Eur J Cardiothorac Surg* 22 (5):673-678.

[87] Etoch, S. W., M. F. Bar-Natan, F. B. Miller, and J. D. Richardson. (1995). Tube thoracostomy. Factors related to complications. *Arch Surg* 130 (5):521-525; discussion 525-526.

[88] Burrows, C. M., W. C. Mathews, and H. G. Colt. (2000). Predicting survival in patients with recurrent symptomatic malignant pleural effusions: an assessment of the prognostic values of physiologic, morphologic, and quality of life measures of extent of disease. *Chest* 117 (1):73-78.

[89] Boujaoude, Z., T. Bartter, M. Abboud, M. Pratter, and W. Abouzgheib. (2015). Pleuroscopic Pleurodesis Combined With Tunneled Pleural Catheter for Management of Malignant Pleural Effusion: A Prospective Observational Study. *J Bronchology Interv Pulmonol* 22 (3):237-243. doi: 10.1097/LBR. 0000000000000186.

[90] Putnam, J. B., Jr., G. L. Walsh, S. G. Swisher, J. A. Roth, D. M. Suell, A. A. Vaporciyan, W. R. Smythe, K. W. Merriman, and L. L. DeFord. (2000). Outpatient management of malignant pleural effusion by a chronic indwelling pleural catheter. *Ann Thorac Surg* 69 (2):369-375.

[91] Kheir, F., K. Shawwa, K. Alokla, M. Omballi, and A. H. Alraiyes. (2016). Tunneled Pleural Catheter for the Treatment of Malignant Pleural Effusion: A Systematic Review and Meta-analysis. *Am J Ther* 23 (6):e1300-e1306. doi: 10.1097/MJT. 0000000000000197.

[92] Freeman, R. K., A. J. Ascioti, M. Dake, and R. S. Mahidhara. (2014). A propensity-matched comparison of pleurodesis or tunneled pleural catheter for heart failure patients with recurrent pleural effusion. *Ann Thorac Surg* 97 (6):1872-1876; discussion 1876-1877. doi: 10.1016/ j.athoracsur.2014.02.027.

[93] Hunt, B. M., A. S. Farivar, E. Vallieres, B. E. Louie, R. W. Aye, E. E. Flores, and J. A. Gorden. (2012). Thoracoscopic talc versus tunneled pleural catheters for palliation of malignant pleural effusions. *Ann Thorac Surg* 94 (4):1053-1057; discussion 1057-1059. doi: 10.1016/j.athoracsur.2012.01.103.

[94] Chen, A., J. Massoni, D. Jung, and J. Crippin. (2016). Indwelling Tunneled Pleural Catheters for the Management of Hepatic Hydrothorax. A Pilot Study. *Ann Am Thorac Soc* 13 (6):862-866. doi: 10.1513/AnnalsATS.201510-688BC.

[95] Haas, K. P., and A. C. Chen. (2017). Indwelling tunneled pleural catheters for the management of hepatic hydrothorax. *Curr Opin Pulm Med* 23 (4):351-356. doi: 10.1097/MCP.0000000000000386.

[96] Sharaf-Eldin, M., A. S. Bediwy, A. Kobtan, S. Abd-Elsalam, F. El-Kalla, L. Mansour, W. Elkhalawany, M. Elhendawy, and S. Soliman. (2016). Pigtail Catheter: A Less Invasive Option for Pleural Drainage in Egyptian Patients with Recurrent Hepatic Hydrothorax. *Gastroenterol Res Pract* 2016:4013052. doi: 10.1155/2016/4013052.

[97] Vial, M. R., D. E. Ost, G. A. Eapen, C. A. Jimenez, R. C. Morice, O. O'Connell, and H. B. Grosu. (2016). Intrapleural Fibrinolytic Therapy in Patients With Nondraining Indwelling Pleural Catheters. *J Bronchology Interv Pulmonol* 23 (2):98-105. doi: 10.1097/ LBR. 0000000000000265.

[98] Light, R. W. (1985). Parapneumonic effusions and empyema. *Clin Chest Med* 6 (1):55-62.

[99] Lemmer, J. H., M. J. Botham, and M. B. Orringer. (1985). Modern management of adult thoracic empyema. *J Thorac Cardiovasc Surg* 90 (6):849-855.

[100] Cameron, R., and H. R. Davies. (2004). Intra-pleural fibrinolytic therapy versus conservative management in the treatment of parapneumonic effusions and empyema. *Cochrane Database Syst Rev* (2):CD002312. doi: 10.1002/14651858. CD002312.pub2.

[101] Tillett, W. S., S. Sherry, and C. T. Read. (1951). The use of streptokinase-streptodornase in the treatment of postneumonic empyema. *J Thorac Surg* 21 (3):275-297.

[102] Huang, D., D. Zhao, Y. Zhou, H. Liu, and X. Chen. (2016). Intrapleural Fibrinolytic Therapy for Residual Coagulated Hemothorax after Lung Surgery. *World J Surg* 40 (5):1121-1128. doi: 10.1007/s00268-015-3378-9.

[103] Zuckerman, D. A., M. F. Reed, J. A. Howington, and J. S. Moulton. (2009). Efficacy of intrapleural tissue-type plasminogen activator in the treatment of loculated parapneumonic effusions. *J Vasc Interv Radiol* 20 (8):1066-1069. doi: 10.1016/j.jvir. 2009.04.067.

[104] Shenoy-Bhangle, A. S., and D. A. Gervais. (2012). Use of fibrinolytics in abdominal and pleural collections. *Semin Intervent Radiol* 29 (4):264-269. doi: 10.1055/s-0032-1330060.

[105] Gervais, D. A., D. A. Levis, P. F. Hahn, R. N. Uppot, R. S. Arellano, and P. R. Mueller. (2008). Adjunctive intrapleural tissue plasminogen activator administered via chest tubes placed with imaging guidance: effectiveness and risk for hemorrhage. *Radiology* 246 (3):956-963. doi: 10.1148/radiol.2463070235.

[106] Rahman, N. M., N. A. Maskell, A. West, R. Teoh, A. Arnold, C. Mackinlay, D. Peckham, C. W. Davies, N. Ali, W. Kinnear, A. Bentley, B. C. Kahan, J. M. Wrightson, H. E. Davies, C. E. Hooper, Y. C. Lee, E. L. Hedley, N. Crosthwaite, L.

Choo, E. J. Helm, 107. F. V. Gleeson, A. J. Nunn, and R. J. Davies. (2011). Intrapleural use of tissue plasminogen activator and DNase in pleural infection. *N Engl J Med* 365 (6):518-526. doi: 10.1056/NEJMoa1012740.

[107] Dikensoy, O., and R. W. Light. (2005). Alternative widely available, inexpensive agents for pleurodesis. *Curr Opin Pulm Med* 11 (4):340-344.

[108] Erasmus, J. J., P. C. Goodman, and E. F. Patz, Jr. (2000). Management of malignant pleural effusions and pneumothorax. *Radiol Clin North Am* 38 (2):375-383.

[109] Lee, Y. C., M. H. Baumann, N. A. Maskell, G. W. Waterer, T. E. Eaton, R. J. Davies, J. E. Heffner, and R. W. Light. (2003). Pleurodesis practice for malignant pleural effusions in five English-speaking countries: survey of pulmonologists. *Chest* 124 (6):2229-2238.

[110] Shaw, P., and R. Agarwal. (2004). Pleurodesis for malignant pleural effusions. *Cochrane Database Syst Rev* (1):CD002916. doi: 10.1002/ 14651858.CD002916. pub2.

[111] Mager, H. J., B. Maesen, F. Verzijlbergen, and F. Schramel. (2002). Distribution of talc suspension during treatment of malignant pleural effusion with talc pleurodesis. *Lung Cancer* 36 (1):77-81.

[112] Dryzer, S. R., M. L. Allen, C. Strange, and S. A. Sahn. (1993). A comparison of rotation and nonrotation in tetracycline pleurodesis. *Chest* 104 (6):1763-1766.

In: Pleural Effusions: Causes, Types and Treatment ISBN: 978-1-53614-683-7
Editor: Rahul Khosla

Chapter 12

PLEURAL MANOMETRY

Kurt Hu[1], MD, Terrill Huggins[2], MD, Malik Khan[1], MD and Amit Chopra[1*], MD

[1]Pulmonary and Critical Care, Albany Medical College, Albany, NY, US

[2]Pulmonary and Critical Care, Medical University of South Carolina, Charleston, SC, US

ABSTRACT

The procedure of measuring the pleural pressure is referred to as pleural manometry. Routine use of pleural manometry is debatable. Currently, the main indication for pleural manometry is to identify unexpandable lung. It may also guide safe fluid removal during large volume (>1L) therapeutic thoracentesis and facilitates future decisions regarding therapy such as pleurodesis which is ineffective in those with unexpandable lung. Pleural manometry can be performed by using various devices such as water manometer, electronic transducer manometer, or digital manometers. Mean pleural pressure is measured during tidal volume breathing over four to five respiratory cycles at the beginning, during each subsequent removal of 250 mL aliquot, and at the end of pleural drainage. As serial aliquots of pleural fluid are withdrawn and serial measurements of pleural pressure are made, the pleural elastance is calculated by dividing the change in pleural pressure (in cmH_2O) by the volume (in liters) of pleural fluid removed. A measurement of $\geq$14.5 cmH_2O/L indicates poor lung expansion with additional fluid removal. With a free-flowing pleural effusion and an expandable lung, the initial pleural pressure is slightly positive and changes minimally as fluid is withdrawn. The pressure-volume curve is flat (monophasic) with a calculated pleural elastance $\leq$14.5 cmH_2O/L throughout the procedure. Lung entrapment is associated with a nearly normal initial pleural pressure followed by a steep decrease in the pressure when minimal fluid remains in the pleural space. The pleural elastance is biphasic with a calculated elastance $\leq$14.5 cmH_2O/L during the initial stages of drainage and a sharp increase exceeding 14.5 cmH_2O/L during the terminal stages of drainage. Trapped lung is

* Corresponding Author Email: ChopraA1@amc.edu.

usually associated with an initial slightly negative pressure. With fluid removal, a rapid decrease in pleural pressure occurs, correlating with a pleural elastance >14.5 cmH_2O/L (often >25 cmH_2O/L) throughout the procedure.

Keywords: unexpandable lung, trapped lung, lung entrapment, pleural elastance, pleural manometry, pleurodesis, malignant pleural effusion

INTRODUCTION

The pleural space is a potential space that exists between the layers of parietal and visceral pleura separating the lung and the chest wall. Normal intra-pleural pressure ranges between -3 to -5 cmH_2O at FRC and between -6 to -10 cmH_2O during inspiration [19]. However, in some pathological states, with the accumulation of fluid or air in the pleural space the pleural pressure may become positive resulting in disturbed respiratory mechanics and collapse of the underlying lung. In certain conditions, removal of fluid or air from the pleural space during thoracentesis can result in significant decline in the pleural pressures. This uncontrolled decrease in the pleural pressure may be associated with some of the complications of procedures involved with removing pleural air or pleural fluid, like chest pain in someone with unexpandable lung and may be one of the underlying mechanisms of re-expansion pulmonary edema.

The procedure of measuring the pleural pressure is referred to as pleural manometry and can be done during pleural drainage. The first person credited with measurement of pleural pressures was a German internist, Heinrich Irenaeus Quincke (1842–1922), who in 1878 performed the first pleural pressure measurement during pleural fluid removal [8]. In the early twentieth century, pleural manometry became an important component in the management of pulmonary tuberculosis and was widely used to collapse the affected lung by creating an artificial pneumothorax [14]. Later on, when anti-tuberculous drugs became available, the use of this collapse therapy and thus pleural manometry was abandoned. In 1980, Light and colleagues used simple U-tube water manometer to measure pleural pressure changes during therapeutic thoracentesis [21]. However, the U-tube water manometer was undampened, which resulted in large continuous oscillations of the water column with respiration and thus only allowed estimation of the mean values of the pleural pressure. This renewed the interest in pleural manometry and became more widely used to study various aspects of the pathophysiology of pleural diseases. In 1997, Lan and colleagues successfully used a 16 Gauge intracatheter needle inserted into the pleural space connected to a central venous pressure monitor to measure pleural elastance [26]. In 2004, Doelken and colleagues proposed a modified version of water manometer with the addition of a resistor to the system, this resulted in a dampened pleural pressure oscillations making for a more accurate measurement of the mean pleural pressure [6]. Around the same time,

Doelken and colleague also developed the first successful electronic manometer, which was capable of measuring accurate and continuous pleural pressure instantaneously [6, 14].

Nowadays, there are multiple different devices available to measure the pleural pressure ranging from simple U-tube water manometers to digital manometers, making pleural manometry an important tool in the armamentarium of the physicians and researchers today.

Pleural Space Mechanics

The pressure inside the pleural space is a result of opposing forces. The parietal pleura lines the entire thoracic cavity along the diaphragm and follows their movement during respiration. During inspiration, the diaphragm and external intercostal muscle contract leading to enlargement of the thoracic and pleural space, which causes the decrease in pleural pressure to about -6 to -10 cmH_2O [19, 31] (Figure 1).

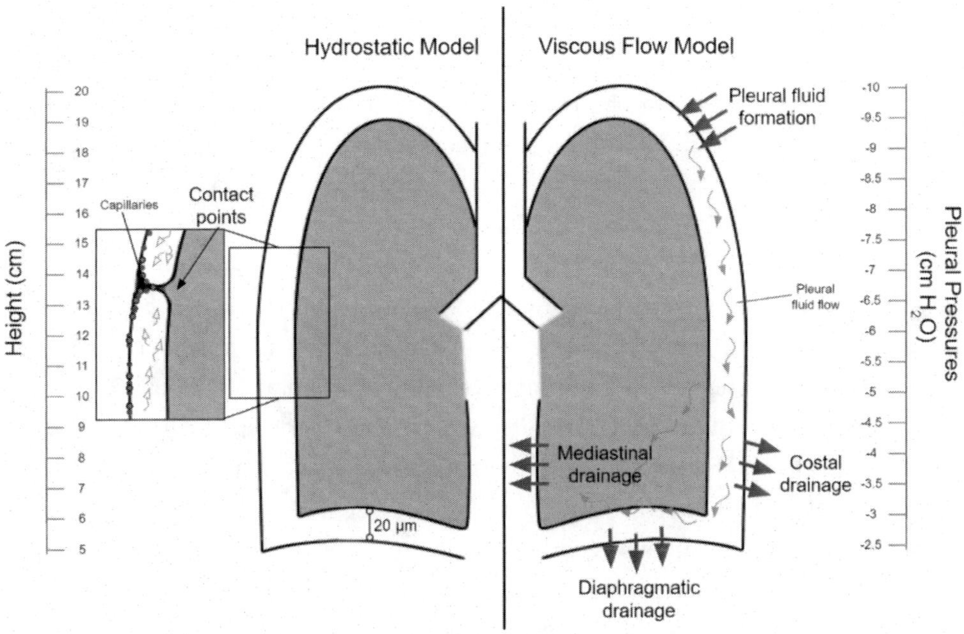

Figure 1. This figure describes the pleural pressure gradient across the vertical height of the thoracic cavity. Pleural pressure becomes more negative with increasing height but at 0.5 cmH_2O per 1 cm of vertical space. The left side figure describes the hydrostatic model of pleural pressure variability. This model describes that a contact point forms from the apposition of the two pleural surfaces when equilibrium is achieved by the absorption of pleural fluid into small capillaries that line the parietal pleura. The right sided figure describes the viscous flow model. The pleural fluid (arrows on-top) that is produced gets absorbed by multiple lymphatic drainage sites along the costal, diaphragmatic, and mediastinal pleura (arrows towards the bottom) which causes this fluid to flow through the pleura. This circulating flow creates a pressure gradient within the pleural space.

The hydrostatic pressure within the normal pleural space is slightly negative, approximately -3 to -5 cmH_2O when measured at functional residual capacity (FRC) [19]. This results from the inward recoil of the lung and outward recoil of the chest wall. The negative pressure is necessary to keep the lung from collapsing inwards under their own elastic recoil [31].

The pleural space doesn't behave just as a simple hydrostatic column of fluid as one may expect. Although the pleural pressure does become more negative with increasing distance from the base to the apex of the lung, it does so more at a rate of approximately 0.5 cmH_2O per 1 cm of vertical distance compared to the expected 1 cmH_2O per 1 cm of vertical distance. There are two competing theories to explain this actuality. One explanation is termed the hydrostatic model, proposed by Setnikar and colleagues and Agostoni and colleagues [1]. They describe the pleural liquid is constantly absorbed into the blood via pleural capillaries, once equilibrium is achieved between oncotic and hydrostatic forces, it causes the creation of points of contact between the parietal and visceral pleura. Therefore, pleural pressure consists of both pleural surface and pleural fluid pressures (Figure 1). However, animal models have suggested this proposal is less likely given that pleural fluid is shown to covers the entire lung as a continuous layer and lacks these points of contacts [2, 18].

The more accepted model suggests the liquid pressure and pleural space pressure are identical. As the pleural fluid flows through the parietal pleura towards the dependent areas of the lung it is removed by the lymphatics. The flow of fluid is maintained by the interplay of multiple factors such as gravity, ventilatory, and cardiogenic forces [2, 18]. As the pleural space widens in the setting of pleural effusion, the resistance to viscous flow decreases and the pleural pressures resemble more that of hydrostatic pressures [14].

The measurement of the pleural pressures in the setting of no pleural effusion is technically challenging because the normal pleural space is approximately 20 μm thick [17]. The introduction of a device would lead to local geometric distortion and the measurement would represent the local deformation forces and not the pleural pressures. Therefore, a small amount of effusion is needed to be present to accurately measure pleural pressures with the pleural catheter technique. The pressures measured is a representation of the actual pressure at the level of catheter insertion and reflects recoil forces of the lung and chest wall and the vertical height of the pleural effusion [6].

The dynamic changes in pleural pressure during respiration is a result from geometric deformation of the pleural space as the lung expands and as the chest wall deforms. As fluid fills the pleural space, pleural pressure increases causing the outward expansion of the chest wall and compression of the lung. Pressure changes during thoracentesis are due to the elastic forces of the lung expanding outwards and chest wall recoiling inwards to a steady state at FRC. Although pressure inside a pleural effusion can be determined by multiple factors, these can be assumed to be relatively constant during fluid drainage.

Therefore, the pleural pressure change is due to fluid removal and can be used to calculate pleural elastance [6].

CLINICAL APPLICATIONS

Pleural manometry can be very helpful in several different clinical situations; however, there is no strong supporting evidence at this time to justify its use on routine basis. The main clinical situations where pleural manometry may be indicated and useful include:

Large Volume Thoracentesis

Large volume thoracentesis is defined as removal of >1 L of pleural fluid. Large volume thoracentesis can be beneficial in certain situations by maximizing symptom relief and minimize the necessity of a second pleural procedure. However, large volume thoracentesis can be associated with increased chest discomfort and potentially can cause a rare but life-threatening complication called as re-expansion pulmonary edema (RPE) (Figure 2). There is no single absolute maximum volume of fluid that can be safely removed during therapeutic thoracentesis. Traditionally, fluid removal was discontinued when the total amount of fluid removed reached 1000 to 1500 mL [27]. However, this practice does not always prevent adverse effects. In fact, many patients do well with removal of more than 1500 mL, while others may experience symptoms, such as chest pain, or complications, such as RPE even at lower volumes.

We suggest using pleural manometry as a guidance to improve the safety of large volume thoracentesis, especially in those patients with suspected unexpandable lung. Fluid removal should be stopped if a) the patient develops symptoms such as chest discomfort b) if no more fluid can be aspirated or c) if the pleural pressure decreases to less than -20 cmH_2O. This approach is based upon the two animal studies which suggested that excessive negative pleural pressure, less than -40 mm of Hg was unsafe and was associated with RPE. Where a pleural pressure of greater than -20 mm of Hg was safe [23, 25]. Using this approach, Doelken and colleagues reported no occurrences of RPE in a large series of 192 patients during pleural manometry guided therapeutic thoracentesis [13]. Using a similar approach, Feller-Kopman and colleagues reported a very low incidence of clinically significant RPE (1/185, 0.5%) during large volume thoracentesis [9]. The mean amount of fluid removed in this study was 1670 mL, ranging from 1000 to 6550 mL. The occurrence of RPE did not correlate with either the volume of pleural effusion drained, pleural pressure, or pleural elastance. However, the prevalence of RPE was extremely low in this series to provide a meaningful correlation.

If pleural manometry is not available then symptoms should be closely monitored. The onset of vague chest discomfort correlates with greater negative pleural pressures. Feller-Kopman and colleagues reported that onset of chest discomfort was associated with lower (more negative) pleural pressures and a greater total change in pleural pressure, while cough did not correlate with lower pressures or the change in pressure [11]. Therefore, the presence of cough should not be an indication for termination of further pleural drainage. In fact, the group with the higher incidence of cough had lower pleural elastances, suggesting expandable lungs. Majority of those who developed chest discomfort had a pleural pressure less than -20 cmH_2O, while only 22% of patients had potentially unsafe decreases in their pleural pressure. This suggests that stopping fluid removal at the onset of chest discomfort avoids "unsafe" pleural pressures in the majority of patients. In a similar study, Khosla and colleagues reported a significant relationship between pleural pressure after pleural fluid drainage and the development of clinical symptoms in 141 patients. Chest pain alone or with other symptoms was significantly more common in patients with pleural pressure below -20 cmH_2O compared to the remaining patients (ATS poster Abstract).

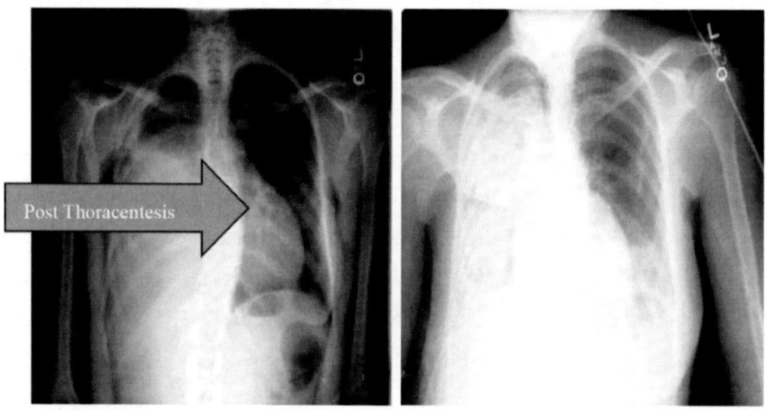

(a) (b)

Figure 2a. CXR showing large right pleural effusion. Figure 2b. CXR after large volume thoracentesis showing re-expansion pulmonary edema on ipsilateral side.

Identification of Unexpandable Lung

Unexpandable lung is defined as a condition in which the lung is unable to conform to the chest wall allowing normal visceral parietal pleural interaction. The unexpandable lung in the setting of malignancy may be the result from atelectasis caused by endo-bronchial obstruction or due to visceral pleural restriction caused by tumor or fibrosis on the visceral pleural surface [29]. An unexpandable lung may present clinically as the inability to completely drain a pleural effusion, typically due to the development of anterior, sub-sternal chest pain associated with negative pleural pressures [7, 13, 16, 24]. Rarely, a post-thoracentesis chest x-ray (CXR) may reveal drainage related pneumothorax (Figure 3) [13]. The reported prevalence of unexpandable lung as detected by CXR was extremely low, 6% in the TIME2 study [4] and 2% in the AMPLE study [30]. Post-pleural drainage CXR is an insensitive tool to detect unexpandable lung. Our unpublished data suggest that the prevalence of unexpandable lung in malignant pleural effusion (MPE) is around 50% which supports the reported outcome of pleurodesis in MPE of 50% at best (Abstract presented at annual CHEST meeting). Pleural manometry remains the gold standard technique to identify unexpandable lung.

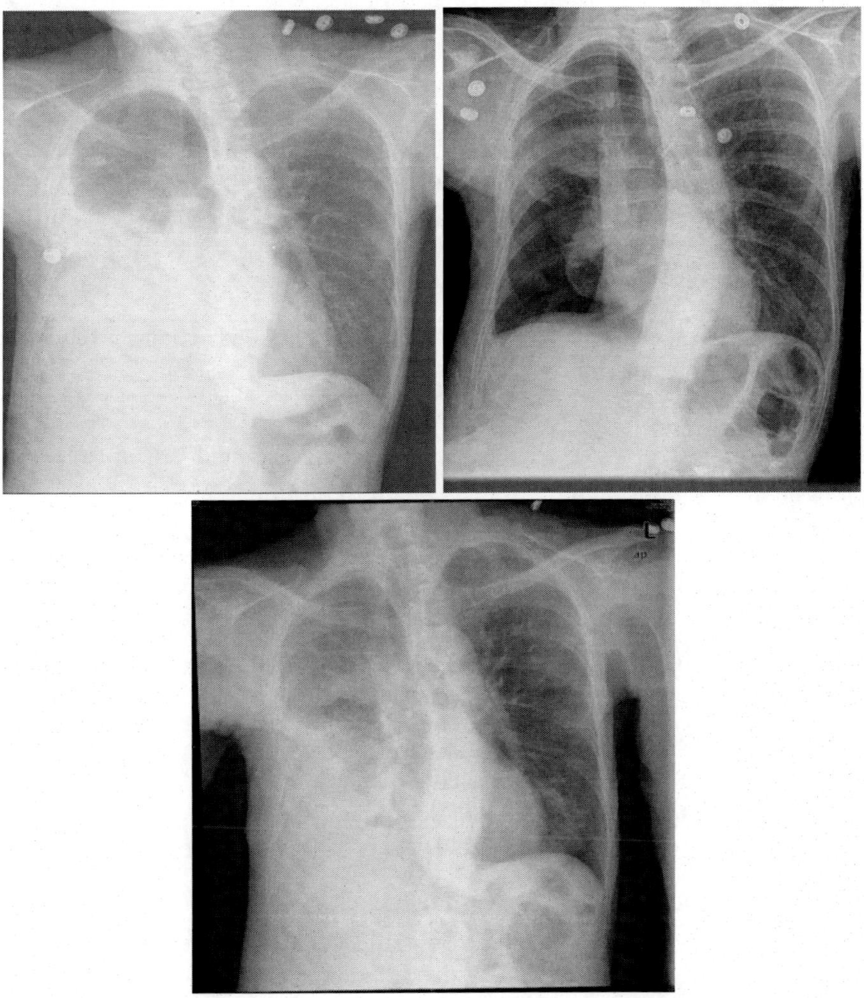

Figure 3a. CXR showing large right pleural effusion. Figure 3b. CXR after large volume thoracentesis showed large loculated basilar pneumothorax without contralateral mediastinal shift. Figure 3c. CXR after one week of pleural fluid drainage showed re-accumulation of pleural effusion.

In the case of expandable lung, pleural fluid drainage will result in a decline of pleural pressure down to a more physiological level (Figure 6). Occasionally, a sharp decline in pleural pressure with minimal fluid drainage will be observed, either immediately in case of a trapped lung or after an initially normal gradual drop in the patient with a lung entrapment (Table 1) [15].

Table 1. Difference between trapped lung and lung entrapment

	Trapped lung	Lung entrapment
Causes	Remote pleural injury such as resolved hemothorax, pleural infection	Active pleural inflammation such as pleural infection, malignant pleural effusion
Clinical Presentation	Asymptomatic, chronic stable persistent effusion without contralateral mediastinal shift	Dyspnea, chest pain Contralateral mediastinal shift may be present
Pressure volume curve	Monophasic, with initial negative pressure and elastance of >14.5cm H2O/L	Biphasic, initial pressure positive with initial elastance <14.5 cm H2O/L followed by high terminal elastance >14.5cm H2O/L
Pleural fluid analysis	Transudate	Exudate
Management	Observation Decortication if disabling symptoms	Treat underlying active disease

Trapped lung is characterized by the presence of a thickened visceral pleural peel as result of remote pleural injury which limits the ability of lung to conform to the chest wall (Figure 4). This process creates a negative intrapleural pressure (*ex vacuo* phenomenon) which results in excessive pleural fluid accumulation. However, this effusion is usually chronic and persistent in nature and doesn't cause dyspnea. Therefore, trapped lung should be considered in patients with a remote pleural injury and in whom a chronic, radiographically stable pleural effusion without obvious cause is encountered [7, 16, 29]. Therapeutic thoracentesis in these cases will not improve the dyspnea. Occasionally, drainage of these persistent pleural effusions may result in unintentional pneumothoraces. Heidecker and colleague described eight unintentional pneumothoraces in 192 patients, who underwent pleural manometry guided therapeutic thoracentesis [13, 16]. All these unintentional pneumothoraces were present in patients with unexpandable lung. Drainage related pneumothorax is caused by nonuniform stress distribution over the visceral pleura that develop during large-volume drainage where the lung cannot conform to the shape of the thoracic cavity in some patients with unexpandable lung. Hypothetically, these drainage related pneumothoraces are thought to result because of an opening of a transient, pressure dependent parenchymal-pleural fistulae. These pneumothoraces are drainage related and not due to penetrating lung trauma or external air introduction. This is evident by the terminal pressure in patients who equilibrated to the normal sub-atmospheric pleural pressure rather than atmospheric pressure (Figure 5) [13]. These pneumothoraces are stable and are not symptomatic or result in tension pneumothoraces and therefore, do not need treatment. These unintentional pneumothoraces cannot be prevented by monitoring symptoms or excessively negative pressure. This is perhaps because regional fistula formation might have occurred even before lowering the pleural pressures or during withdrawal of the last aliquot. This excessive pressure drop may not be detected with pleural manometry due to the entry of air into the pleural space before the last measurement.

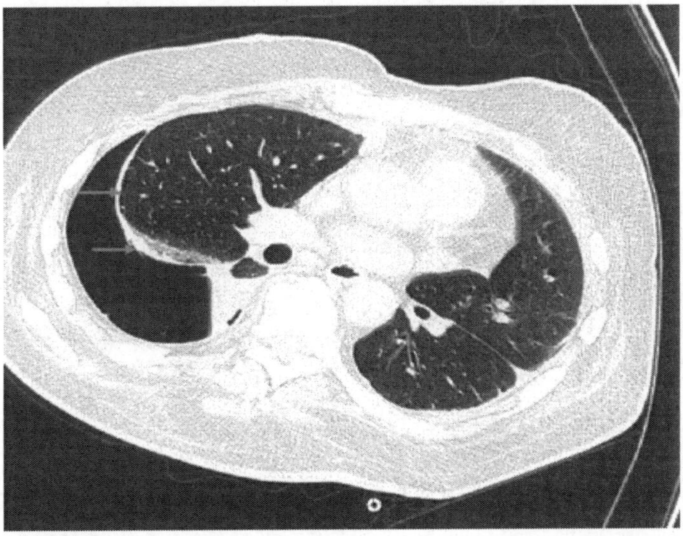

Figure 4. Cross section of chest CT scan showing thickened (arrow) right pleural peel from remote pleural injury in a patient with unexpandable lung.

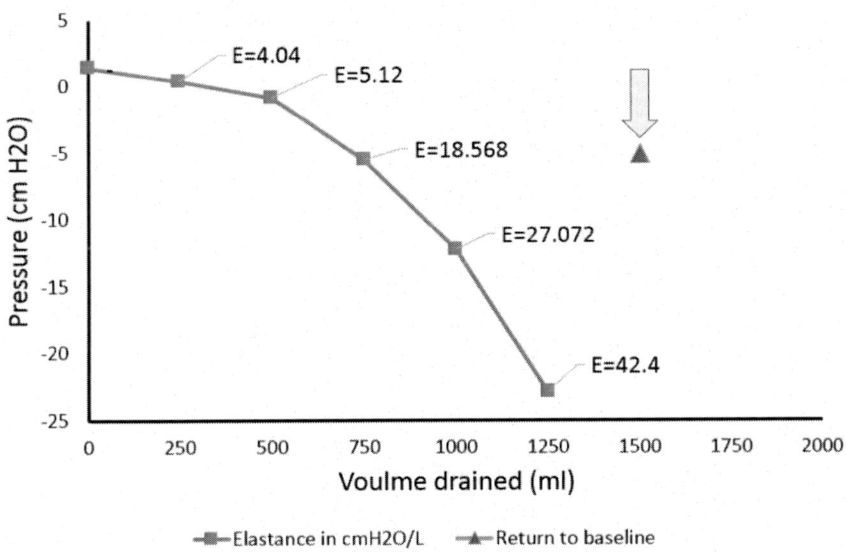

Figure 5. Biphasic P/V curve in patient with lung entrapment who developed pneumothorax after thoracentesis. Note the rise in pressure to a sub-atmospheric physiological pressure level at the end of the procedure (arrow). This rise is due to the drainage related pneumothorax that relieved the tension across the lung by opening of a pressure-dependent transient parenchymal-pleural fistula.

Whereas, lung entrapment implies an active pleural fluid formation process which may result in patient symptoms through increasing pleural pressures, potentially amenable to pleural interventions. An unexpandable lung may be encountered in a variety of clinical scenarios and establishing the presence or the absence of an active inflammatory or malignant process is paramount in the management of this condition. The presence of active pleural disease usually requires addressing the underlying process, as well as the potential clinical implications of an unexpandable lung. In the absence of an active process with an unexpandable lung, assessment and management is primarily concerned with the physiologic consequences of the unexpandable lung [5].

Guidance for Pleurodesis

Pleural apposition is a prerequisite in achieving successful pleurodesis in MPE. Unexpandable lung is an absolute contraindication for the pleurodesis. Post pleural drainage CXR is an insensitive tool to identify unexpandable lung (please see above). Pleural manometry can accurately identify the presence of unexpandable lung. That being said there is paucity of research study evaluating systematically the role of pleural manometry in guiding pleurodesis success rate. Lan and colleagues suggested that pleural elastance $\geq$19 cmH_2O was associated with 100% failure of pleurodesis in patients with malignant pleural effusions [26]. However, pleural elastance was calculated with initial drainage of 0.5 L which limits its applications as it provides insufficient data to identify unexpandable lungs. In our experience and from our unpublished data, most of the patients with MPE with abnormal elastance curve have a biphasic pleural elastance curve with terminal pleural elastance $\geq$14.5 cmH_2O/L. At present, there is no strong evidence to support pleural manometry guided pleurodesis approach. However, there is a randomized feasibility trial underway, looking at the elastance directed outcome of talc pleurodesis vs indwelling pleural catheter in the management of malignant pleural effusion. Hopefully, this trial will shed some light in this area.

Measurement and Techniques

Pleural pressure measurement is typically done in conjunction with the pleural fluid drainage. Ideally, pleural pressures should be measured sequentially during the pleural fluid drainage throughout the procedure as the pleural elastance may change during the drainage. Pleural pressure can be measured in the sitting or supine position. The manometer is attached to a stopcock on the pleural catheter to allow repeated measures of pleural pressure during fluid removal. The catheter insertion site serves as a reference point for the pressure measurements. The initial mean pleural pressure is measured just after insertion of the thoracentesis catheter into the pleural space and withdrawal of an initial sample of pleural fluid. We typically calculate the initial mean of four to five measurements of pleural pressure during tidal volume breathing, assessed over four to five respiratory cycles. This method requires use of an electronic hemodynamic transducer system with the capability to record tracings for review after the procedure. Subsequent pleural pressures are recorded in similar way after every 100 mL to 250 mL aliquots of pleural fluid drainage until the termination of the procedure [8, 6, 12, 32].

Pleural drainage is typically terminated when there is either: a) cessation of further drainage b) the mean pleural pressure decreases to -20 cmH_2O or lower (an arbitrary number suggested by animal data that further removal of fluid may increase the risk of re-expansion pulmonary edema) or c) inability to tolerate further drainage because of chest pain [6, 9, 10, 14]. Terminal pleural pressures should be measured cautiously as local deformation forces around the catheter can result in excessively negative pleural pressure and therefore we recommend that the closing pressure should be measured when at least 50 mL of pleural fluid is present as demonstrated by ultrasound or additional drainage [6, 14].

Interpretations of Pleural Pressures: The Pressure/Volume (P/V) Curve

Pleural elastance, in units of cmH_2O/L, is the measurement of the elastic properties of the lung and pleura. It is the measurement of the "stiffness," i.e., the ability to return to its original shape. This is calculated as the change in pleural pressure divided by the change in volume [15]. A large change in pleural pressure from a small change in pleural fluid volume yields a higher pleural elastance. Huggins and colleagues proposed the value of 14.5 cmH_2O/L as the upper limit for a normal pleural elastance [29, 16]. Determination of pleural elastance is visually aided by creating a pressure/volume (P/V) graph. This is done by placing the mean pleural pressure on the y-axis and the change in volume on the x-axis (Figure 6). The slope between points represent the inverse of elastance and the trajectory of the slope can be used to differentiate normal expandable lung, lung entrapment, or trapped lung.

Pleural fluid drainage in a normal expandable lung usually starts off with positive pleural pressure and gradually decreases and appears flat with a slight downward slope on the pressure/volume curve (Figure 6). This is a monophasic curve with a pleural elastance usually less than 14.5 cmH_2O/L [15, 16, 29]. This small change in pressure compared to a large removal of volume represents a normal lung elastance, with mean pleural pressure usually approaching the normal -3 to -5 cmH_2O, at the end of drainage. Monophasic curves can typically be seen in pleural effusions caused by hepatic hydrothorax or congestive heart failure [10, 15, 29]. There can be a sharp decline in pleural pressure towards the end of complete drainage consequently from local deformation forces acting on the catheter. Thus, the last pressure measurement needs to be validated by showing that there is fluid left by ultrasound or that at least 50 mL of additional pleural fluid can be removed (see below).

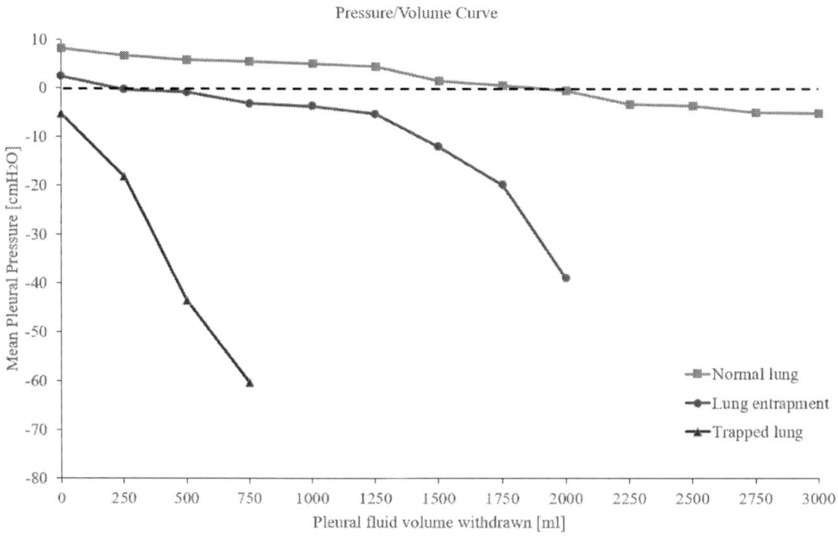

Figure 6. Three types of pressure/volume (P/V) curves. First P/V curve represents an expandable lung, the curve is monophasic with an elastance of 5 cmH_2O/L. Second P/V curve represents lung entrapment, the curve represents normal elastance of 6 cmH_2O/L until 1250 ml is removed, and the slope becomes very steep as the lung is unexpandable from this point with an elastance of 45 cmH2O/L. Lower P/V represents trapped lung, the initial mean pressure is negative and the curve is very steep with an elastance of 73 cmH_2O/L.

Pleural fluid drainage from a trapped lung, comparatively, usually starts off with a negative pleural pressure (Figure 6). As fluid is drained, there is a monophasic sharp decline in pressure representing a high pleural elastance [10, 16]. This is a thickened pleura with high elastance which resists expansion [16]. This produces a space of constant negative pressure during the entire respiratory cycle and draws fluid into the negative pleural space described as effusion *ex vacuo* and therefore the effusion is always transudative in nature.

Another commonly seen P/V curve is produced by lung entrapment (Figure 6). Pleural pressures start positive and will initially follow a flat monophasic curve, with a normal elastance, and abruptly become steeper as the volume, where the lung can no longer expand, is reached. This results in two different elastance curves known as a biphasic curve with terminal pleural elastance $\geq$14.5 cmH_2O (Figure 6) [6, 16, 29, 32]. The lung is unable to fully expand due to active pleural inflammation from malignancy or infection. Other causes of lung entrapment are due to lung parenchymal restriction such as from endobronchial blockage, interstitial lung disease, or lymphangitic carcinomatosis. These curves can be biphasic but at times monophasic with a pleural elastance >14.5 cmH_2O/L [10]. These pleural effusions are generally exudative and will produce symptoms and can progress to trapped lung if not treated.

Biphasic pleural elastance can also be seen patients with trapped who develops pleural effusion from additional competing mechanism such as congestive heart failure. The P/V curve will appear like that of lung entrapment with an initial flat appearance followed by a steep decline, however the effusion is generally transudative in nature [3].

CURRENT MEASUREMENT TOOLS

Pleural pressure measurement technique has evolved in last two decades from simple un-dampened U-shape water manometer to digital pleural manometer. At present there are three different ways of measuring pleural pressure.

Water Column Manometer

A U-shaped undampened water manometer made from intravenous tubing and syringe aspiration system is a part of a standard thoracentesis kit. First use of this simple U-tube manometer was described by Richard Light in 1980 [21]. U-shape manometer was made of plastic tube which was attached to Abrams needle using a three-way stop cock. However, there were significant variability observed between patients. Lan described pleural pressure measurement by using commercially available central venous pressure measurement tubing [26]. However, the pleural measurements by these undampened system had some obvious limitations. One of the major limitations was large pressure swings in patients with dyspnea and large amplitude pressure oscillations towards the end of the procedure. Doelken modified the water manometer by interposing a resistor made of 22 gauge needle between the two limbs (intravenous tubing) of U-shape manometer which dampened the water manometer and thereby minimizing these pressure oscillations (Figure 7). With this dampened water manometer, the reading will oscillate around 2-4 cm of H_2O around the mean pleural pressures [6].

Electronic Manometer

Electronic hemodynamic transducers, which is routinely used in intensive care unit (ICU) to measure vascular pressures can be used to measure pleural pressures. The major limitation is that ICU the electronic hemodynamic transducer is not designed to measure negative pressures. To compensate, the height of the zero-reference level (i.e., at the point of catheter insertion) of the pressure transducer is lowered such that pleural pressures are recorded as positive numbers and then later corrected by subtracting the number of centimeters that the manometer is below the point of the needle insertion (actual zero).

Another step required is that the electronic transducers records in mmHg and therefore, transducer pressures need to be converted to cmH_2O (1 mmHg = 1.36 cmH_2O) [26].

Considering these limitation, Doelken and colleagues described the first successful use of electronic manometer [6]. Doelken used a hemodynamic transducer with a signal conditioner and a personal computer data acquisition system (Figure 7). This system is capable of displaying pressure signal precisely, instantaneously, and at a very high frame rate of up to 3200 frames per second. The electronic manometer also has a very low inertia and a high frequency of measurements (50 Hz) allowing for reliable measurements of the pleural pressure even during a cough. However, this technique requires cessation of drainage during the pressure measurement but this technique is as accurate as the over dampened water manometer. Doelken showed a very strong correlation between pleural pressures measured by the over dampened water manometer versus the electronic transducer system. However this device is not commercially available for routine usage. Recently, Salamonsen and colleagues described a continuous way of measuring pleural pressure during pleural drainage [28]. The author described a manometer set consisting of a small-bore catheter, a pressure transducer, and an urodynamic computer for continuous measurements of pleural pressure during the fluid drainage. The author separated the pressure measuring circuit from the drainage kit in order to continuously measure the pressure without having to cease the drainage. With this technology, the author was not only able to measure pleural pressures but was also able to display the pleural elastance in real time with the ability to measure pleural volume drainage simultaneously.

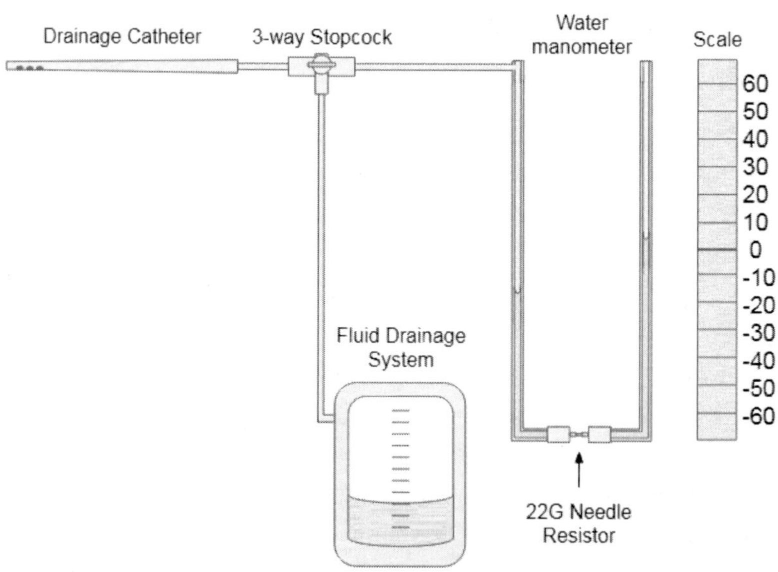

Figure 7. This is a cartoon that represents a dampened U-shaped water manometer. There is a resistor, in this case a 22 gauge needle placed in between the two arms of the water columns in order to reduce the oscillations to allow for easy reading and recording of the pleural pressures.

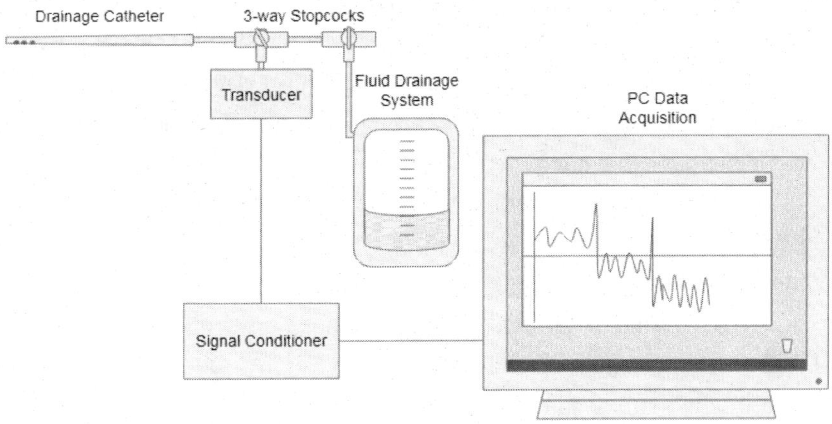

Figure 8a. This is a cartoon representation of our electronic manometer. It uses an electronic hemodynamic transducer connected at to a signal carrier modulator that transforms the analog signal it receives from the hemodynamic transducer into digital signal that can be displayed on a PC. It is connected via a series of 3-way stopcocks for easy drainage of the pleural fluid and measurement of the pleural pressure without the need to disconnect and reconnect the system multiple times. One can measure pleural pressure after each set volume removal which can be stored for later analysis.

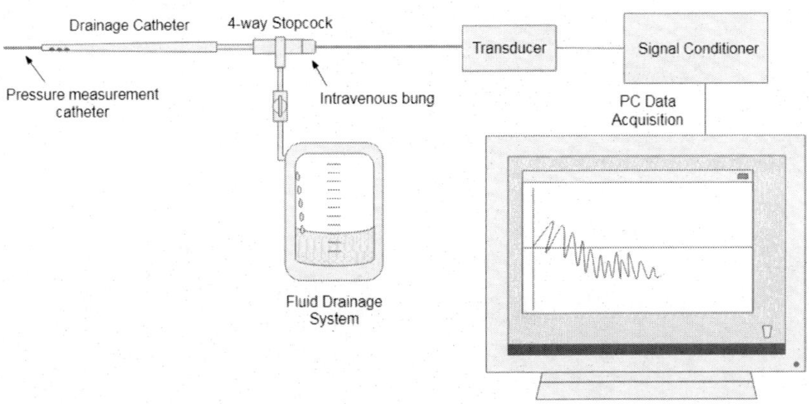

Figure 8b. This is a cartoon representation of a modification of the electronic manometer. Compared to the one in Figure 8 A, this is connected via a 4-way stopcock with an intravenous bung. This allows for a thin catheter to be passed through the drainage catheter and measure pleural pressures at the same time as pleural drainage occurs. One can measure pleural pressure in real time as well as storing data for later analysis using this setup.

Digital Pleural Manometer

Recently a group from Johns Hopkins, USA, described the use of the first handheld digital pleural manometer (DPM) (Figure 9) [20]. This device is compact and easy to use. It can be easily attached in-line to a pleural catheter during pleural fluid removal. The author compared the accuracy of pleural measurement by DPM, undampened U-tube water manometer, and electronic transducer manometer. The authors found a strong linear correlation between the elastance calculated for the digital manometer and the electronic transducer ($r = 0.9582$, $p < 0.001$) [20]. In contrast, the measurements made with the U-tube manometer correlated neither with the digital manometer nor the electronic transducer measurements. Results of this study differed from Doelken's observation where he found the U-tube water manometer and electronic manometer have a strong correlation between measurements of pleural pressures [6]. The differences in the results were likely due to Lee using an undampened water manometer system. The author's conclusion of this study was that the DPM is as accurate as an electronic manometer in evaluating pleural pressures. Currently, DPM is commercially available in USA for single use for $70. The disadvantage of this technique include a low sampling time (the sampling time is only for 3 seconds, so if a patient is breathing less than 20 breaths per minute, the entire respiratory cycle is not sampled), the ability to estimate the mean pressure due to a wide pressure oscillation during respiration (which is especially true toward the end of drainage). Recently, Rocket medical (UK) has developed an improved single use handheld DPM which allows for continuous pleural pressure measurements [22]. Pleural pressure is measured once per second and is mechanically dampened to display a mean pleural pressure on a re-usable digital display unit, based on the preceding 5 seconds of data. There is a randomized feasibility trial underway using this tool looking at the elastance directed outcome of talc pleurodesis vs indwelling pleural catheter in the management of malignant pleural effusions [22].

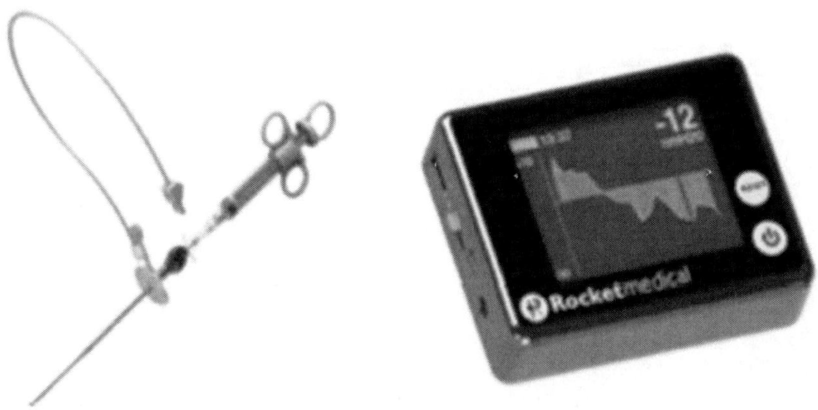

Figure 9. Digital pleural manometer by Rocket medical with re-usable monitor.

Conclusion

Pleural manometry is a potentially useful tool which can improve the safety of pleural procedures and at the same time provide useful clinical data in the management of patients with pleural disorders. Now with the development of widely available digital pleural manometers, the usage has become easier and more user friendly. However, the routine application of pleural manometer is still debatable. There are ongoing future large studies looking at clinical utility of this technique. At this time pleural manometry is recommended at specialized centers where clinicians are experienced with the use and interpretation of pleural manometry.

REFERENCES

[1] Agostoni, Emilio. 1972a. "Mechanics of the Pleural Space." *Physiological Reviews* 52 (1): 57–128.

[2] Albertine, Kurt H, Jeanine P Wiener-Kronish, Jacob Bastacky, and Norman C Staub. 1991b. "No Evidence for Mesothelial Cell Contact across the Costal Pleural Space of Sheep." *Journal of Applied Physiology* (Bethesda, Md. : 1985) 70 (1): 123–34. https://doi.org/10.1152/jappl.1991.70.1.123.

[3] Chopra, Amit, Rahul Argula, Christopher Schaefer, Marc A Judson, and Terrill Huggins. 2016c. "The Value of Sound Waves and Pleural Manometry in Diagnosing a Pleural Effusion with the Dual Diagnosis." *Thorax* 71 (11): 1064 LP-1065. http://thorax.bmj.com/content/71/11/1064.abstract.

[4] Davies, Helen E, Eleanor K Mishra, Brennan C Kahan, John M Wrightson, Andrew E Stanton, Anur Guhan, Christopher W H Davies, Jamal Grayez, Richard Harrison, and Anjani Prasad. 2012d. "Effect of an Indwelling Pleural Catheter vs Chest Tube and Talc Pleurodesis for Relieving Dyspnea in Patients with Malignant Pleural Effusion: The TIME2 Randomized Controlled Trial." *Jama* 307 (22): 2383–89.

[5] Doelken, Peter. 2008e. "Clinical Implications of Unexpandable Lung Due to Pleural Disease." *The American Journal of the Medical Sciences* 335 (1): 21–25. https://doi.org/https://doi.org/10.1097/MAJ.0b013e31815f1a44.

[6] Doelken, Peter, John T. Huggins, Nicholas J. Pastis, and Steven A. Sahn. 2004f. "Pleural Manometry: Technique and Clinical Implications." *Chest* 126 (6): 1764–69. https://doi.org/10.1378/CHEST.126.6.1764.

[7] Doelken, Peter, and Steven A Sahn. 2001g. "Trapped Lung." In *Seminars in Respiratory and Critical Care Medicine*, 22:631–36. Copyright© 2001 by Thieme Medical Publishers, Inc., 333 Seventh Avenue, New York, NY 10001, USA. Tel.:+ 1 (212) 584-4662.

[8] Feller-Kopman, David. 2007h. "Therapeutic Thoracentesis: The Role of Ultrasound and Pleural Manometry." *Current Opinion in Pulmonary Medicine* 13 (4): 312–18. https://doi.org/10.1097/MCP.0b013e3281214492.

[9] Feller-Kopman, David, David Berkowitz, Phillip Boiselle, and Armin Ernst. 2007i. "Large-Volume Thoracentesis and the Risk of Reexpansion Pulmonary Edema." *The*

Annals of Thoracic Surgery 84 (5): 1656–61. https://doi.org/https://doi.org/10.1016/j.athoracsur.2007.06.038.

[10] Feller-Kopman, David, Michael J Parker, and Richard M Schwartzstein. 2009j. "Assessment of Pleural Pressure in the Evaluation of Pleural Effusions." *Chest* 135 (1): 201–9. https://doi.org/10.1378/chest.08-1788.

[11] Feller-Kopman, David, Allan Walkey, David Berkowitz, and Armin Ernst. 2006k. "The Relationship of Pleural Pressure to Symptom Development During Therapeutic Thoracentesis." *Chest* 129 (6): 1556–60. https://doi.org/https://doi.org/10.1378/chest.129.6.1556.

[12] Grabczak, Elzbieta M, Rafal Krenke, Monika Zielinska-Krawczyk, and Richard W Light. 2018l. "Pleural Manometry in Patients with Pleural Diseases – the Usefulness in Clinical Practice." *Respiratory Medicine*. https://doi.org/https://doi.org/10.1016/j.rmed.2018.01.014.

[13] Heidecker, Jay, John T Huggins, Steven A Sahn, and Peter Doelken. 2006m. "Pathophysiology of Pneumothorax Following Ultrasound-Guided Thoracentesis." *Chest* 130 (4): 1173–84. https://doi.org/https://doi.org/10.1016/S0012-3692(15)51155-0.

[14] Huggins, John T, and Peter Doelken. 2006n. "Pleural Manometry." *Clinics in Chest Medicine* 27 (2): 229–40. https://doi.org/10.1016/j.ccm.2005.12.007.

[15] Huggins, John T, Peter Doelken, and Steven A Sahn. 2010o. "The Unexpandable Lung." *F1000 Medicine Reports* 2 (October): 77. https://doi.org/10.3410/M2-77.

[16] Huggins, John T, Steven A Sahn, Jay Heidecker, James G Ravenel, and Peter Doelken. 2007p. "Characteristics of Trapped Lung: Pleural Fluid Analysis, Manometry, and Air-Contrast Chest CT." *Chest* 131 (1): 206–13. https://doi.org/https://doi.org/10.1378/chest.06-0430.

[17] Lai-fook, Stephen J. 2004q. "Pleural Mechanics and Fluid Exchange." *Physiological Reviews* 84 (2): 385–410. https://doi.org/10.1152/physrev.00026.2003.

[18] Lai-Fook, Stephen J, and Mark R Kaplowitz. 1985r. "Pleural Space Thickness in Situ by Light Microscopy in Five Mammalian Species." *Journal of Applied Physiology* (Bethesda, Md. : 1985) 59 (2): 603–10. https://doi.org/10.1152/jappl.1985.59.2.603.

[19] Lai-Fook, Stephen J, and Joseph R Rodarte. 1991s. "Pleural Pressure Distribution and Its Relationship to Lung Volume and Interstitial Pressure." *Journal of Applied Physiology* 70 (3): 967–78. https://doi.org/10.1152/jappl.1991.70.3.967.

[20] Lee, Hans J, Lonny Yarmus, David Kidd, Ricardo Ortiz, Jason Akulian, Christopher Gilbert, Andrew Hughes, Richard E Thompson, Sixto Arias, and David Feller-Kopman. 2014t. "Comparison of Pleural Pressure Measuring Instruments." *Chest* 146 (4): 1007–12.

[21] Light, Richard W, Stephen G Jenkinson, Vu-Dinh Minh, and Ronald B George. 1980u. "Observations on Pleural Fluid Pressures as Fluid Is Withdrawn during

Thoracentesis." *American Review of Respiratory Disease* 121 (5): 799–804. https://doi.org/10.1164/arrd.1980.121.5.799.

[22] Martin, Geoffrey A, Selina Tsim, Andrew C Kidd, John E Foster, Philip McLoone, Anthony Chalmers, and Kevin G Blyth. 2018v. "Pre-EDIT: Protocol for a Randomised Feasibility Trial of Elastance-Directed Intrapleural Catheter or Talc Pleurodesis (EDIT) in Malignant Pleural Effusion." *BMJ Open Respiratory Research* 5 (1): e000293.

[23] Miller, Warren C, Richard Toon, Herman Palat, and John Lacroix. 1973w. "Experimental Pulmonary Edema Following Re-Expansion of Pneumothorax." *American Review of Respiratory Disease* 108 (3): 664–66. https://doi.org/10.1164/arrd.1973.108.3.664.

[24] Moore, Patrick J, and Paul A Thomas. 1967x. "The Trapped Lung with Chronic Pleural Space, a Cause of Recurring Pleural Effusion." *Military Medicine* 132 (12): 998–1002.

[25] Pavlin, Janet, and Frederick W Cheney. 1979y. "Unilateral Pulmonary Edema in Rabbits after Reexpansion of Collapsed Lung." *Journal of Applied Physiology* 46 (1): 31–35. https://doi.org/10.1152/jappl.1979.46.1.31.

[26] R, Lan, Lo S, Chuang M, Yang C, Tsao T, and Lee C. 1997z. "Elastance of the Pleural Space: A Predictor for the Outcome of Pleurodesis in Patients with Malignant Pleural Effusion." *Annals of Internal Medicine* 126 (10): 768–74. https://doi.org/10.7326/0003-4819-126-10-199705150-00003.

[27] Roberts, Mark E, Edmund Neville, Richard G Berrisford, George Antunes, and Nabeel J Ali. 2010aa. "Management of a Malignant Pleural Effusion: British Thoracic Society Pleural Disease Guideline 2010." *Thorax* 65 (Suppl 2): ii32-ii40.

[28] Salamonsen, Matthew, Robert Ware, and David Fielding. 2014ab. "A New Method for Performing Continuous Manometry during Pleural Effusion Drainage." *Respiration* 88 (1): 61–66.

[29] T., Huggins John, Maldonado Fabien, Chopra Amit, Rahman Najib, and Light Richard. 2017ac. "Unexpandable Lung from Pleural Disease." *Respirology* 23 (2): 160–67. https://doi.org/10.1111/resp.13199.

[30] Thomas, Rajesh, Edward Fysh, Nicola Smith, Pyng Lee, Benjamin C. H. Kwan, Elaine Yap, Fiona C. Horwood, et al. 2017ad. "Effect of an Indwelling Pleural Catheter vs Talc Pleurodesis on Hospitalization Days in Patients with Malignant Pleural Effusion: The Ample Randomized Clinical Trial." *JAMA* 318 (19): 1903–12. http://dx.doi.org/10.1001/jama.2017.17426.

[31] Troyer, André De, and Theodore A. Wilson. 2016ae. "Action of the Diaphragm on the Rib Cage." *Journal of Applied Physiology* 121 (2): 391–400. https://doi.org/10.1152/japplphysiol.00268.2016.

[32] Zielinska-Krawczyk, Monika, Rafal Krenke, Elzbieta M Grabczak, and Richard W Light. 2018af. "Pleural Manometry–historical Background, Rationale for Use and Methods of Measurement." *Respiratory Medicine* 136: 21–28. https://doi.org/https://doi.org/10.1016/j.rmed.2018.01.013.

In: Pleural Effusions: Causes, Types and Treatment
Editor: Rahul Khosla
ISBN: 978-1-53614-683-7

Chapter 13

PLEURAL EFFUSION CASES: PART 1

Akshay Bhatnagar[1,2*], MD, Kewakebt Lemma[1], MD and Rahul Khosla[2], MD

[1]Pulmonary, Critical Care, and Sleep Medicine,
The George Washington University, Washington DC, US
[2]Pulmonary & CCM Section,
Veterans Affairs Medical Center, Washington DC, US

ABSTRACT

In this chapter five interesting cases have been presented for the reader to review and recap important topics presented in the book thus far.

Keywords: chylothorax, hemothorax, exudative pleural effusion, rheumatoid pleural effusion

CASE 1

42 years old female with a past medical history significant for right breast invasive ductal carcinoma treated with chemotherapy, radiation therapy, and right-sided mastectomy with axillary node dissection, followed by breast reconstructive surgery. Chest x-ray (CXR) prior to reconstructive surgery is displayed below (Figure 1a).

Soon after reconstructive surgery, patient presented with increasing dyspnea and upper body swelling and was diagnosed by chest x-ray (Figure 1b) with a new right-sided pleural effusion.

*Corresponding Author Email: Akshay.virginia@gmail.com.

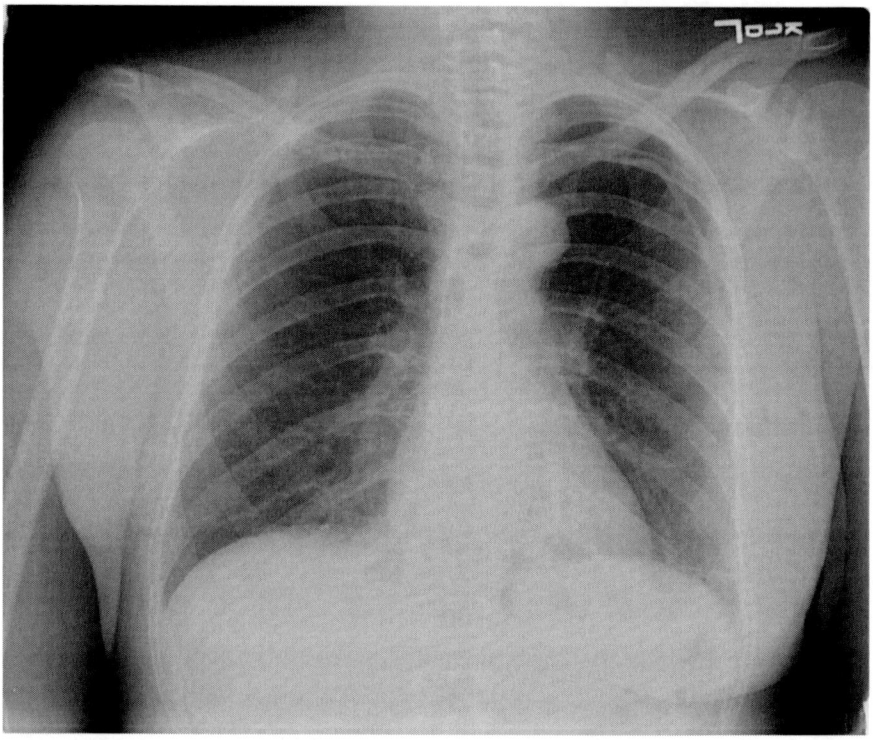

Figure 1a. CXR prior to surgery.

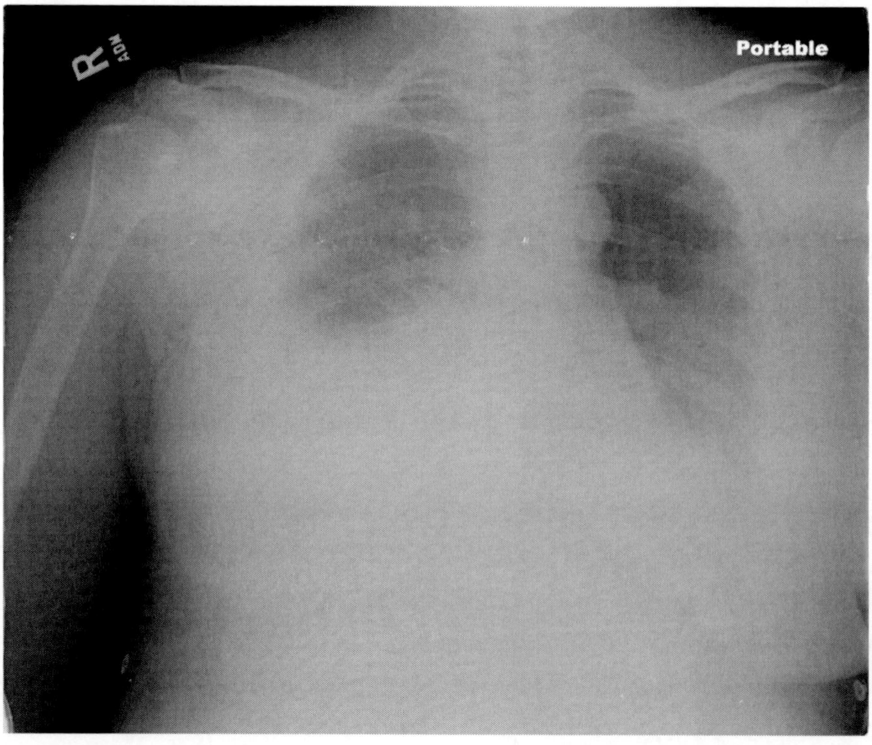

Figure 1b. CXR after surgery.

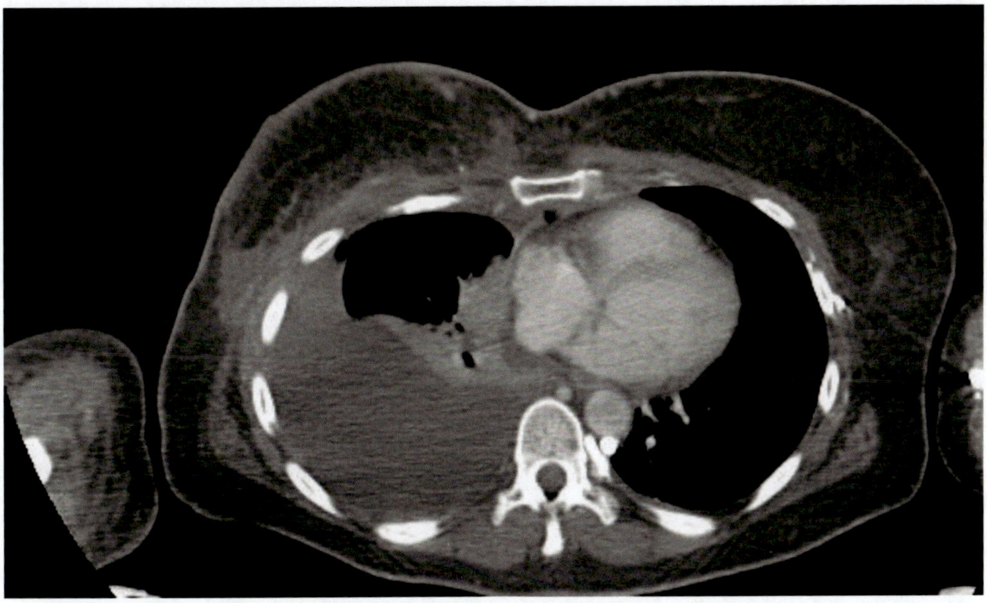

Figure 1c. CT after surgery.

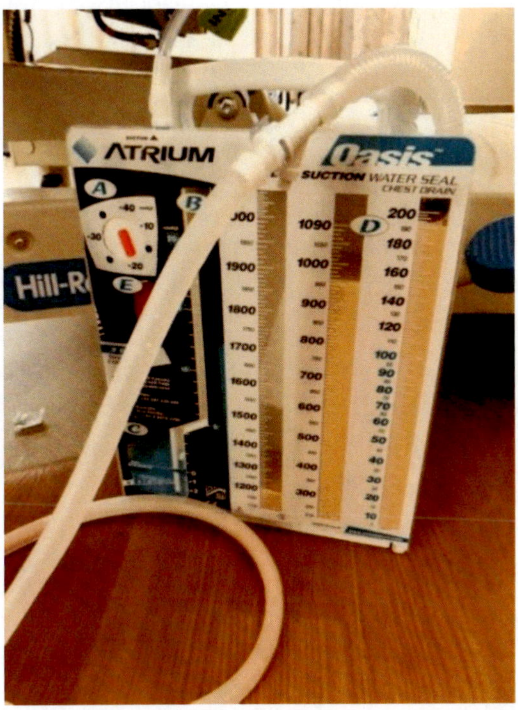

Figure 1d. Chylous effusion.

Computed tomography (CT) scan (Figure 1c) confirmed a moderate-sized right-sided pleural effusion with mild compressive atelectasis. CT scan also demonstrated an obstruct-tion of the brachiocephalic vein secondary to thrombosis and systemic anticoagulation was initiated.

Thoracentesis was performed and one liter of milky fluid was removed. Pleural fluid analysis demonstrated negative cytology, negative culture and gram stain, pH 7.48, glucose 115mg/dL, protein 2.9 g/dL, amylase 43, LDH 135 mU/mL, triglyceride 451 mg/dL, and cholesterol 87 mg/dL. Pleural fluid cell differential demonstrated total non-RBC cells 225/cm^2, RBC 540/cm^2, segmented cells 18%, lymphocytes 71%, and monocytes 11%. Chest tube was placed to drain chylous effusion [Figure 1d] for a symptomatic effusion with rapid re-accumulation.

Upper extremity venogram demonstrated superior vena cava (SVC) occlusion with drainage through the azygous vein. Angioplasty was performed with complete resolution of the occlusion.

Thus, clinical history, imaging, and laboratory analysis confirmed the diagnosis of right-sided chylothorax. This was likely secondary to SVC syndrome with resulting venous backflow and obstruction of lymphatics, along with possible injury, in setting of recent surgery, to the right lymphatic duct.

Normalization of the venous occlusion did not result in resolution of lymphatic drainage into the pleural space and thus a right-sided video-assisted thoracoscopic surgery (VATS) with pleurodesis and indwelling pleural catheter insertion was performed.

CASE 2

85 years old male with a past medical history significant for non-Hodgkin's lymphoma (marginal zone lymphoma) treated with rituximab, stage III chronic kidney disease, and stage II diastolic heart failure, presented with dyspnea. CT scan demonstrated bilateral L> R pleural effusions (Figure 2a).

Given the bilateral nature of the pleural effusions, the patient was initiated on diuretic therapy as the pleural effusions were felt to be secondary to a combination of diastolic heart failure and chronic kidney disease. He continued to complain of dyspnea on exertion despite an increase in his diuretic dose. Subsequent CXR (Figure 2b) demonstrated persistent bilateral, now R> L, pleural effusions.

The patient was scheduled for a right-sided thoracentesis. Ultrasound was used to localize the most appropriate drainage site and demonstrated a moderate sized right anechoic pleural effusion (Figure 2c).

Thoracentesis was performed and two liters of serous fluid removed. Pleural fluid analysis demonstrated negative cytology, negative culture and gram stain, pH 7.50, glucose 109 mg/dL, protein 5.0 g/dL, LDH 101 mU/mL, amylase 101 U/L, and adenosine deaminase 9.5 U/L. Pleural fluid cell differential demonstrated total non-RBC cells 1341/cm^2, RBC 1917/cm^2, lymphocytes 38%, and monocytes 54%.

Post-thoracentesis CXR (Figure 2d) demonstrated resolution of right-sided pleural effusion.

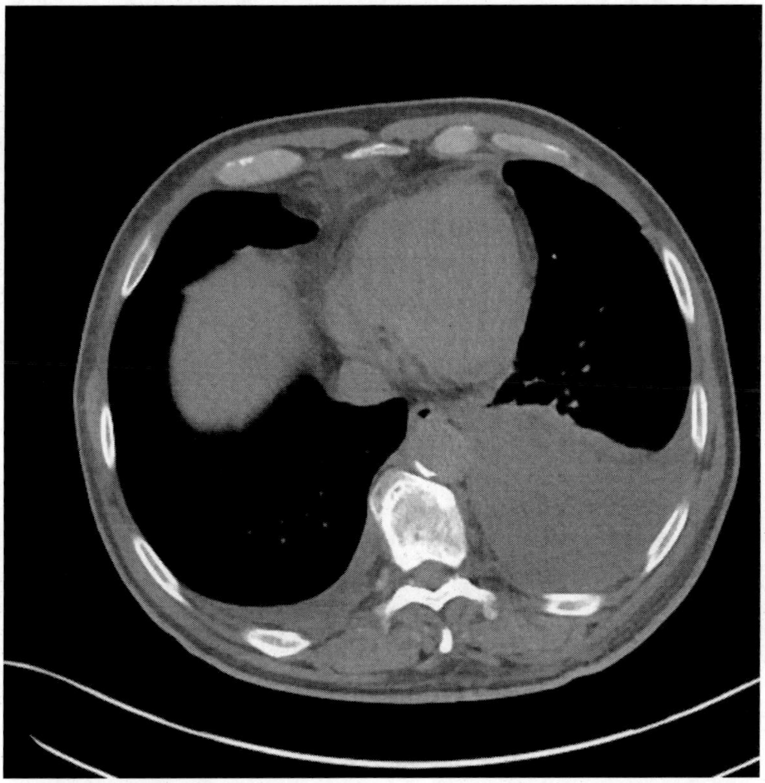

Figure 2a. CT scan with new L> R pleural effusion.

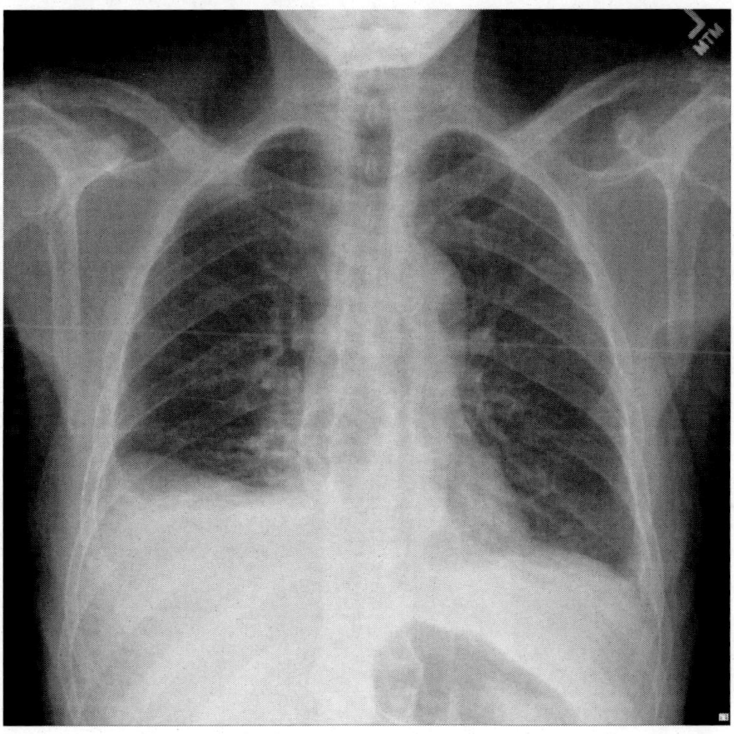

Figure 2b. CXR with persistent bilateral R> L pleural effusions following diuresis.

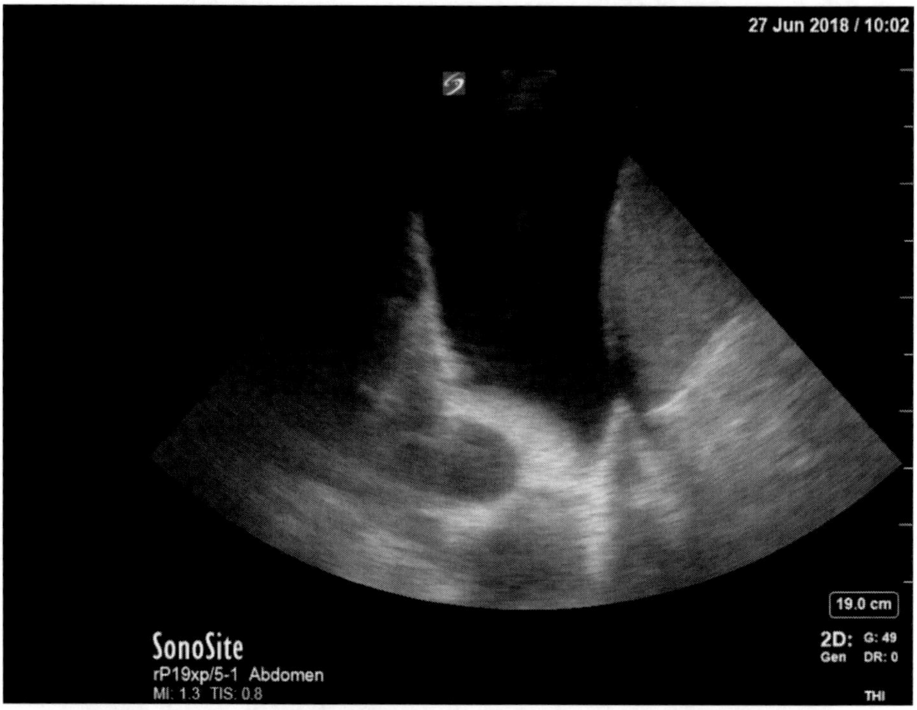

Figure 2c. Ultrasound of right-sided pleural effusion with diaphragm seen on right.

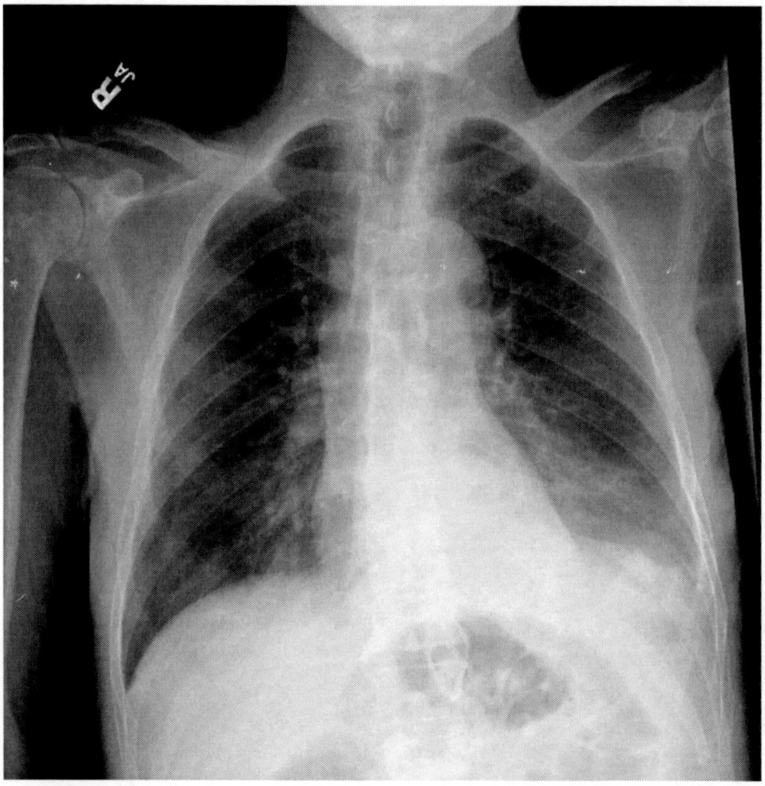

Figure 2d. Post-thoracentesis CXR.

Patient had significantly improved dyspnea following thoracentesis. The exudative nature of the pleural fluid was attributed to aggressive diuresis leading to increased pleural fluid protein concentration. Recommendations were made for continued management and optimization of his diastolic heart failure and chronic kidney disease.

Case 3

63-year-old female with a past medical history significant for long-standing rheumatoid arthritis (RA) on leflunomide who presented with left knee pain, dry cough, and dyspnea. No signs or symptoms suggestion an infection. Based on arthrocentesis, knee pain was attributed to RA flare. Initial CXR (Figure 3) demonstrated predominantly right-sided significant-sized pleural effusion.

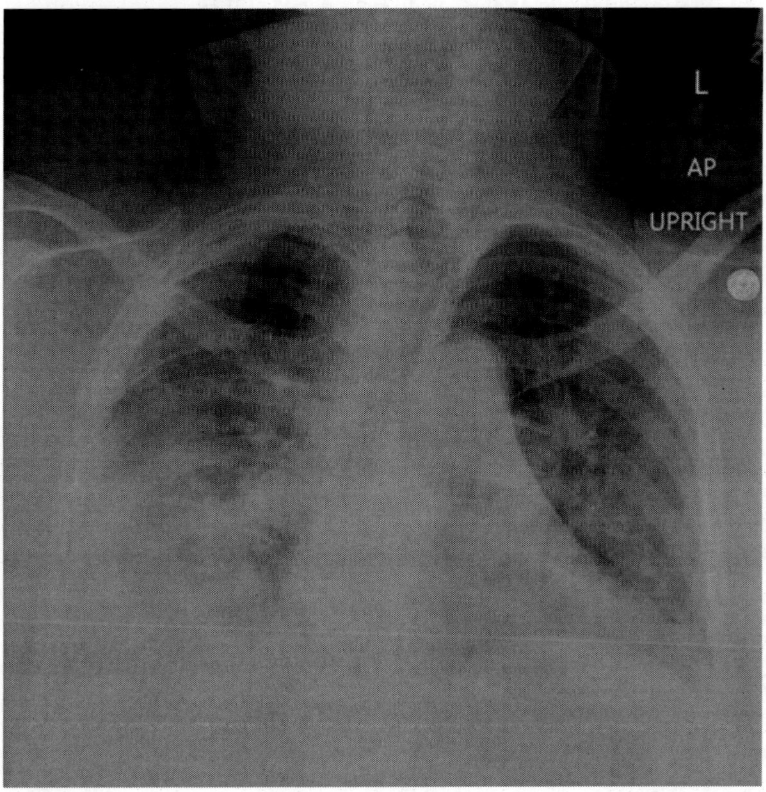

Figure 3. CXR with significant right-sided pleural effusion.

Thoracentesis was performed and two liters of serous fluid removed. Pleural fluid analysis demonstrated negative cytology, negative culture and gram stain, pH 7.20, glucose < 2 mg/dL, protein 4.4 g/dL, and LDH > 2500 mU/mL. Pleural fluid cell differential demonstrated total non-RBC cells 1500/cm^2, lymphocytes 11%, neutrophils 84%, and monocytes 5%.

Given that her acute joint pain was attributed to an RA flare, and based on the pleural fluid analysis, it was determined that her acute pleural pathology was secondary to rheumatoid pleural disease. Patient was started on a steroid taper with subsequent improvement in her respiratory and joint symptoms.

CASE 4

69 years old male with no significant past medical history presented with progressive exertional dyspnea. In addition to his respiratory symptoms he reported a weight loss of 20 pounds over a period of three months. A CXR was obtained which demonstrated a large left-sided pleural effusion (Figure 4a).

He underwent a therapeutic and diagnostic thoracentesis with 1.4 liters of bloody fluid removed. Pleural fluid analysis demonstrated negative culture and gram stain, pH 7.10, LDH 561 mU/mL and protein 4.4 g/dL consistent with an exudative effusion. Pleural fluid cell differential demonstrated 72% lymphocytes. Following thoracentesis, he underwent CT scan of the chest. (Figures 4b).

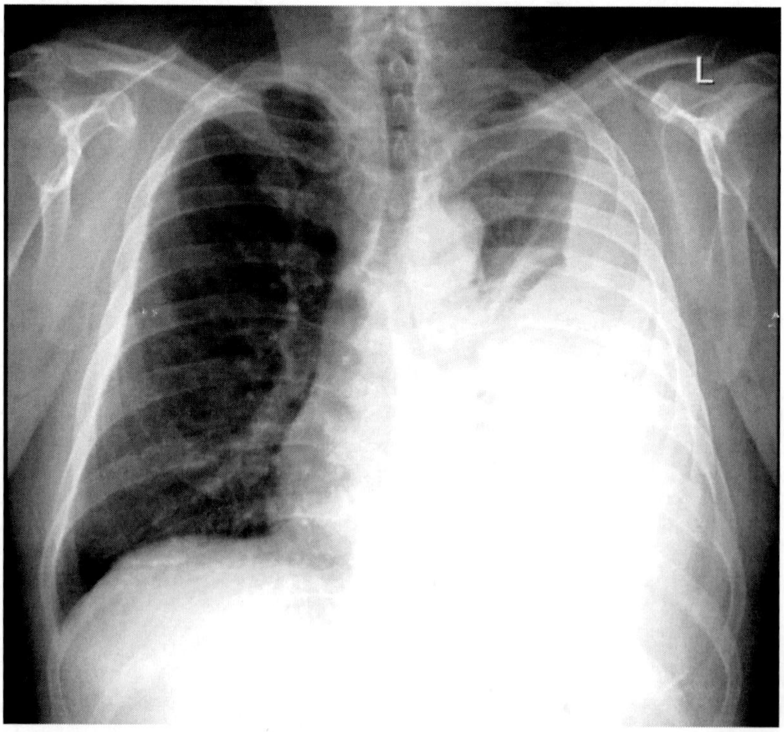

Figure 4a. CXR with left-sided pleural effusion.

Post-thoracentesis, fluid re-accumulated and the left lung remained atelectatic. The lung parenchyma was thus unable to be fully examined for the presence of any pulmonary lesions or masses. The pleural fluid was sent to cytopathology and demonstrated atypical cells with enlarged nuclei. Immunohistochemical staining was positive for CK7, consistent with metastatic adenocarcinoma, presumed to be of lung origin. The patient underwent a bronchoscopy and an extrinsic compression of the left main bronchus was identified with no endobronchial lesions. Biopsies were obtained and consistent with adenocarcinoma of lung origin. He was referred to oncology for further evaluation and treatment.

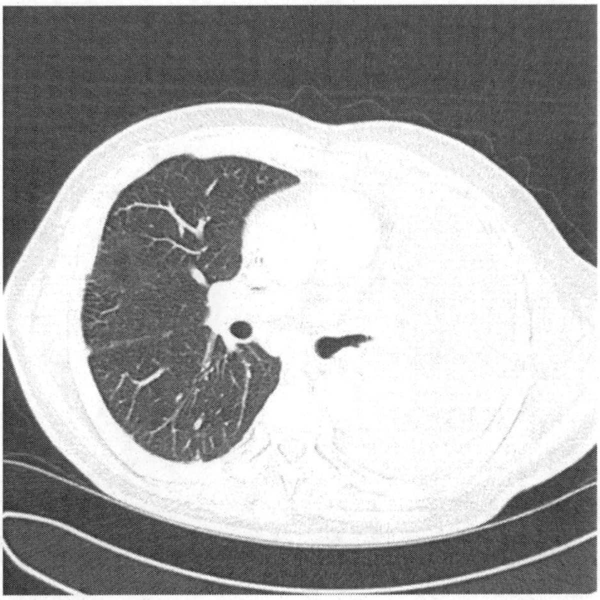

Figure 4b. CT chest (lung window).

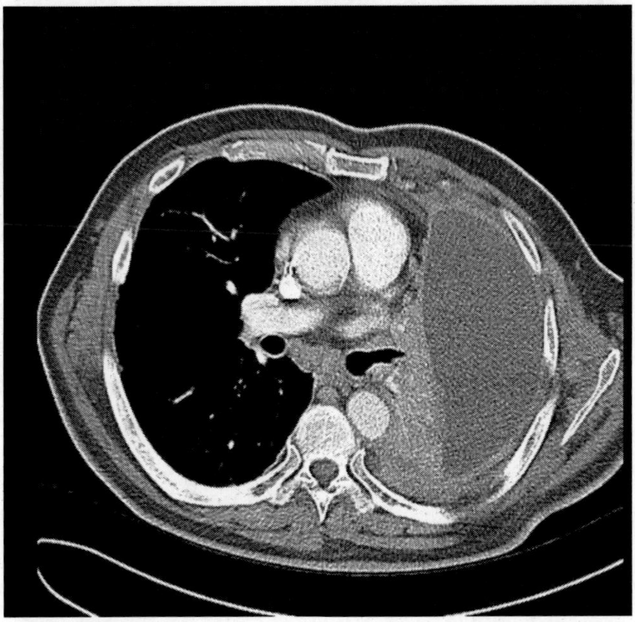

Figure 4c. CT chest (soft tissue window).

CASE 5

74 years old male with a past medical history significant for uncontrolled hypertension and severe chronic obstructive pulmonary disease presented with sudden onset of sharp anterior chest pain radiating to the mid-scapular region and an initial systolic blood pressure of 210 mm Hg.

Workup for acute coronary syndrome was negative. The patient was clinically and radiographically diagnosed with non-ruptured aortic dissection involving only the proximal portion of the descending aorta with no end-organ compromise. Given this, along with the presence of a significant pulmonary co-morbidity, medical management with impulse control was decided upon rather than surgical intervention.

Several hours later, the patient began complaining of increased dyspnea, worsening back pain, and lightheadedness. Vital signs demonstrated relative hypotension and increased tachycardia. Physical exam was notable for new dullness to percussion at the left lung base. Ultrasound (Figure 5) demonstrated a left-sided complex heterogeneously echogenic pleural effusion.

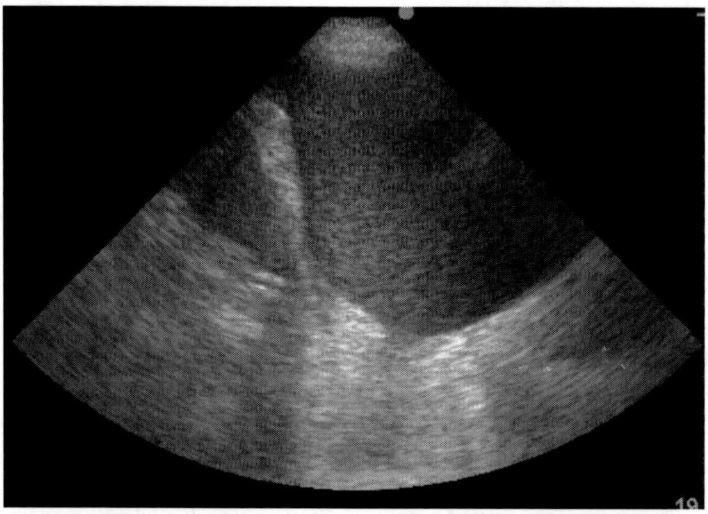

Figure 5. Ultrasound imaging demonstrating complex left-sided pleural effusion.

Urgent diagnostic thoracentesis was performed. Pleural fluid analysis demonstrated negative cytology, negative culture and gram stain, pH 7.25, protein 3.2 g/dL, and LDH 142 mU/mL. Pleural fluid cell differential was notable for significantly elevated RBC count with pleural fluid hematocrit 64% of peripheral blood hematocrit.

Given these results and the appearance of the fluid, a diagnosis of non-traumatic left-sided hemothorax was made, likely secondary to aortic rupture. Patient's hemodynamics were stabilized and CT scan confirmed the diagnosis. He was then taken to the operating room for definitive surgical management.

Conclusion

Clinicians will encounter patients with chylothorax, hemothorax, malignant pleural effusion, rheumatoid pleural effusion and pleural effusions in patients with chronic kidney disease.

In: Pleural Effusions: Causes, Types and Treatment
Editor: Rahul Khosla
ISBN: 978-1-53614-683-7

Chapter 14

PLEURAL EFFUSION CASES: PART 2

Ivana Milojević*[1,2,*]*, MD and Rahul Khosla*[2]*, MD
[1]Pulmonary, Critical Care, and Sleep Medicine,
The George Washington University,
Washington DC, US
[2]Pulmonary & CCM Section, Veterans Affairs Medical Center,
Washington DC, US

ABSTRACT

In this chapter five interesting cases have been presented for the reader to review and recap important topics presented in the book thus far.

Keywords: Parapneumonic, empyema, yellow nail syndrome

CASE 1

A 58-year-old frail, schizophrenic woman, active smoker with 30-pack-year history presented with cough productive of purulent sputum, dyspnea, pleuritic chest pain, fever, and chills. Medical history was significant for seizure disorder, cervical spinal stenosis, and dysphagia. On exam she was febrile, tachycardic, and hypoxic, with decreased breath sounds on the right. Laboratory data revealed leukocytosis of 42,000/mm^3. Initial chest X-ray is shown in figure 1a.

* Corresponding Author Email: milojevic.ivana@gmail.com.

CT chest without contrast revealed a moderate right-sided loculated pleural effusion with consolidation and atelectasis of the right middle and lower lobes (Figure1b).

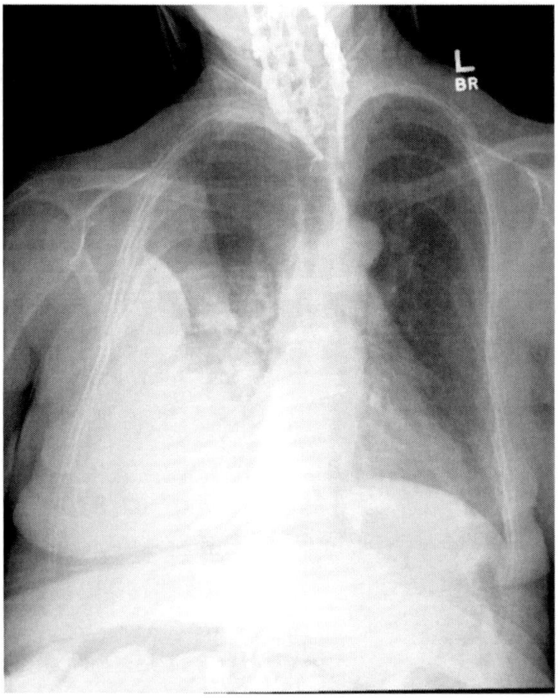

Figure 1a. Initial anteroposterior portable chest radiograph.

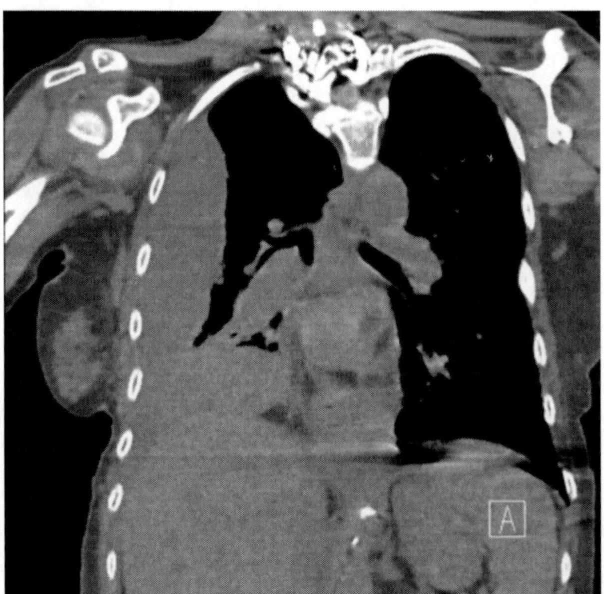

Figure 1b. Computerized tomography of the chest without contrast, coronal cut, soft tissue window.

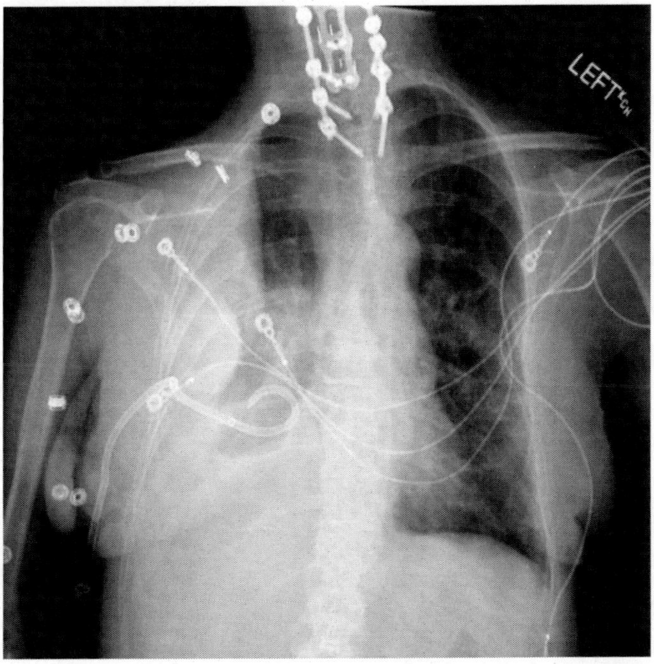

Figure 1c. Anteroposterior portable chest radiograph after pigtail catheter placement.

Table 1.1. Pleural fluid laboratory values

Fluid appearance		Hazy, yellow
Biochemistry		
pH		7.26
Glucose		20 mg/dL
Protein		4.0 g/dL
Protein (serum)		5.8 g/dL
LDH		4565 U/L
LDH (serum)		277 U/L
Cell count		
RBC		800/mm^3
Non-RBC		3051/mm^3
Diff	Seg	98%
	Mono	1%
	Lymph	1%
Micro		
Gram stain		negative
Bacterial culture		negative
AFB smear/culture		negative
Fungal culture		negative

She was diagnosed with aspiration pneumonia complicated by parapneumonic effusion, and broad spectrum antibiotics were started. Sputum and blood cultures remained negative. 14 Fr pigtail catheter was placed (Figure 1c) followed by intrapleural administration of tissue plasminogen activator (t-PA) and Dnase per MIST2 protocol.

Pleural fluid characteristics were consistent with empyema (Table 1.1).

She subsequently developed hemoptysis. CT chest with intravenous contrast showed a loculated right pleural effusion with near collapse of the right middle and right lower lobe, with tip of the pigtail catheter in the atelectatic lung parenchyma of the right lower lobe (Figure 1d, 1e).

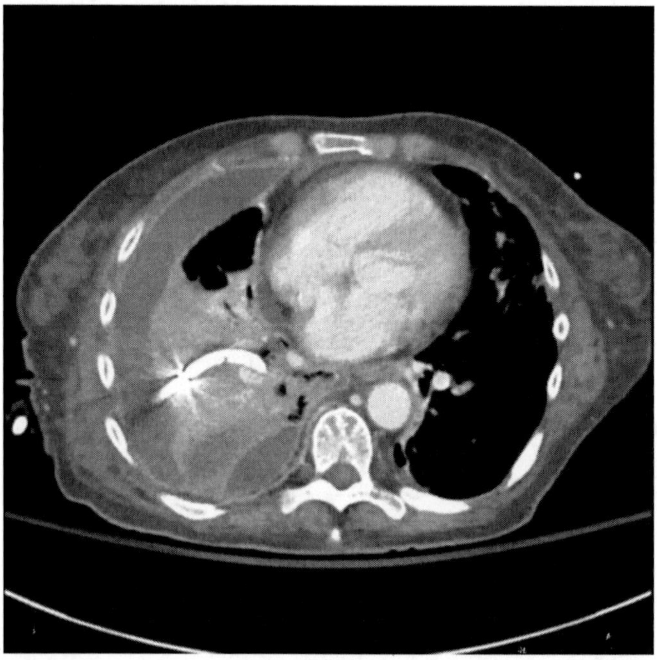

Figure 1d. Computerized tomography of the chest with intravenous contrast for hemoptysis work-up, axial cut, soft tissue window.

The pigtail catheter was removed without complications, which lead to resolution of hemoptysis. She was deemed high risk for video-assisted thoracoscopic surgical intervention. Another 14 Fr pigtail catheter was placed in the right anterior chest (Figure 1f) followed by initiation of MIST2 protocol, which resulted in immediate drainage of 1,500mL of purulent material.

As her clinical condition improved, chest X-ray showed significant resolution of effusion (Figure 1g).

The pigtail catheter was removed. She completed a four-week course of total antibiotic therapy.

A follow-up chest X-ray done six months later showed complete resolution (Figure 1h).

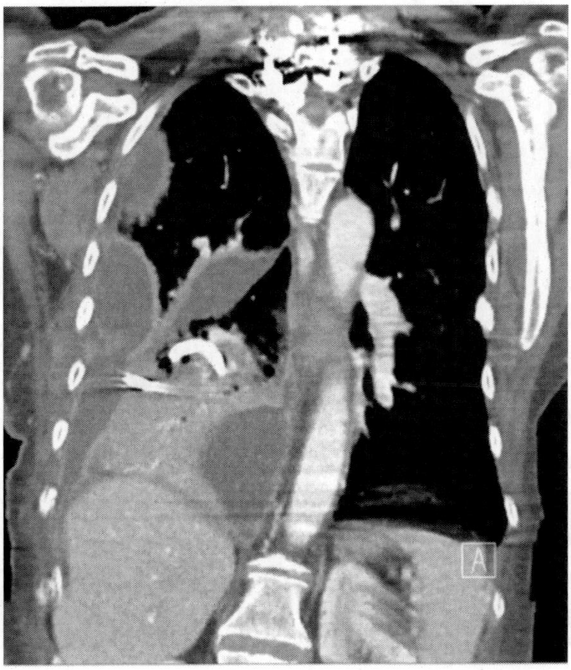

Figure 1e. Computerized tomography of the chest with intravenous contrast for hemoptysis work-up, coronal cut, soft tissue window.

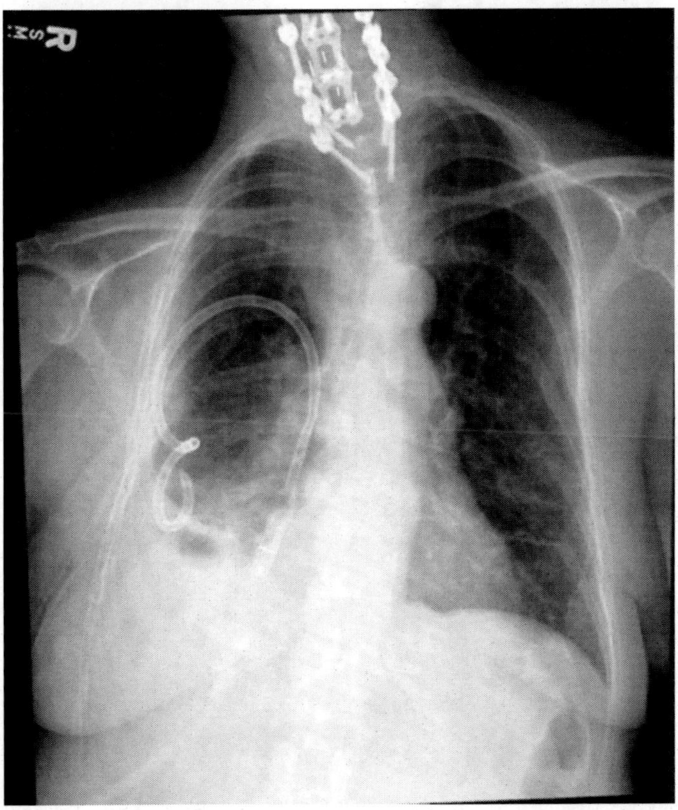

Figure 1f. Anteroposterior portable chest radiograph after second pigtail catheter placement.

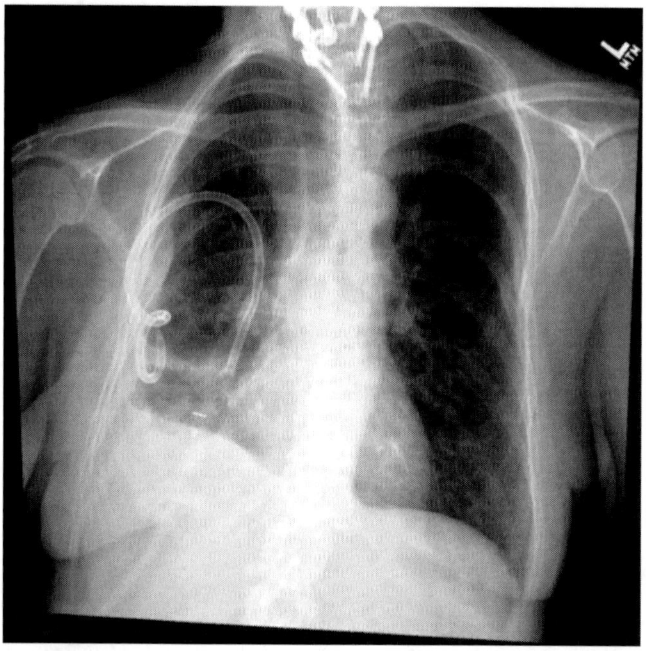

Figure 1g. Anteroposterior portable chest radiograph prior to second pigtail catheter removal.

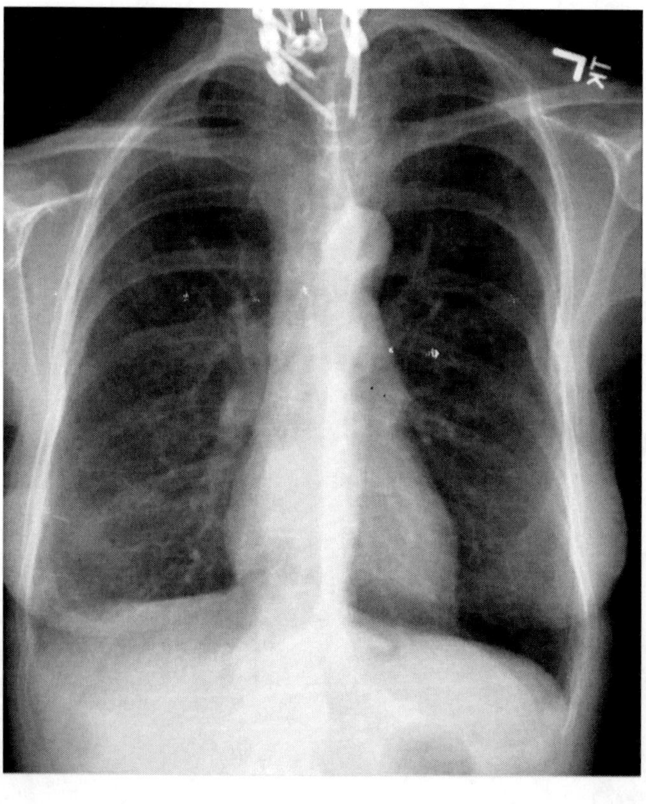

Figure 1h. Follow-up posteroanterior chest radiograph after 6 months.

CASE 2

A 64-year-old alcoholic male presented with sharp, right-sided pleuritic chest pain and weight loss. On exam he was emaciated, with a BMI of 15, tachycardic, and had decreased breath sounds on the right. Laboratory tests revealed hyponatremia, leukocytosis with left shift, normocytic anemia, and thrombocytosis. Chest X-ray showed a pleural effusion associated with a mid and lower zone parenchymal process on the right (Figure 2a).

CT chest with intravenous contrast demonstrated pleural thickening, a loculated right pleural effusion, right lower lobe infiltrate, and atelectasis (Figure 2b and 2c).

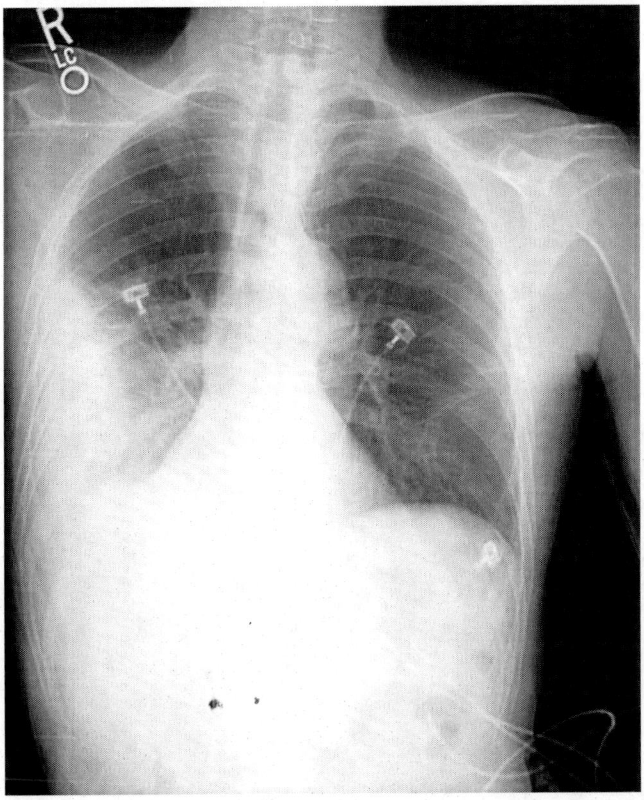

Figure 2a. Initial portable anteroposterior chest radiograph.

A right hilar mass could not be excluded. Thoracentesis resulted in aspiration of 20 mL of pus (Figure 2d). Pleural fluid studies are shown in Table 2.1.

Broad spectrum antibiotics with anaerobic coverage were started. Blood cultures remained negative. Patient underwent video assisted thoracoscopic surgical exploration and ultimately required a utility thoracotomy due to the severity and organization of empyema. Lung abscess with necrotic tissue in the basilar segments was diagnosed intraoperatively. Putrid odor suggested an anaerobic infection. Lung abscess was debrided and marsupialized into the pleural space. Extensive decortication and peel removal with dissection of adhesions was performed. Postoperative chest X-ray findings are shown in figure 2e.

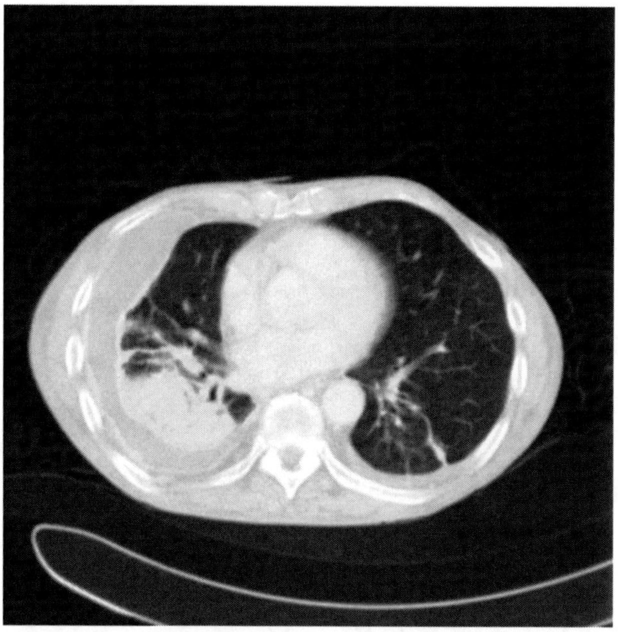

Figure 2b. Computerized tomography of the chest with intravenous contrast, axial cut, lung window.

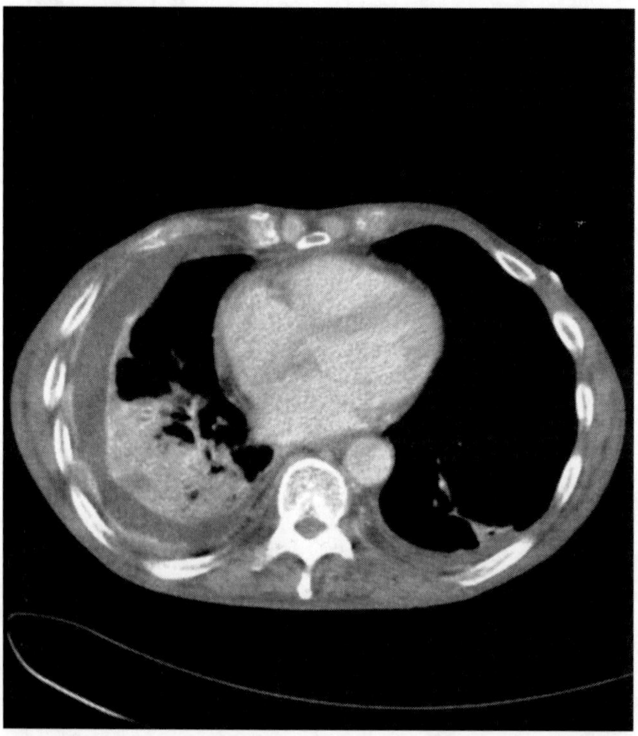

Figure 2c. Computerized tomography of the chest with intravenous contrast, axial cut, soft tissue window.

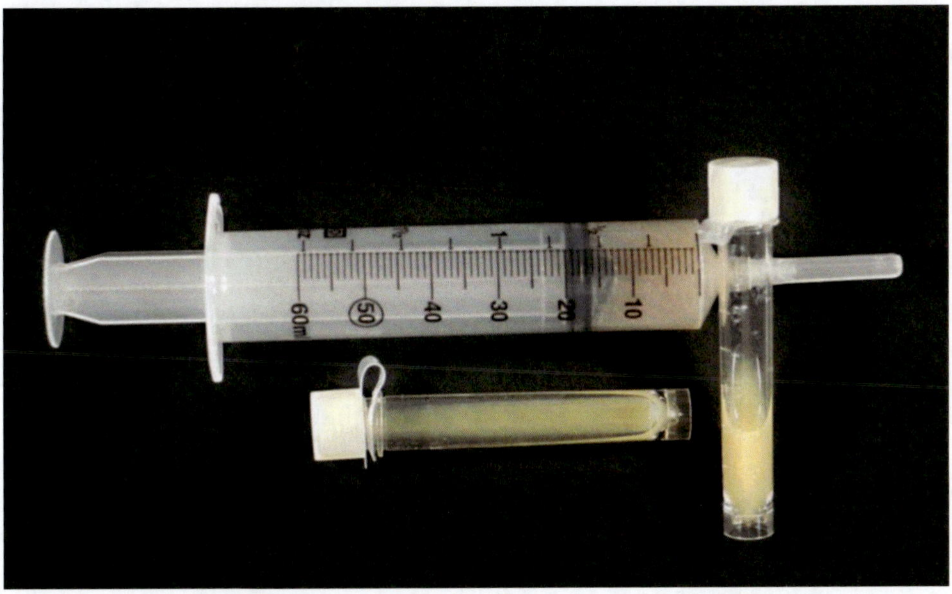

Figure 2d. Appearance of aspirated pleural fluid.

Table 2.1. Pleural fluid laboratory values

Fluid appearance		Cloudy, faint yellow
Biochemistry		
pH		6.37
Protein		3.8 g/dL
Protein (serum)		5.7 g/dL
LDH		14029 mU/ml
Cell count		
RBC		
Non-RBC		82000/mm^3
Diff	Seg	94%
	Mono	2%
	Lymph	4%
Micro		
Gram stain		negative
Bacterial culture		Fusobacterium sp.

Pleural fluid culture obtained during thoracentesis grew Fusobacterium sp. while operative cultures remained negative. Bronchoscopy did not identify an endobronchial lesion. Patient clinically improved to be discharged on oral antibiotics (Figure 2f) and was eventually lost to follow-up.

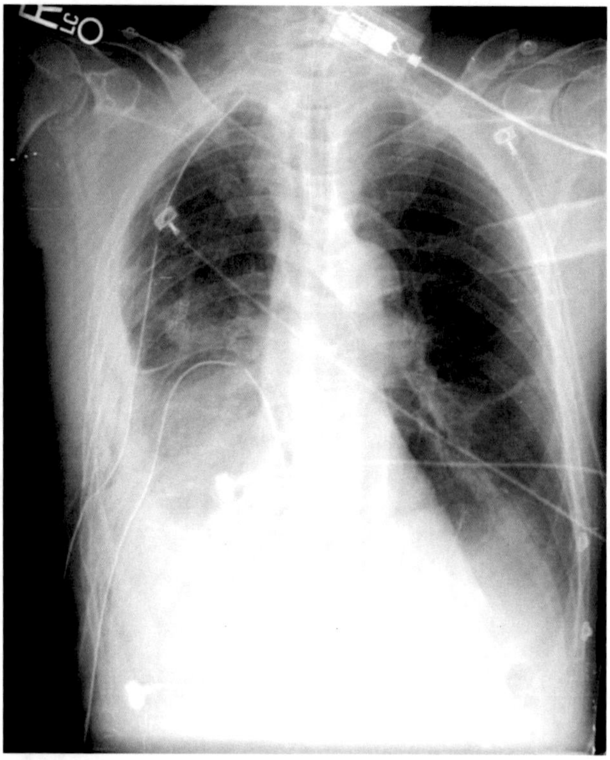

Figure 2e. Post-operative portable anteroposterior chest radiograph.

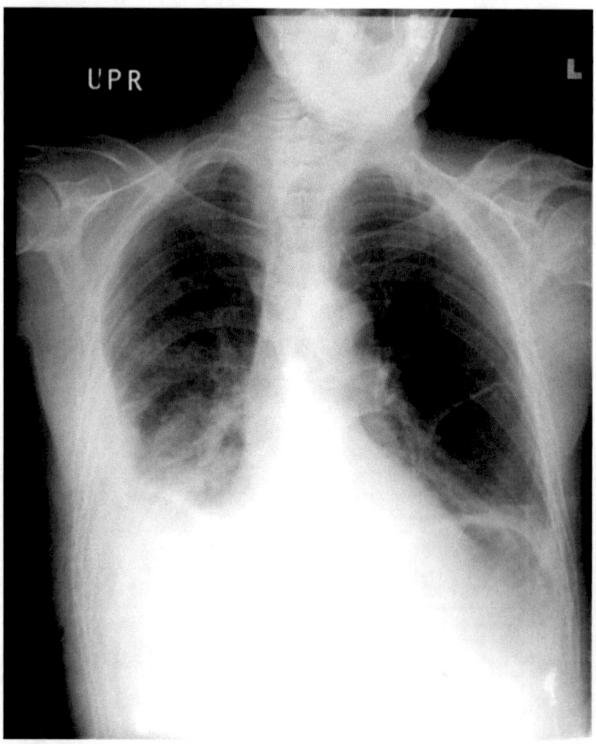

Figure 2f. Portable anteroposterior chest radiograph on discharge.

CASE 3

A 69-year-old man, former smoker with 25-pack-year history presented with dyspnea on exertion, fatigue, and 20lb weight loss. Family history was positive for various malignancies including lung cancer in his father and two paternal uncles. A large left pleural effusion was apparent on chest X-ray. CT without contrast confirmed a massive loculated effusion with compressive atelectasis. An underlying mass within compressed lung was suspected but not clearly visualized. Thoracentesis yielded hemorrhagic, exudative fluid without evidence of infection. Cytologic exam was consistent with metastatic adenocarcinoma of unknown primary origin and he was transferred to a tertiary facility to complete the workup. Repeat thoracentesis of the anterior fluid pocket with pleural manometry accomplished drainage of 1,400 mL of hemorrhagic fluid with recorded pleural pressure at the end of procedure of - 35cm H_2O. Lung re-expansion did not occur post-procedure (Figure 3a). Pleural fluid studies are listed in table 3.1.

Cytologic immunopattern was suggestive of adenocarcinoma (CK7, CK 5/6 and CEA positive; CK20 and TTF-1 negative), although primary origin of the cancer remained unclear.

Lung cancer was favored over upper gastrointestinal tract, gallbladder or breast adenocarcinoma. CT chest with intravenous contrast failed to demonstrate primary lung tumor (Figure 3b and 3c).

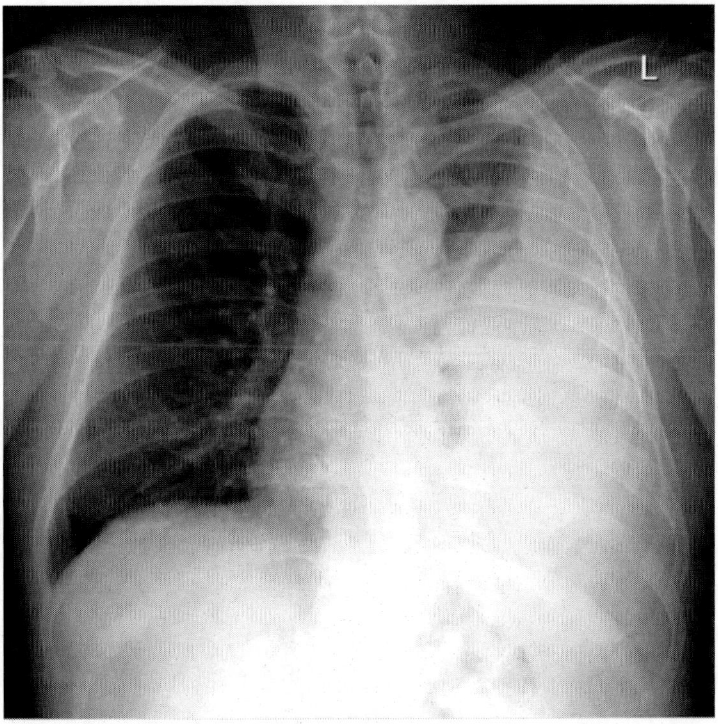

Figure 3a. Posteroanterior chest radiograph post second thoracentesis.

Table 3.1. Pleural fluid laboratory values

Fluid appearance		hemorrhagic
Biochemistry		
Glucose		112 mg/dL
Protein		4.4 g/dL
Protein (serum)		6.8 g/dL
LDH		561 mU/ml
LDH (serum)		173 mU/ml
Cell count		
RBC		264,200/mm^3
Non-RBC		2,800/mm^3
Diff	Seg	60%
	Mono	8%
	Lymph	30%
	Eos	2%
Micro		
Gram stain		negative
Bacterial culture		negative
AFB smear/culture		negative

FDG-avid lesion (SUV 7.4) in the atelectatic left lower lobe was identified on PET/CT, along with left hilar and mediastinal FDG-avid lymph nodes (2-3 SUV) and left pleural surface FDG uptake (Figure 3d).

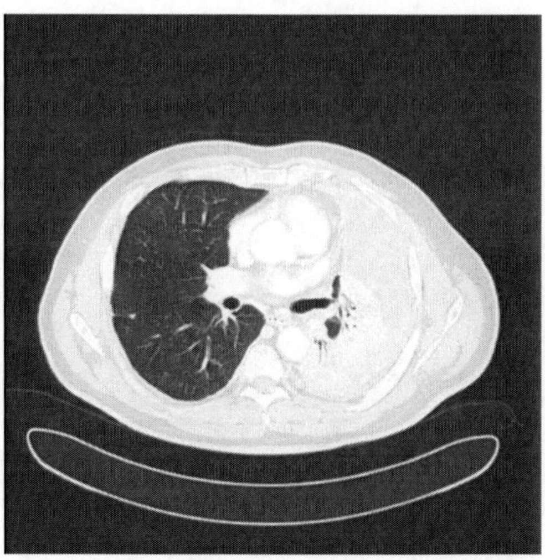

Figure 3b. Computerized tomography of the chest with intravenous contrast, axial cut, lung window.

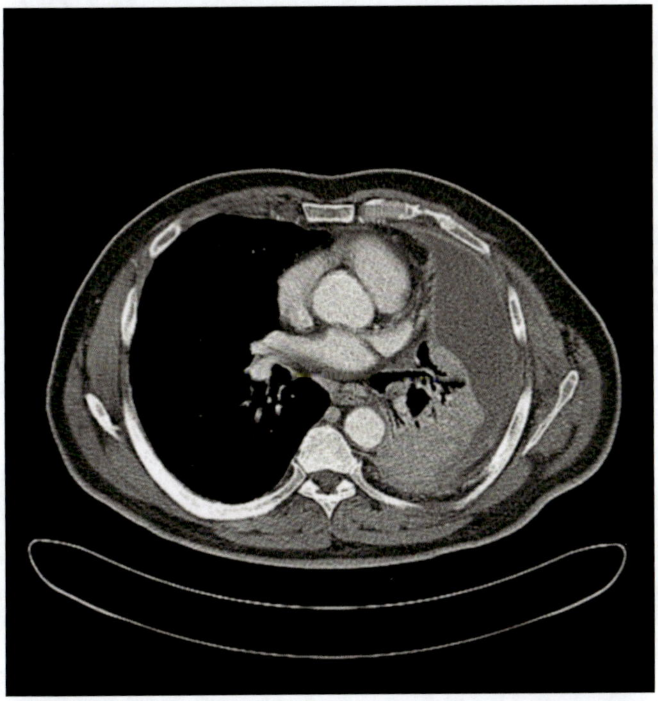

Figure 3c. Computerized tomography of the chest with intravenous contrast, axial cut, soft tissue window.

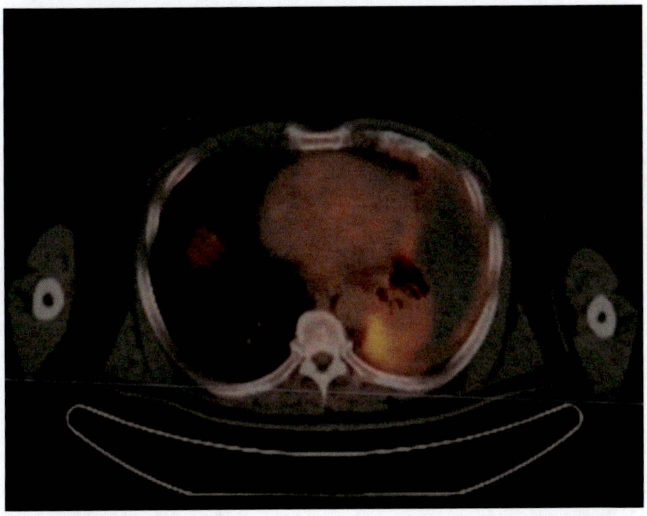

Figure 3d. Positron emission tomography of the chest demonstrating FDG-avid lesion in the left lower lobe.

No distant metastasis or other lesions were seen. Repeat therapeutic thoracentesis targeting the fluid pocket in the left lung base resulted in removal of 1,000mL of dark, hemorrhagic fluid with measured pleural pressure at the end of procedure of -21 cmH_2O.

No lung re-expansion or significant symptomatic improvement was observed. Bronchoscopy demonstrated external compression to the entry of the left lower lobe bronchus, but no endobronchial lesion. Patient completed staging with brain MRI which showed no evidence of metastatic disease. Treatment with carboplatin/gemcitabine and bevacizumab was started.

CASE 4

75-year-old man status post esophagectomy for stage I moderately differentiated esophageal adenocarcinoma, and total thyroidectomy followed by iodine ablation therapy for stage II papillary thyroid cancer, was diagnosed with a massive right-sided non-metabolically active pleural effusion on a surveillance PET/CT scan. PET/CT was also indicative of recurrent esophageal disease at the anastomotic site and new osteoblastic metastases. After developing progressive dyspnea he was admitted to the hospital for work-up and management of the effusion. Chest X-ray findings are shown in figure 4a.

Thoracentesis resulted in drainage of 2800 ml of clear, faint yellow fluid. Pleural fluid laboratory values are shown in table 4.1.

Low amylase level in pleural fluid was considered to have practically excluded a fistula between gastrointestinal tract and pleural space. Thoracentesis was complicated by a small apical pneumothorax (Figure 4b).

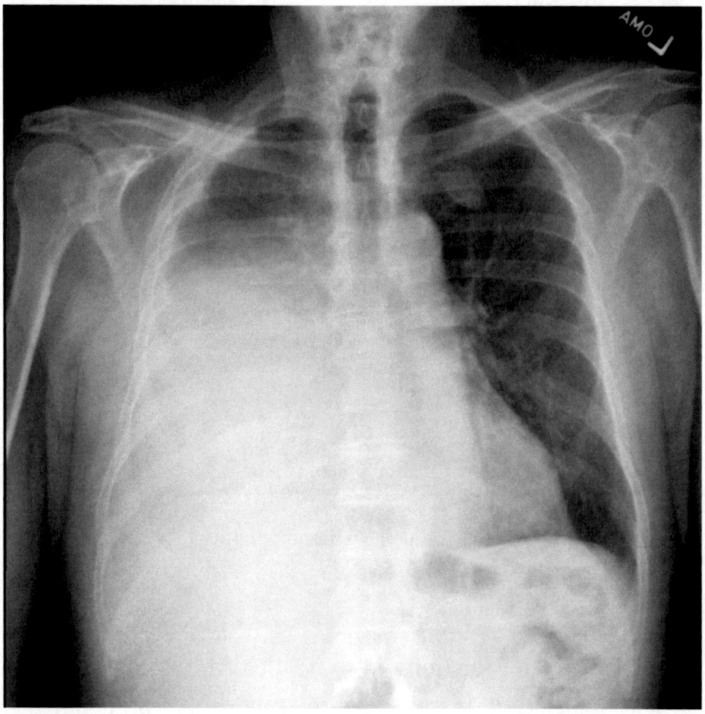

Figure 4a. Initial posteroanterior chest radiograph: large right-pleural effusion.

Table 4.1. Pleural fluid laboratory values

Fluid appearance		clear, faint yellow
Biochemistry		
pH		7.34
Amylase		41 U/L
Cholesterol		70 U/L
Protein		4.6 g/dL
Protein (serum)		5.9 g/dL
LDH		110 U/L
LDH (serum)		109 U/L
Cell count		
RBC		71/mm^3
Non-RBC		68/mm^3
Diff	Seg	11%
	Mono	25%
	Lymph	23%
	Mesothelial	41%
Micro		
AFB smear/culture		negative

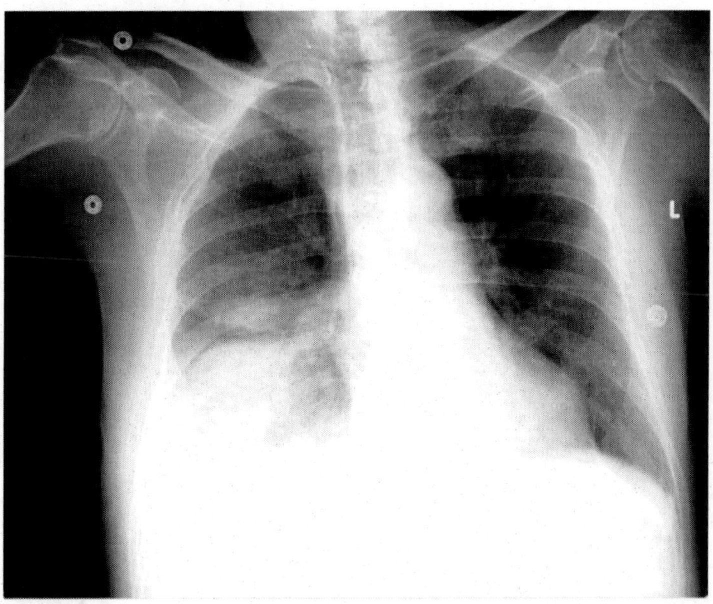

Figure 4b. Anteroposterior chest radiograph post thoracentesis: small right apical air collection, right lower lung zone airspace disease.

CT scan with intravenous contrast demonstrated right-sided hydropneumothorax with atelectasis/infiltrate in the right middle and lower lobes (Figure 4c, 4d and 4e).

Since patient was clinically improved with stable size pneumothorax, trapped lung pathophysiology was suspected and he was initially managed conservatively. Cytology returned consistent with metastatic adenocarcinoma (Figure 4f and 4g).

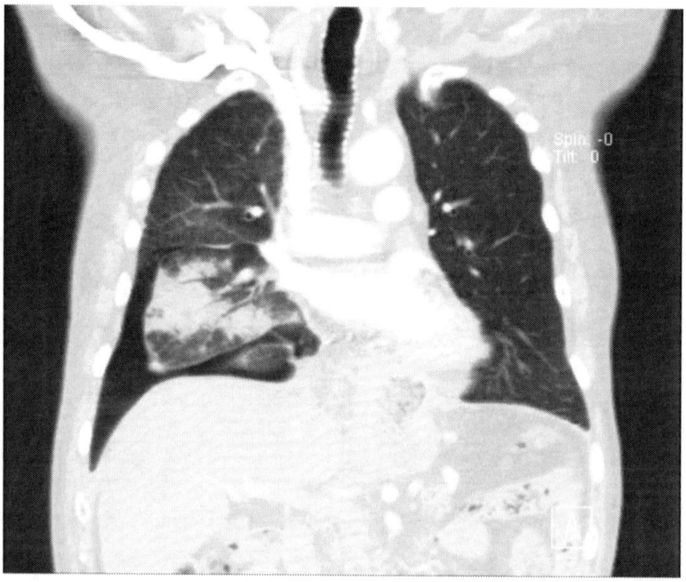

Figure 4c. Computerized tomography of the chest with intravenous contrast, coronal cut, lung window: pneumothorax.

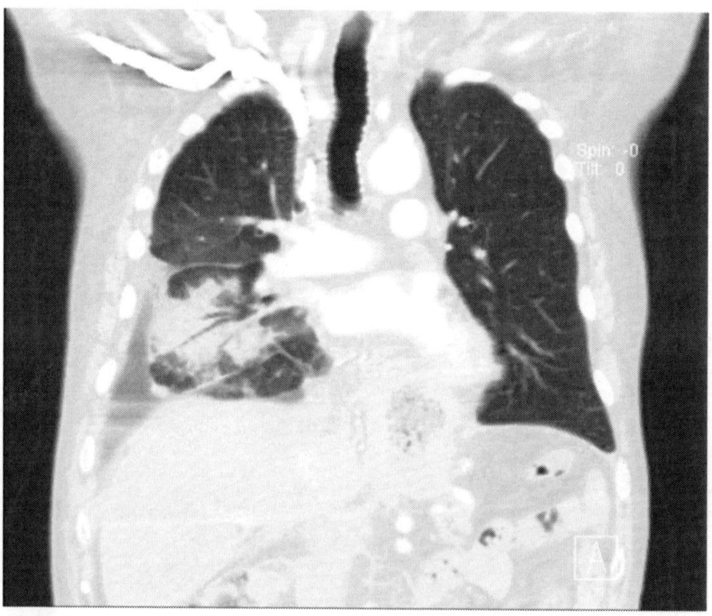

Figure 4d. Computerized tomography of the chest with intravenous contrast, coronal cut, lung window: air-fluid interface.

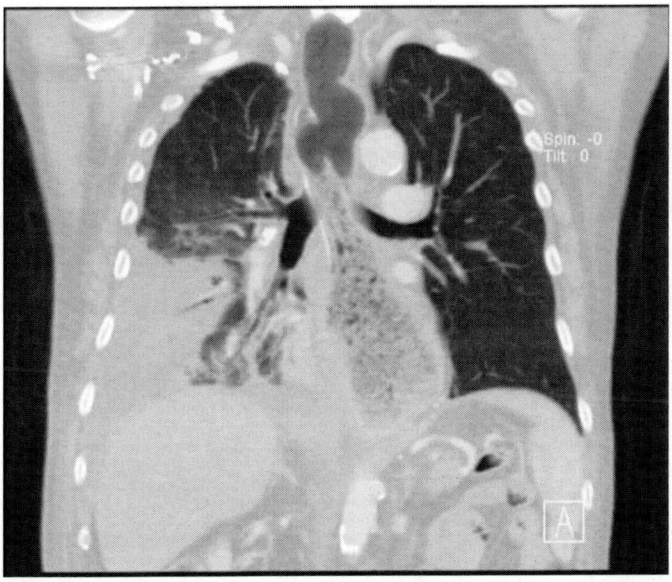

Figure 4e. Computerized tomography of the chest with intravenous contrast, coronal cut, lung window: pleural effusion; surgical changes of gastric pull through.

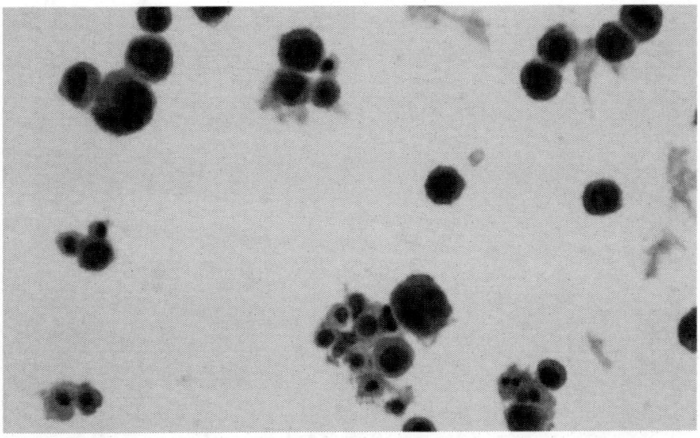

Figure 4f. ThinPrep™, Papanicolaou stain, 100X: large atypical cells with few mesothelial cells.

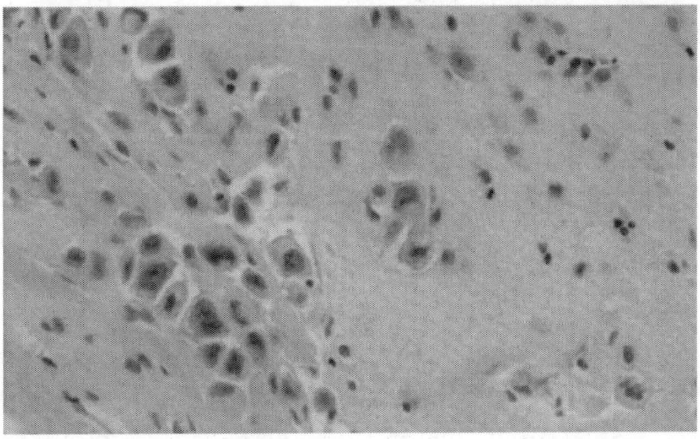

Figure 4g. Cell block, H&E stain, 40X: large atypical cells on the background of inflammatory and mesothelial cells.

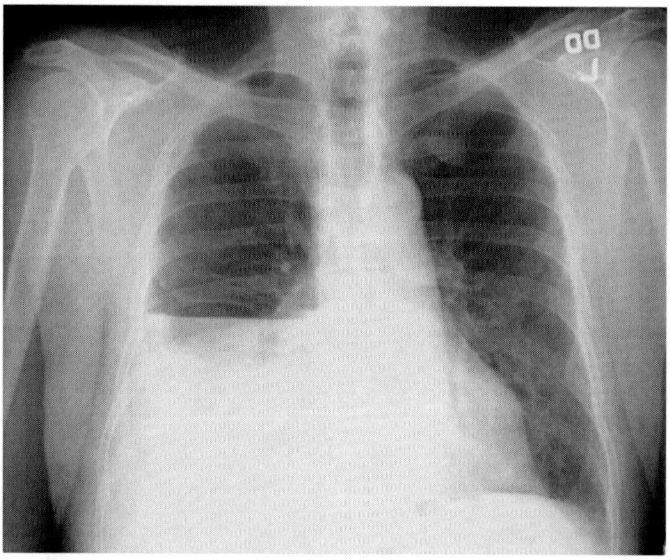

Figure 4h. Posteroanterior chest radiograph: hydropneumothorax.

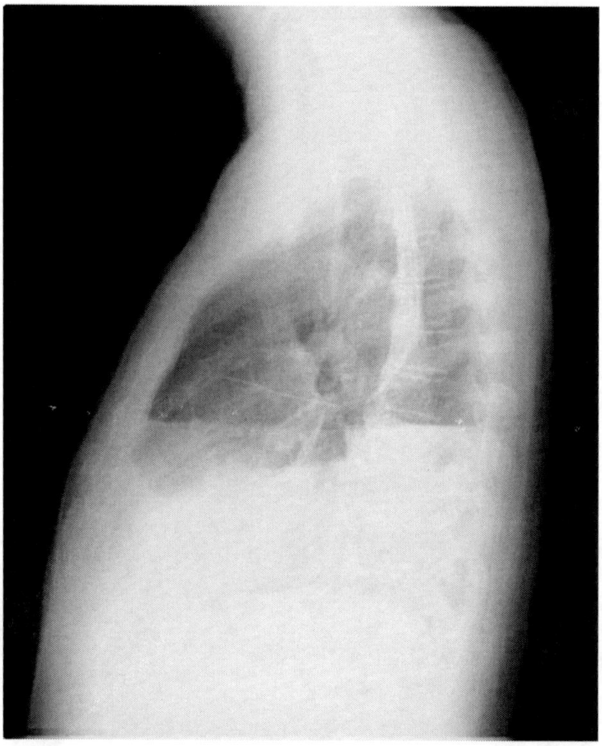

Figure 4i. Lateral chest radiograph: hydropneumothorax.

Immunological stains revealed that atypical cells were positive for monoclonal CEA and CD15, weakly positive for calretinin, and negative for CK5/6. Five days after the thoracentesis, chest X-ray exhibited classical findings of right hydropneumothorax with significant fluid reaccumulation (Figure 4h and 4i) while patient was increasingly short of breath.

PleurX™ catheter was placed and post procedural imaging showed complete resolution of the right pleural effusion with persistence of the small loculated pneumo-thorax without air leak (Figure 4j).

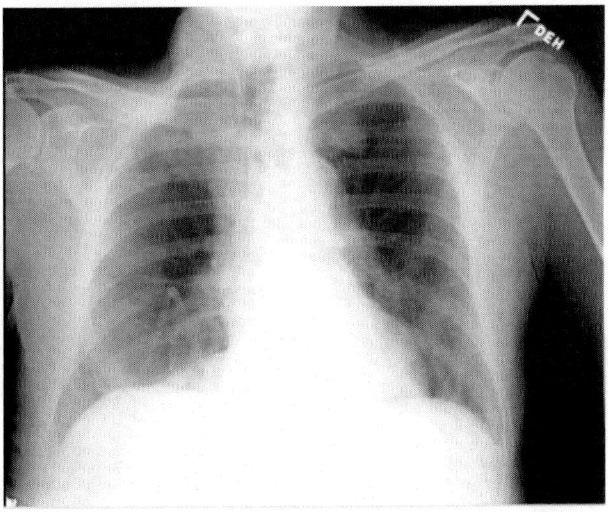

Figure 4j. Anteroposterior chest radiograph after PleurX™ catheter placement.

This clinical scenario was interpreted as a more definitive evidence of non-expandable lung and pleurodesis was not recommended. Follow-up chest X-ray two weeks later demonstrated two different air-fluid levels: one due to small hydropneumothorax in the right lung base and the other inferior to the right hilum secondary to gastric pull through procedure (Figure 4k). Patient ultimately decided to pursue palliative treatment.

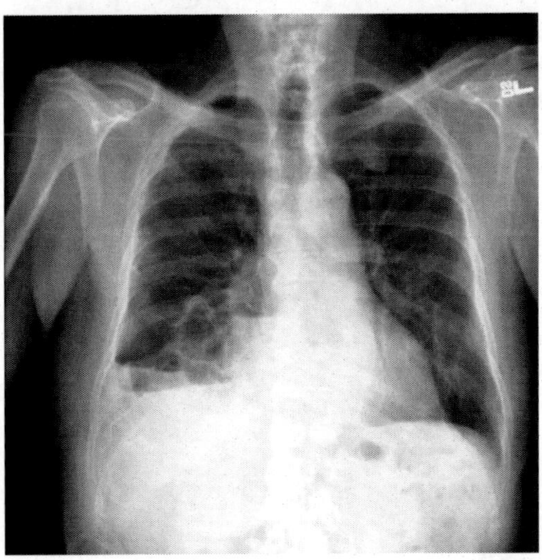

Figure 4k. Posteroanterior chest radiograph: two different air fluid levels.

CASE 5

A 78-year-old Caucasian woman with *yellow nail syndrome* was followed in pulmonary clinic for over a decade. She had atopic asthma since childhood, and had experienced several episodes of nut anaphylaxis. In her 50s she started developing arthritic deformities of both feet (Figure 5a), which eventually rendered her wheelchair-dependent and obese.

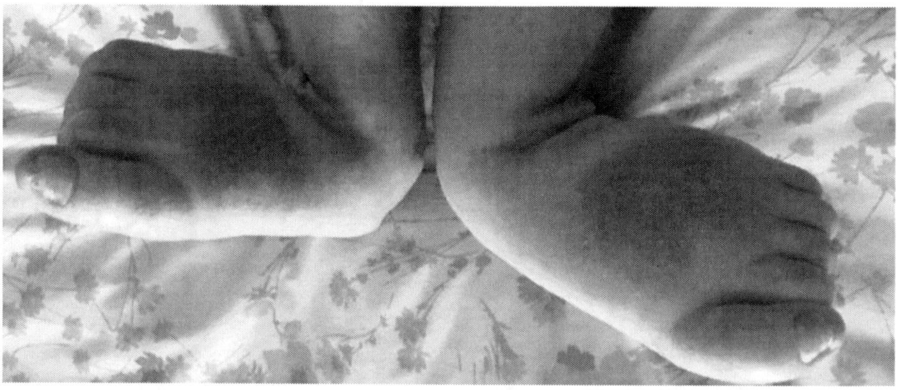

Figure 5a. Feet deformity and swelling, thickened yellow nails, skin hyperpigmentation.

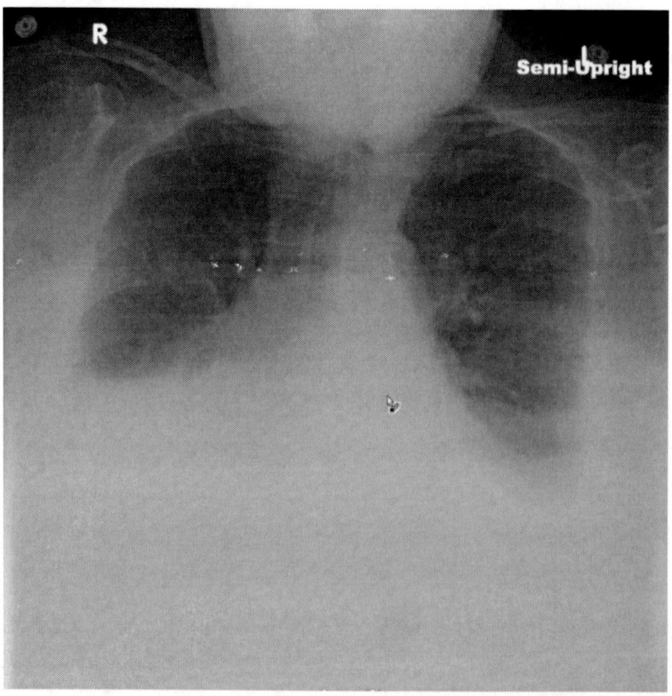

Figure 5b. Anteroposterior chest radiograph: bilateral pleural effusions.

In her early 60s she was diagnosed with *yellow nail syndrome* on the basis of recurrent pleural effusions (Figure 5b), lower extremity lymphedema, and yellow nail plate discoloration with increased nail thickness and onycholysis (Figure 5c).

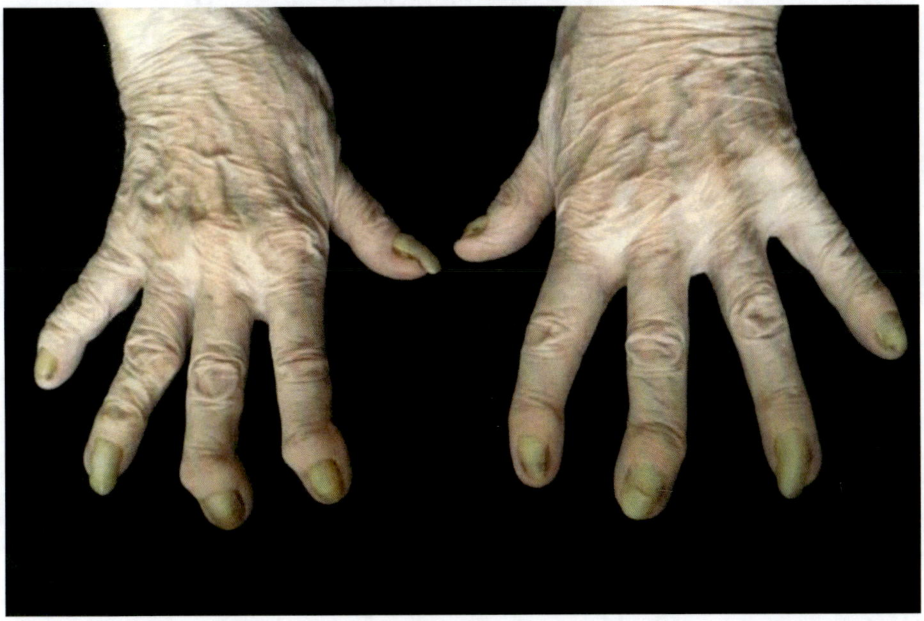

Figure 5c. Yellow nails and arthritic deformities of the hands.

Table 5.1. Pleural fluid laboratory values

Fluid appearance		clear, yellow
Biochemistry		
pH		7.37
Glucose		117 mg/dL
Protein		4.3 g/dL
Protein (serum)		5.5 g/dL
Cell count		
RBC		2222/mm³
WBC		934/mm³
Diff	Seg	11%
	Mono	5%
	Lymph	84%
Meso		present
Micro		
Gram stain		negative
Bacterial culture		negative

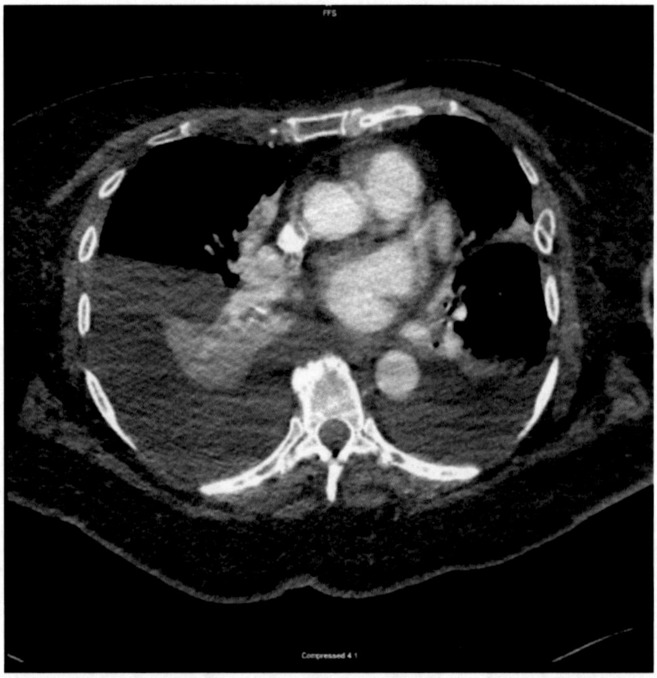

Figure 5d. Computerized tomography of the chest with intravenous contrast, axial cut, soft tissue window.

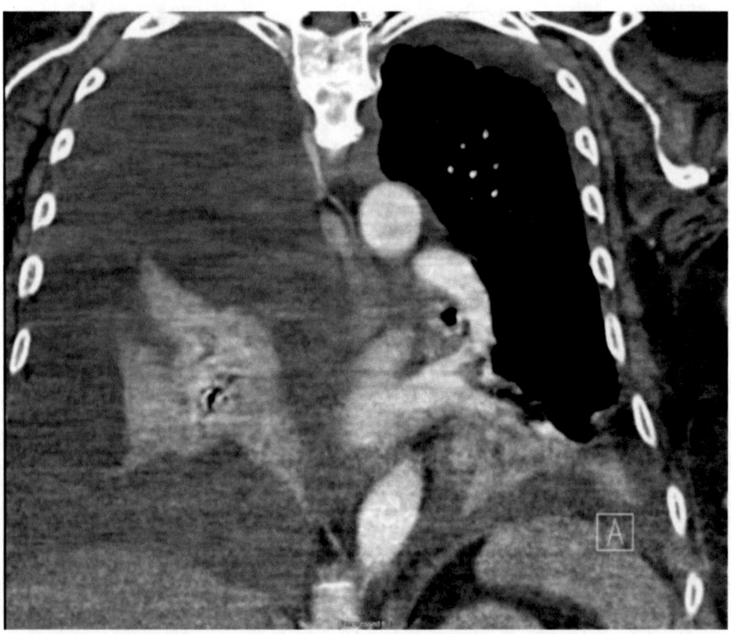

Figure 5e. Computerized tomography of the chest with intravenous contrast, coronal cut, soft tissue window.

CT scans of the chest re-demonstrated effusions (Figure 5d and 5e), but there were no bronchiectasis or other significant lung parenchymal abnormalities. Pleural fluid studies were as shown in table 5.1.

After the initial thoracentesis, pleural effusions were managed conservatively. Lymphedema was treated with diuretics as needed and compression stockings, along with multiple courses of antibiotics for superimposed cellulitis. Her nails were thick and brittle, challenging to cut safely, but had ultimately stopped growing. Despite significant debility, she has done well over the years.

CONCLUSION

These five cases are a combination of common and uncommon causes of pleural effusions that one may encounter in practice.

About the Editor

Dr. Rahul Khosla, MD, MBA is an Associate Professor in the Department of Medicine at The George Washington University, Washington DC and the Chief of Pulmonary and Critical Section at the Washington, DC Veterans Affairs Medical Center. He completed his medical school education at Maulana Azad Medical College, New Delhi, India. After graduating from the internal medicine residency program, University of Rochester, Rochester NY, he completed his pulmonary medicine fellowship at Baylor College of Medicine, Houston Texas followed by a fellowship in critical care medicine at University of Medicine and Dentistry of New Jersey, Camden NJ. He is also trained in sleep medicine and interven-tional procedures in pulmonary medicine. He received his Master's in Business Administration degree from George Washington University. He is currently the Chief of Pulmonary and Critical care Section at the Washington, DC Veterans Affairs Medical Center. His clinical and research interests are in the use of ultrasound in pulmonary and critical care medicine. He is also interested in pleural space diseases and the use of procalcitonin as a diagnostic and prognostic marker. He has an avid interest in cricket and also enjoys tennis, hiking and cooking.

List of Contributors

Georges Al-Helou, MD

Dr. Georges Al-Helou was born in Lebanon and grew up in Gold Coast, Australia. He graduated with a Bachelor in Biology with high distinction from the American University of Beirut in Lebanon. He then attended, and graduated with distinction from the American University of Beirut medical school. Following this, he worked for a year in clinical research at the Chronic Care Center and the American University of Beirut with a focus on iron chelation therapy and systemic iron overload. He then moved to the United States where he did his residency in internal medicine and fellowship in pulmonary critical care at the George Washington University in Washington D.C. He is currently an attending in pulmonary and critical care medicine at the Nanticoke Memorial Hospital in Seaford, De.

Ramasubramanian Baalachandran, MD

Ram Baalachandran graduated from Kilpauk Medical College, India. He finished post-graduation in Anesthesiology before moving to the United States of America. He completed his residency in internal medicine from University of Arizona and is a second year fellow in Pulmonary and critical care medicine at University of Maryland.

Venkata Bandi, MD

Dr. Bandi is Professor of Medicine at Baylor College of Medicine and the Chief of the Pulmonary, Critical Care, and Sleep Section at the Michael E. DeBakey VA Medical Center in Houston, Texas. He earned his medical degree at Guntur Medical College in Andhra, India. He completed residency at St Luke's Hospital in St. Louis, Missouri before fellowship training in Pulmonary/Critical Care at Baylor College of Medicine. He has completed additional training in Lung Transplant and Interventional Pulmonology.

Amandeep S. Bawa

Dr. Amandeep Singh Bawa is an Assistant Professor in the Department of Medicine at The George Washington University, Washington DC. He is currently the MICU director at the

DC VA Medical Center at Washington, DC. He graduated from the prestigious University College of Medical Sciences, New Delhi, India in 1997. He finished his Internal Medicine residency followed by a year of Chief Residency at the Queens Hospital Center in affiliation with Icahn School of Medicine at Mount Sinai, New York in 2002. He subsequently completed his Pulmonary and Critical Care Medicine Fellowship at The George Washington University, Washington, DC in 2005. He has been actively involved in the education and training of medical students, residents and fellows since then. He is ABIM board certified in Internal Medicine, Pulmonary diseases, Critical Care medicine and Sleep medicine.

Akshay Bhatnagar, MD

Dr. Akshay Bhatnagar grew up in Northern Virginia, right outside Washington, D.C. He graduated with a major in Biochemistry and a minor in History from the University of Virginia in Charlottesville, Virginia. After working in a medical research laboratory for a year after graduation at the University of Virginia, he obtained a Master of Science degree in Biomedical Sciences from Eastern Virginia Medical School (EVMS) in Norfolk, Virginia. He then attended, and graduated from, EVMS for medical school. Following this, he completed a three-year residency program in Internal Medicine at Cleveland Clinic. He then moved back to Washington, D.C. and currently he is in his second year of a Pulmonary and Critical Care fellowship program at George Washington University.

Lindsey B. Black, MS, CRNP

Mrs. Black graduated from Liberty University with her BSN in 2010. She started her nursing career working as a medical surgical nurse for two years in Charlotte, NC. She then entered a master's degree in Acute Care Nurse Practitioner program at University of Maryland. During her graduate studies she worked at Shock Trauma at University of Maryland on the Multi Trauma Critical Care Unit. She graduated in May 2015 with a Master's of Science and became dual certified as an Adult Acute Care Nurse Practitioner and also as an Adult Gerotonolgy Clinical Nurse Specialist. She started her advanced practitioner role utilizing her dual degree as a CNS/NP on a thoracic surgery and oncology unit in a community hospital in Maryland. She then returned to University of Maryland as a Thoracic Surgery NP. She is the Assistant Director of the Lung Cancer Screening Program with University of Maryland Medical Center. Currently she is completing a Registered Nurse First Assist program. Lindsey is interested in the surgical care of lung and esophageal cancer patients, especially post-esophagectomy quality of life. In her spare time, she enjoys raising her two young boys with her husband in rural Howard County, Maryland.

Stephen Bujarski, MD

Dr. Bujarski is an Assistant Professor of Medicine at Baylor College of Medicine in Houston, Texas. He also serves as an Associate Program Director for the Pulmonary/ Critical Care Fellowship. He received his undergraduate education at Washington University in St. Louis before obtaining his medical degree from the University of Nebraska. He completed Internal Medicine Residency at the University of Illinois at Chicago and Pulmonary/Critical Care Fellowship at Baylor College of Medicine.

Amit Chopra, MD

Amit Chopra, MBBS, FCCP is a Pulmonary Critical Care Physician, practicing at Albany Medical College. Dr. Chopra received his MBBS degree in 2005 from Maulana Azad Medical College, New Delhi, India. He received his Pulmonary and Critical care training from Montefiore Medical Center. Dr. Chopra is currently directing pleural services at Albany Medical College. Dr. Chopra has contributed extensively in pleural diseases. He has special interest in pleural manometry.

Janaki Deepak, MD

Dr. Janaki Deepak graduated from Seth GS Medical college, Mumbai India with honors. She then went on to complete my radiology residency from King Edward Memorial Hospital Mumbai India and was practicing as a radiologist. On arrival in the US, she then went on to do my internal medicine residency at Medstar Harbor Hospital and fellowship in Pulmonary and Critical Care at University of Maryland School of Medicine.She is board certified in internal medicine, pulmonary medicine and critical care medicine. She has won teaching awards at my residency and also received the Lockard Conley award for teaching and mentoring from the American College of Physicians. She is actively involved with student, resident and fellow education. She has been serving as a small group leader for both ICM 1 and ICM II since 2008. In addition I am the co director of the Pulmonary Unit for the second year medical students. I also run the pulmonary physiology course for the graduate students. She is the site director for University of Maryland for the summer and winter education blocks for the pulmonary and critical care fellows in the Baltimore, DC area and also the Director of the Pulmonary Lung Mass Clinic in the Baltimore VA hospital. From a clinical standpoint her focus on interest is in assessment of smoking related health and prevention of smoking related lung disease including COPD .She is in the process of setting up a smoking risk assessment and treatment clinic and is also interested in assessing patients for lung cancer screening and in follow up of lung nodules.

Montserrat Diaz-Abad, MD

Dr. Montserrat Diaz-Abad is an assistant Professor in the Department of Medicine, Division of Pulmonary and Critical Care Medicine at University of Maryland School of Medicine in Baltimore, Maryland, U.S.A. She graduated from medical school from

Instituto Tecnologico de Santo Domingo, in Santo Domingo, Dominican Republic, and completed residency in Internal Medicine followed by fellowship training in Pulmonary, Critical Care and Sleep Medicine at Temple University Hospital in Philadelphia, Pennsylvania, U.S.A. She currently directs the Sleep Medicine Fellowship Program at University of Maryland. Research interests include chronic respiratory failure, noninvasive ventilation and sleep respiratory disorders.

Van K. Holden, MD

Dr. Van K. Holden is an Assistant Professor of Medicine in the section of Interventional Pulmonology at the University of Maryland School of Medicine in Baltimore, Maryland. She completed her Internal Medicine residency at Rutgers-Robert Wood Johnson University Hospital in New Brunswick, New Jersey. She subsequently completed a Pulmonary and Critical Care Medicine fellowship at the University of Maryland Medical Center, followed by an Interventional Pulmonology fellowship at the Beth Israel Deaconess Medical Center and Massachusetts General Hospital combined program. Afterwards, she returned to Maryland as a faculty member. Her clinical interests include minimally invasive diagnostic techniques for parenchymal lung lesions, therapeutic airway interventions, and management of pleural disease. Dr. Holden also enjoys teaching and serves as Associate Program Director of the PCCM fellowship program.

Kurt Hu, MD

Kurt Hu, MD is a Pulmonary Critical Care Fellow at Albany Medical Center. Dr. Hu received his MD degree in 2012 from American University of the Caribbean School of Medicine, Sint Marteen. He received his Internal Medicine training from Allegheny General Hospital in Pittsburgh, Pennsylvania. Dr. Hu is currently finishing up his fellowship and has a strong interest in academic medicine. His special interests include pleural physiology, pleural disease, and thoracic ultrasound.

J. Terrill Huggins, MD

J. Terrill Huggins, MD is a Professor of Medicine in the Division of Pulmonary, Critical Care, Allergy and Sleep Medicine at the Medical University of South Carolina (MUSC). He received a Bachelors of Science degree from Wake Forest University and Doctorate of Medicine from MUSC in 1997. Dr. Huggins has contributed extensively in areas of pleural disease, with numerous publications, monographs, and book chapters related to this field. Dr. Huggins would like to acknowledge his former mentor and a true pioneer in our current understanding of pleural disease, Dr. Steven A. Sahn.

Ari J. Isaacson, MD

Dr. Ari J. Isaacson completed his Diagnostic Radiology residency and Vascular & Interventional Radiology fellowship at the University of North Carolina after 3 years of service as a flight surgeon in the US Navy. In 2013, he stayed in Chapel Hill and joined the faculty as an assistant professor. Dr. Isaacson's clinical interests include arterial embolization, interventional oncology and vascular imaging. Chief among his research interests is prostatic artery embolization, a new minimally invasive treatment for benign prostatic hyperplasia. He is the principal investigator for an ongoing clinical trial being performed at UNC with FDA oversight. Dr. Isaacson has received multiple grants to study both embolization and novel nanoparticle treatment of liver cancer. He also enjoys teaching and mentoring students and residents and is the faculty advisor for the UNC School of Medicine Interventional Radiology Interest Group.

Katie R. Jeans, MD

Dr. Jeans is currently one of the Chief Fellows of the Pulmonary/Critical Care Fellowship Program at Baylor College of Medicine in Houston, Texas. She is a graduate of Louisiana State University for both undergraduate education and medical school. She completed Internal Medicine Residency at Baylor College of Medicine, where she has remained for fellowship training.

Or Kalchiem-Dekel, MD

Dr. Or Kalchiem-Dekel completed his residency in Internal Medicine in Soroka University Medical Center, affiliated with Ben-Gurion University, in Israel. He is a current pulmonary and critical care fellow in the collaborative training track between the National Institute of Heart, Lung, and Blood at the National Institutes of Health and the University of Maryland School of Medicine. His main interest lies in translational research, applying novel approaches to defining gene signatures and protein expression in cells and tissues obtained via interventional pulmonology modalities. His current focus is on the role of apolipoproteins in inflammatory pathways in asthma, with emphasis on patients undergoing bronchial thermoplasty. Additionally, he is currently involved in multiple other clinical research projects in the field of interventional pulmonology. In his spare time, Dr. Kalchiem-Dekel enjoys playing modern board games with his children and listening to Israeli oldies.

Donald R. Lazarus, MD

Dr. Lazarus is an Assistant Professor of Medicine at Baylor College of Medicine in Houston, Texas. He is the Medical Director for Bronchoscopy and Interventional Pulmonology at the Michael E. DeBakey VA Medical Center. After undergraduate and medical education at Texas A&M University, he completed Internal Medicine Residency at Walter Reed Army Medical Center in Washington, D.C. He later completed Pulmonary/Critical Care training at Baylor College of Medicine and a Fellowship in Interventional Pulmonology at the University of Texas M. D. Anderson Cancer Center.

Kewakebt Lemma, MD

Dr. Lemma is a senior fellow in pulmonary and critical care medicine at the George Washington University in Washington, DC. She earned her medical degree at the University of Louisville School of Medicine in Louisville, KY before completing Internal Medicine residency training at the Wake Forest University Hospital in Winston-Salem, NC.

Ivana Milojević, MD

Dr. Milojević is a senior fellow in pulmonary and critical care medicine at the George Washington University in Washington, DC. She earned her medical degree at the Belgrade University School of Medicine, Serbia, before completing internal medicine residency training at the Johns Hopkins University/Sinai Hospital in Baltimore, MD, where she also served as Chief Resident.

Warren Naselsky, MD

Dr. Warren Naselsky is an integrated cardiothoracic surgery resident at University of Maryland Center in Baltimore, Maryland. He completed his undergraduate and medical school studies at the University of North Carolina at Chapel Hill where he graduated with highest honors with distinction. His previous research studies include the immunologic pathogenesis of asthma and the pathophysiology of ventilator induced lung injury. His most recent research study, funded by a grant from the American Association for Thoracic Surgery (AATS), investigated the novel use of photodynamic therapy for the treatment of malignant pleural mesothelioma. Outside of that, Dr. Naselsky is fluent in Chinese and enjoys studying the language in his spare time.

Edward M. Pickering, MD

Dr. Edward M. Pickering is an Assistant Professor of Medicine at University of Maryland School of Medicine in Baltimore, Maryland. He completed his Internal Medicine residency at the University of Connecticut and a fellowship in Pulmonary and Critical Care at the University of Maryland Medical Center. After completing his fellowship, he joined the faculty at the University of Maryland where he completed additional training in Interventional Pulmonology. Dr. Pickering's clinical interests include minimally invasive diagnostic and therapeutic procedures for benign and malignant diseases of the thorax as well as device development. He has served as the sub-investigator on a number of clinical trials and is enrolled in the University of Maryland School of Medicine Certificate Program in Clinical Research. He also has a joint appointment with the Baltimore VA Medical Center as the Director of Interventional Pulmonology. Dr. Pickering is a rabid basketball fan and enjoys watching/following his World Champion Golden State Warriors.

Amrik S. Ray, MD

Dr. Amrik S. Ray is a fellow in Interventional Pulmonology at University of Maryland School of Medicine in Baltimore, Maryland. He completed residency in internal medicine at the University of Louisville in Louisville, Kentucky and a fellowship in pulmonary & critical care medicine at Yale University in New Haven, Connecticut. He has interests in malignant pleural effusion management and endobronchial ultrasound. He has done research in these areas while at Yale University. Dr. Ray enjoys spending his free time with his family and dog, exploring local restaurants and hiking.

Ashutosh Sachdeva, MBBS, FCCP

Dr. Ashutosh Sachdeva is an Assistant Professor of Medicine at University of Maryland School of Medicine in Baltimore, Maryland. He completed his Internal Medicine residency and fellowship in Pulmonary and Critical Care at Saint Louis University Hospital, Saint Louis, Missouri. He then went on to complete advanced fellowship in Interventional Pulmonology at Virginia Commonwealth University Health Sciences, in Richmond, Virginia. Currently, he is the Chief, section of Interventional Pulmonology and has established a comprehensive Interventional Pulmonology Program at University of Maryland Medical Center. He is a full-time faculty in the Division of Pulmonary and Critical Care at University of Maryland School of Medicine. In his spare time, he enjoys traveling and watching movies with his family.

Justin Segraves, MD

Dr. Segraves is currently a second year Pulmonary/Critical Care Fellow at Baylor College of Medicine in Houston, Texas. He completed medical school at New York Medical College and residency at the Mayo Clinic before fellowship training.

Kavita Vyas, MD

Dr Vyas is an Assistant Professor of Medicine at George Washington University in Washington DC and the Washington DC VA Medical Center. She received her undergraduate education at University of Illinois before obtaining her medical degree from Ross University. She completed her Internal Medicine Residency and Pulmonary/Critical Care Fellowship at the Medical College of Wisconsin.

Hyeon Yu, MD

Dr. Hyeon Yu is an associate professor of Radiology at the University of North Carolina at Chapel Hill. He completed his residency of Diagnostic Radiology at the Chung-Ang University Hospitals in Seoul, South Korea and 2-year fellowship of Vascular & Interventional Radiology at the University of North Carolina at Chapel Hill. After finishing his fellowship he joined the faculty at the University of North Carolina in 2010. His main interest lies in the interventional management of complications associated with portal hypertension and interventional oncology including chemoembolization, radioembolization, and thermal ablation therapy of liver malignancies. He is currently conducting multiple clinical researches as the principal investigator and participating in multidisciplinary clinical trials as a coinvestigator. He is also a scientific committee member of the Radiological Society of North America and contributing to academic journals as a manuscript reviewer.

INDEX

A

B

C

N

O

P

Q

R

S

PULMONARY EMBOLISM: CAUSES, SYMPTOMS AND TREATMENT

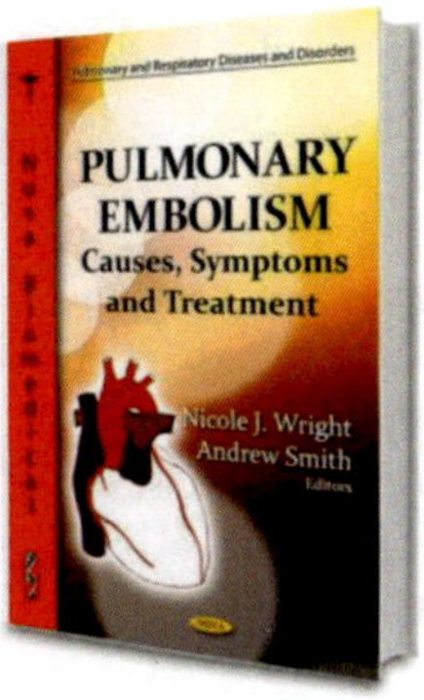

EDITORS: Nicole J. Wright and Andrew Smith

SERIES: Pulmonary and Respiratory Diseases and Disorders

BOOK DESCRIPTION: In this book, the authors discuss the causes, symptoms and treatment for pulmonary embolism. Topics include parenteral anticoagulant therapy; incidence and predictors in acute intraoperative pulmonary thromboembolism; surgical management of PE; technical and clinical aspects of MRI for pulmonary embolism; and radiological imaging with cement as a causative factor in PE.

HARDCOVER ISBN: 978-1-62081-258-7
RETAIL PRICE: $182

HYPOXIA: CAUSES, TYPES AND MANAGEMENT

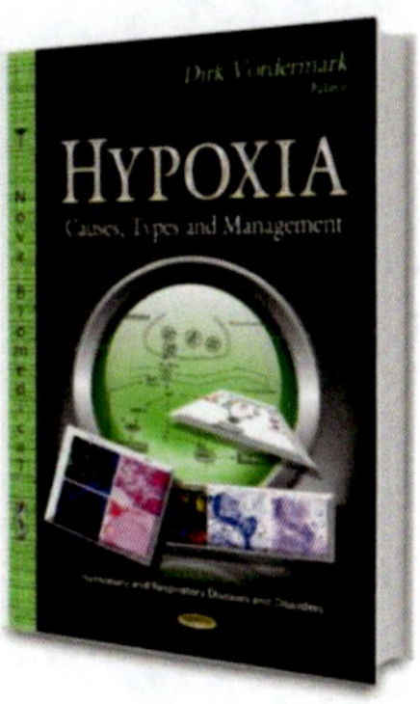

EDITOR: Dirk Vordermark (Martin Luther University Halle-Wittenberg, Halle/Saale, Germany)

SERIES: Pulmonary and Respiratory Diseases and Disorders

BOOK DESCRIPTION: This book contains contributions from an international group of authors covering a wide range of situations in benign as well as malignant diseases, in which understanding the role of hypoxia may lead to novel diagnostic and therapeutic strategies.

HARDCOVER ISBN: 978-1-62081-769-8
RETAIL PRICE: $270

Chronic Obstructive Pulmonary Disease: New Research

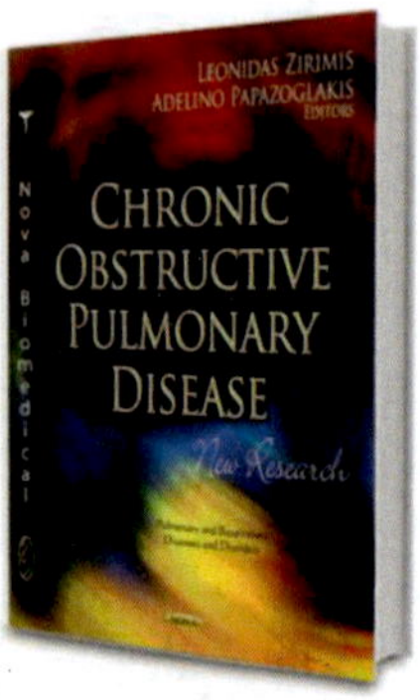

Editors: Leonidas Zirimis and Adelino Papazoglakis

Series: Pulmonary and Respiratory Diseases and Disorders

Book Description: In this book, the authors present current research on COPD including the clinical effects of continuous positive airway pressure therapy for COPD patients; anxiety and depression in patients with COPD; the role of non-invasive mechanical ventilation in the management of acute COPD; the immunology of COPD; multi-drug resistant bacteria in severe acute exacerbations of COPD requiring mechanical ventilation; and dietary prevention of COPD.

Hardcover ISBN: 978-1-62081-848-0
Retail Price: $182

Pneumothorax: Classification, Treatment and Prognostic Factors

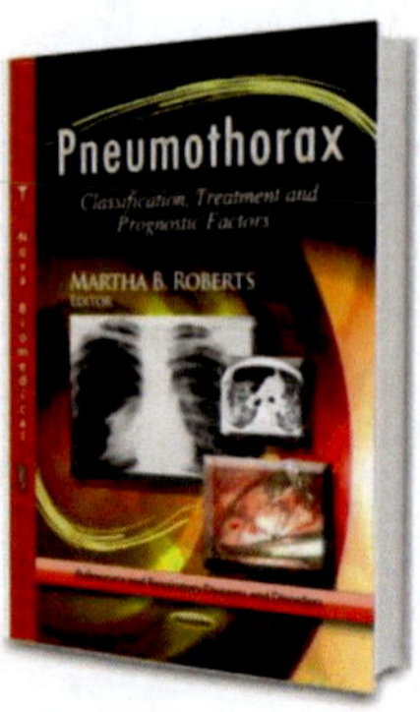

Editor: Martha B. Roberts

Series: Pulmonary and Respiratory Diseases and Disorders

Book Description: In this book, the authors present current research and an overview in the study of the classification, treatment and prognostic factors of pneumothorax. Topics include the treatment of primary spontaneous pneumothorax; the pathology of pneumothorax and multiple pulmonary cysts associated with Birt-Hogg-Dube syndrome; and management of pneumothorax in the single lung.

Softcover ISBN: 978-1-62618-562-3
Retail Price: $98